UNEQUAL OPPORTUNITY

UNEQUAL OPPORTUNITY

Health Disparities Affecting Gay and Bisexual Men in the United States

Edited by

Richard J. Wolitski

Ron Stall

Ronald O. Valdiserri

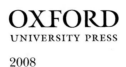

OXFORD

UNIVERSITY PRESS

2008

OXFORD
UNIVERSITY PRESS

Oxford University Press, Inc., publishes works that further
Oxford University's objective of excellence
in research, scholarship, and education.

Oxford   New York
Auckland   Cape Town   Dar es Salaam   Hong Kong   Karachi
Kuala Lumpur   Madrid   Melbourne   Mexico City   Nairobi
New Delhi   Shanghai   Taipei   Toronto

With offices in
Argentina   Austria   Brazil   Chile   Czech Republic   France   Greece
Guatemala   Hungary   Italy   Japan   Poland   Portugal   Singapore
South Korea   Switzerland   Thailand   Turkey   Ukraine   Vietnam

Copyright © 2008 by Oxford University Press, Inc.

Published by Oxford University Press, Inc.
198 Madison Avenue, New York, New York 10016
www.oup.com

Oxford is a registered trademark of Oxford University Press

The findings and conclusions in this volume are those of the chapter authors
and do not necessarily represent the views of the editors, the U. S. Centers
for Disease Control and Prevention, or the U. S. Department of Veterans Affairs.

Library of Congress Cataloging-in-Publication Data

Unequal opportunity : health disparities affecting gay and bisexual men in the United States /
edited by Richard J. Wolitski, Ron Stall, and Ronald O. Valdiserri.
   p. cm.
Includes bibliographical references and index.
ISBN 978-0-19-530153-3
1. Gays—Medical care—United States.   2. Bisexuals—Medical care—United States.
3. Health services accessibility—United States.   4. Discrimination in medical care—United States.
[DNLM: 1. Health Status—United States.   2. Homosexuality, Male—United States.   3. Bisexuality—
United States.   4. Prejudice—United States.   5. Sexually Transmitted Diseases—United States.
6. Socioeconomic Factors—United States.   WA 300 U517 2007]
I. Wolitski, Richard J.   II. Stall, Ron, 1954–   III. Valdiserri, Ronald O., 1951–
RA564.9.H65U94 2007
362.1086'64—dc22   2007017174

9 8 7 6 5 4 3 2 1

Printed in the United States of America
on acid-free paper

This volume is dedicated to the health and well-being of sexual minorities in the United States and throughout the world.

Contents

Contributors

JOSEPH A. CATANIA, PhD, College of Health and Human Sciences, Oregon State University

KYUNG-HEE CHOI, PhD, MPH, Center for AIDS Prevention Studies, University of California, San Francisco

SUSAN D. COCHRAN, PhD, MS, Departments of Epidemiology, School of Public Health, University of California, Los Angeles (UCLA) and the UCLA Center for Research, Education, Training, and Strategic Communications on Minority Health Disparities

RAFAEL M. DÍAZ, MSW, PhD, César E. Chávez Institute, San Francisco State University

CLAUDE EARL FOX, MD, MPH, Miller School of Medicine, University of Miami

MARK FRIEDMAN, PhD, School of Public Health, University of Pittsburgh

ARNOLD H. GROSSMAN, PhD, ACSW, LMSW, Department of Applied Psychology, Steinhardt School of Culture, Education, and Human Development, New York University

GREGORY M. HEREK, PhD, Department of Psychology, University of California, Davis

VICKIE M. MAYS, PhD, MSPH, Departments of Psychology and Health Services, University of California, Los Angeles (UCLA) School of Public Health and the UCLA Center for Research, Education, Training and Strategic Communications on Minority Health Disparities

DAVID G. OSTROW, MD, PhD, David Ostrow and Associates, Chicago, IL; and the Chicago Multicenter AIDS Cohort Study, Howard Brown Health Center, Chicago, IL

JOCELYN D. PATTERSON, MPH, Division of HIV/AIDS Prevention; National Center for HIV/AIDS, Viral Hepatitis, STD, and TB Prevention; Centers for Disease Control and Prevention

JOHN L. PETERSON, PhD, Department of Psychology, Georgia State University

DAVID W. PURCELL, PhD, Division of HIV/AIDS Prevention; National Center for HIV/AIDS, Viral Hepatitis, STD, and TB Prevention; Centers for Disease Control and Prevention

RAJEEV RAMCHAND, PhD, RAND Health, RAND, Arlington, Virginia

GARY REMAFEDI, MD, MPH, Youth and AIDS Projects and Department of Pediatrics, University of Minnesota

SCOTT D. RHODES, PhD, MPH, Departments of Social Sciences and Health Policy, Division of Public Health Sciences, and Internal Medicine and the Maya Angelou Research Center on Minority Health, Wake Forest University Health Sciences

CHARLES SIMS, MA, Department of Psychology, University of California, Davis

PILGRIM S. SPIKES, JR., PhD, Division of HIV/AIDS Prevention; National Center for HIV/AIDS, Viral Hepatitis, STD, and TB Prevention; Centers for Disease Control and Prevention.

RON STALL, PhD, MPH, Department of Behavioral and Community Health Sciences, Graduate School of Public Health, University of Pittsburgh

PATRICK S. SULLIVAN, DVM, PhD, Division of HIV/AIDS Prevention; National Center for HIV/AIDS, Viral Hepatitis, STD, and TB Prevention; Centers for Disease Control and Prevention

RONALD O. VALDISERRI, MD, MPH, Office of Public Health and Environmental Hazards, U.S. Department of Veterans Affairs

RICHARD J. WOLITSKI, PhD, Division of HIV/AIDS Prevention; National Center for HIV/AIDS, Viral Hepatitis, STD, and TB Prevention; Centers for Disease Control and Prevention

LELAND J. YEE, PhD, MPH, Department of Epidemiology, Graduate School of Public Health, University of Pittsburgh

PART I

INTRODUCTION

1

Health Disparities Affecting Gay and Bisexual Men in the United States: An Introduction

Richard J. Wolitski, Ronald O. Valdiserri, and Ron Stall

America is known as the land of opportunity—a meritocracy, where one can start life with little or nothing, and with hard work, determination, and a little ingenuity can go from rags to riches. America is also a land that was founded on the principle of equality. The principle that "all men are created equal" is the bedrock of our government and our society. Sadly, the reality is that America is not a land of equal opportunity for everyone. Long-standing economic and social inequalities have systematically denied racial and ethnic minorities, women, the disabled, the aged, and others from getting and keeping their share of the American dream. These inequities are visible in many aspects of contemporary life. In 2005, working women earned 23% less than their male counterparts;[1] a larger percentage of blacks (25%) and Hispanics (22%) were living in poverty compared to non-Hispanic whites (8%);[1] and fewer blacks (48%), Hispanics (50%), and Asian/Pacific Islanders (60%) owned their own homes, compared to non-Hispanic whites (73%).[2]

Economic and social disadvantage are often closely associated with inequities in physical and mental health, access to health care, and the quality and length of life.[3–8] Lower earnings make it more difficult for people to afford healthy diets and lifestyles, quality housing in safe neighborhoods, health insurance, and high-quality medical care, including vaccinations, other preventive services, and medications to treat existing conditions. Economic disadvantage, stigma, and discrimination also increase stress and diminish the ability of individuals to cope with stress, which in turn contribute to poor physical and mental health.[9–12] Stress can affect health directly (for example, creating anxiety, affecting the immune system, increasing risk of hypertension, heart attack and other health problems) and can also affect health indirectly when individuals adopt or continue unhealthy behaviors in an effort to cope with challenging life circumstances (e.g., use of tobacco, alcohol, or drugs) or are unable to access preventive care and high-quality medical treatment in a timely manner.[9,13]

As a result, multiple health disparities adversely impact the health of economically and socially disadvantaged groups in the United States. Although health disparities have been shown to exist for many different groups, the greatest amount of information is available concerning the health disparities experienced by racial and ethnic minorities. Compared to whites, members of some racial and ethnic minority groups experience reduced life expectancy and higher rates of infant mortality, certain types of cancer, diabetes, hypertension, sexually transmitted infections, HIV and AIDS, hepatitis, tuberculosis, and other health problems, including poorer mental health.[14–17] In addition to increased incidence and prevalence of disease, racial and ethnic minorities often have poorer access to quality health care and have lower survival rates compared to whites.[3,6,18,19]

Like racial and ethnic minorities, sexual minorities also experience a wide range of health disparities. However, gay, lesbian, bisexual, and transgender persons are frequently invisible in research that seeks to measure health disparities because questions about sexual orientation and gender identity are often not included in these studies. As a result, the specific needs and experiences of sexual minorities are often neglected in public health efforts to improve the health and well-being of disadvantaged groups. There are no easy answers as to why the specific experiences of gay, lesbian, bisexual, and transgender persons are so often neglected in research, policy, and programmatic efforts addressing health disparities. We suspect that there are many reasons for this: the historical invisibility of sexual minorities; a failure on the part of some to recognize that sexual minorities are differentially vulnerable to multiple health threats; a reluctance to consider sexual minorities as "authentic" minorities; and negative societal attitudes toward homosexuality that may have caused some to be indifferent to these issues or to opine that the "immoral" lifestyles of sexual minorities are the root cause of their poor health outcomes.

In recent years, however, increased attention has been given to the health-related issues of sexual minorities. A growing number of studies have examined disparities among sexual minorities and have documented significant differences in rates of disease, mental health problems, and risk behaviors that can lead to poor health.[20–22] Although there are notable exceptions,[10,23–27] sexual orientation has not yet been fully integrated into research and theory regarding health disparities, nor has it been consistently addressed in public health efforts to eliminate inequities in health and health care.

This chapter provides an introduction to key issues related to health disparities experienced by gay, bisexual, and other men who have sex with men (MSM). It begins by considering the various ways that this population has been defined, which have important implications for interpreting prior research and describing the size and characteristics of this population. We then argue that the issues faced by MSM should be considered as part of broader efforts to document, understand, and eliminate health disparities in the

United States. Finally, we provide an overview of the issues that will be examined in the chapters that follow and articulate the overarching aims of this volume.

Like the remainder of this volume, this chapter focuses specifically on the health of gay, bisexual, and other MSM in the United States. Given this explicit focus, there is a danger that some readers may incorrectly assume that we are either unaware or unconcerned about the social and health-related disparities experienced more generally by sexual minorities and more specifically by lesbian women and transgender persons. This is not the case. We chose to limit our focus to MSM because we did not believe that we could adequately address the health care needs of lesbians and other sexual minorities in a single volume. Others have documented multiple health disparities experienced by lesbian and bisexual women, but much work remains to be done in this important and understudied area.[28–36] Even less is known about the prevalence of various health problems among transgender men and women, but alarmingly high rates of HIV infection and other disparities also have been documented among transgender persons.[37–41]

It is likely that many of the disparities experienced by members of all sexual minority groups share a common etiology that is driven, at least in part, by the direct and indirect effects of stigma and discrimination. Similarly, although MSM around the world may have much in common, those living outside the United States are affected by different cultural, societal, and historical influences; they receive care from different health care systems, and they are afforded different legal rights and protections. Given the complexity of these issues, we did not believe that we could adequately address all of these issues in this volume. We hope that this work will provide an impetus for increased examination of health issues among sexual minorities and for greater attention to the need to prevent and eliminate health disparities experienced by all sexual minorities in the United States and other parts of the world.

Gay, Bisexual, and Other Men Who Have Sex with Men

Although men with same-gender partners have become increasingly visible in contemporary society in recent decades, these men often remain uncounted and invisible in many large-scale surveys that seek to describe the demographic characteristics and health-related needs of Americans. Even when efforts have been made to document the size of this population and its health-related needs, methodological issues have presented challenges to the use and interpretation of these data. A fundamental issue is the multitude of definitions that have been used to assess sexual orientation. Studies of homosexual and bisexual men have used different definitions of sexual orientation that define homosexuality and bisexuality in terms of three basic aspects: (1) sexual desire or attraction, (2) sexual behavior, and (3) sexual identity. Although these three aspects of sexual orientation are often used interchangeably, each represents a distinct construct that has its own meaning and implications for research and practice.[42–45]

People differ in the degree to which they are sexually attracted to members of their own or the opposite gender. Measures of *sexual attraction* assess responses toward members of the same or opposite gender using (1) self-report measures of sexual or romantic attraction/desire or sexual fantasy or (2) physiological measures of sexual arousal. Individuals may be sexually attracted to only members of the opposite gender, the same gender, both genders, or neither gender.[46] Although most assessments of sexual attraction rely on self-report measures, these measures do not always correspond to physiological measures of sexual arousal that are taken while individuals view erotic images of men or women.[47]

Same-gender attraction often leads to same-gender *sexual behavior*, but individuals' sexual behavior is not necessarily consistent with their degree of attraction to partners of a given gender. Individuals' ability and willingness to act on their sexual attraction to same- or opposite-gender partners can be affected by many factors, including cultural norms regarding sexual relationships, familial expectations, personal beliefs and attitudes, and the availability of partners. Behavioral definitions of sexuality are based on the gender of persons with whom individuals report having had sexual relations. These definitions rely on self-reports of same-gender sexual relations and typically classify individuals as homosexual, bisexual, or heterosexual, based on the gender of their sex partners. Men who report only male sex partners are classified as homosexual, those reporting only female partners are classified as heterosexual, and those reporting both male and female partners during a specified period of time are classified as bisexual. In public health, another behaviorally defined category, MSM, is also commonly used. This classification combines behaviorally homosexual and bisexual men into a single category and is often used when same-gender behavior may place men at increased risk of HIV or other sexually transmitted infections. Although defining sexual orientation based on sexual behavior seems rather straightforward, definitions that do so vary considerably, based on the recall period that is used (e.g., during a respondent's lifetime, since age 18, the past 5 years, the past year), making comparisons across studies difficult.

Sexual identity refers to the label that individuals use to describe their sexual orientation to themselves or others. These labels may, or may not, correspond with individual's sexual attraction or behavior. Most definitions of sexual identity classify individuals into one of the three standard classifications of sexual orientation: homosexual (gay), heterosexual (straight), and bisexual. Many studies also include a fourth category (e.g., questioning, don't know, not sure), reflecting the fact that having a well-defined sexual identity is often a developmental process that is affected not only by attraction and sexual behavior, but also by contextual influences, group affiliation, and social and cultural norms.[48,49] For example, men whose sexual behavior with other men is primarily determined by external forces that limit the availability of female partners (e.g., incarceration, military service, same-gender boarding school) or is driven by drug dependency or economic need may not identify as gay or bisexual even if they report having had sex with other men.[50–53]

Size of the Population

As Kinsey, Laumann, and others have pointed out, accurately assessing the size of the gay/homosexual/MSM population is difficult, if not impossible.[43,44,54] Challenges to estimating the size of this group include the multidimensional nature of sexual orientation, the stigma associated with homosexuality, the reluctance of some individuals to disclose same-gender behavior, variability in the expression of sexual orientation within different subgroups, and the developmental course of human sexual relationships and identity over a lifetime.

Most systematic efforts to document the prevalence of homosexuality among American men have been based wholly, or in part, on behavioral definitions of sexual orientation. Kinsey and colleagues[54] reported that 37% of men had one or more sexual experiences with other men between adolescence and old age. These investigators also reported that 10% of men were "more or less exclusively homosexual" for at least three years between the ages of 16 and 55, and that 4% were exclusively homosexual throughout their lives. The findings reported by Kinsey and colleagues have been strongly criticized in part because they were based on a nonprobability sample that cannot be assumed to be representative of men in the United States. Some of these criticisms include questions about the overrepresentation of white men recruited from urban areas, the inclusion of men recruited from homosexual social networks, and the recruitment of some participants from prisons and other institutional settings in which female partners were not readily available.[43,55]

Despite the limitations of this research, Kinsey and colleagues' work was groundbreaking and represented the first systematic large-scale effort to assess same-gender behavior and attraction in the United States. Since the late 1980s, more rigorously designed studies that are based on representative samples of the United States as a whole have reported somewhat lower rates of same-gender behavior. These studies report that 2.6%[56] to 9.1%[43] of men in the United States report having had sex with a male partner since puberty or during adulthood. The majority of these estimates cluster somewhere between 4 and 6 percent.[43,55–57] Applying these figures to the Census Bureau's estimate that 108.4 million men 18 years of age or older were living in the United States in July 2005[58] suggests that roughly somewhere between 4.3 and 6.5 million men in this country have had sex with a man during adulthood.

Not all of these men are currently sexually active or have had sex with a man in the recent past. Studies that have assessed more recent sexual behavior (e.g., the past 12 months or the past 5 or 10 years) find that fewer men report recent male partners.[55,56,59,60] For example, data from the 1998–2002 General Social Surveys (GSS) indicated that 2.6% to 6.4% of male respondents had sex with a male since adulthood, but fewer (2.0% to 4.6%) reported having had sex with a male in the last five years. Even fewer men, 1.4% to 3.6%, had sex with a man in the last year.[56]

Estimates of the size of the MSM population that are based on sexual behavior provide different results from those that are based on sexual attraction or sexual identity. Typically, studies that compared these three types of measures have found that a larger percentage of men report same-gender attraction than report same-gender behavior, and that even fewer men have a gay or bisexual sexual identity. For example, the 1992 National Health and Social Life Survey (NHSLS) found that 7.7% of men reported same-gender attraction or found other men sexually appealing (desire), 4.9% reported same-gender sexual behavior since age 18, and 2.8% currently identified themselves as homosexual or bisexual.[43] Among men participating in the NHSLS who reported any aspect of having a same-gender orientation (i.e., either same-gender desire, behavior, or identity), most reported same-gender desire (76%), 52% reported same-gender behavior during adulthood, and 27% identified themselves as homosexual or bisexual. Of men who reported same-gender desire, most (60%) had not acted on this desire as adults. This discrepancy likely reflects norms supporting heterosexuality and discouraging homosexuality in American culture. Across the three measures of sexual orientation, only 24% of men with any evidence of a same-gender orientation reported a consistent orientation; that is, same-gender desire, sex with one or more male partners, and same-gender identity. These men represented only 2.4% of all men who participated in the NHSLS.

As this discussion illustrates, there is more than one way to define the population of men with same-gender sex partners. The different definitions that have been used to define this population capture different aspects of these men's experience and may lead to different conclusions about the presence of health disparities and their underlying causes. It is possible that a behavioral definition of MSM may best permit the identification of disparities that are associated with sexual transmission of viruses or other pathogens, whereas a behavioral definition might fail to capture disparities that are a result of the stigma and discrimination faced by openly gay men or the stress experienced by some individuals whose identity is inconsistent with their sexual behavior or attraction.

Although we acknowledge the potential challenges and limitations associated with various definitions of same-gender sexual orientation, we also recognize that this is a relatively young area of inquiry. As such, we have chosen not to limit the focus of this volume to any one definition of sexual orientation, but have attempted to be clear in how the population and specific study samples are defined and discussed. The use of the term MSM reflects reliance on a behavioral definition of sexual orientation that includes gay, bisexual, and otherwise identified men who have had sex with men during a given time period. The terms *gay, homosexual,* and *bisexual* have been applied to both behavioral definitions and those based on self-identification in the literature and in this volume. The reader should not assume that use of these three terms represents one type of definition or the other. To minimize confusion, we have tried, as have the contributing authors, to be clear when discussing issues related to sexual identity or samples that were defined by the self-reported sexual identity or orientation of study participants.

Subgroup Differences

Sexual attraction, identity, and behavior may have different patterns or may be expressed differently within various subgroups of MSM, given the influence that development, culture, norms, and group affiliation have on these components of sexual orientation. Age, race and ethnicity, and urban versus rural residence are among the demographic variables that have been found to be associated with one or more aspects of sexual orientation.

Age

There do not appear to be significant age-related differences in lifetime experience of same-gender sex among men, but younger men are more likely than older men to report recent same-gender sexual activity. An analysis of data from the GSS found that age (as defined by birth cohort) was not associated with significant differences in same-gender sex in adulthood.[56] Among those who were born prior to the 1920s, 4.3% reported having had sex with a man after the age of 18, compared to 5.5% of those born in the 1930s, 5.1% of those born in the 1950s, and 5.0% of those born in the 1970s and later. Recent sexual behavior is associated with age-related differences. An analysis that combined data from the GSS and the NHSLS found that 3.0% of men aged 18–29 had same-gender sex partners in the past year compared to 3.5% of those aged 30–39 years, 2.1% of those 40–49 years of age, and 1.4% of those 50–59 years of age.[43] The factors underlying this age-related decline in same-gender sex are not clear. These data may represent an actual reduction in same-gender sex, a general decline in sexual activity associated with aging, or a greater reluctance among older men to disclose recent same-gender sexual relationships.

In recent times, adolescents and young men may be having same-gender sexual relationships and developing a gay or bisexual identity at a younger age than earlier generations. For example, in a 2003 study, younger gay, lesbian, and bisexual men and women (ages 18–24 years) from New York and Los Angeles reported coming out at significantly earlier ages and initiating same-gender sexual relations at an earlier age than their older peers.[61] Younger men appear to be more likely than older men to develop a gay or bisexual identity. Among male participants in the 1992 NHSLS, men in their forties (2.2%) and in their fifties (0.5%) were less likely to report a homosexual or bisexual identity than were men in their late teens or twenties (2.9%) or in their thirties (4.2%).[43] These differences in recent sexual behavior and sexual identity reflect other differences in the experiences of younger and older

MSM that are associated with myriad social, physical, psychological, and financial differences. These differences affect health disparities within these groups and may require different approaches to preventing and treating the health problems of younger and older men. Remafedi[A] addresses issues affecting younger MSM in Chapter 10, and Grossman considers issues specific to older MSM in Chapter 11.

Race/Ethnicity

The relatively small numbers of racial/ethnic minorities and MSM in population-based samples make it difficult to accurately assess racial/ethnic differences in same-gender sex. Most studies have found no clear differences in rates of same-gender sex during adulthood by race or ethnicity.[43,57,62] Two studies that found racial/ethnic differences had dissimilar results. White men participating in the 1990–1991 National AIDS Behavioral Survey, which focused on major metropolitan areas, were more significantly likely to report same-gender sex in the prior five years than were men who described themselves as black (9.1% vs. 3.1%), Hispanic (2.7%) or Asian/other (2.2%).[55] In contrast, the nationally representative National Survey of Men, conducted in 1991, found that Hispanic men were more likely to report same-gender sex in the last 10 years than were other men (4.8% vs. 2.0%).[59] Taken as a whole, currently available studies do not provide compelling evidence that race/ethnicity is associated with substantial differences in the prevalence of same-gender sex in contemporary American society.

Available data do not indicate that the prevalence of same-gender sex differs substantially by race/ethnicity in America, but good data on this issue are limited. However, MSM from different racial/ethnic groups do vary in terms of how they identify their sexual orientation. Most studies that have compared sexual identity among MSM have found that white men are more likely to identify themselves as gay or homosexual than are men from other racial/ethnic groups, particularly black MSM.[43,63–67] Among 203 HIV-seropositive MSM who donated blood in 1988 and 1989, 54% of white men identified as gay, compared to 34% of blacks and 49% of Hispanics. Hispanics in this study were most likely to identify as heterosexual (34%) compared to blacks (23%) and whites (21%).[66] Social class does affect the adoption of a gay identity, but racial and ethnic differences in sexual identity among MSM persist when social class is controlled.[68] The reasons for these racial/ethnic differences are not fully known. They may reflect differences in the prevalence of opposite-gender sexual relationships, familial and cultural expectations, or the association of the term *gay* with a predominately white community with which some racial/ethnic minority MSM do not identify.[53,69–73]

It is clear that sexual orientation has the potential to interact with race/ethnicity in ways that may differentially impact health across racial/ethnic groups. It is also true that racial and ethnic minorities often have life experiences and perspectives that are distinct from those of white MSM. These include different cultural, familial, and social influences, as well as the need to confront additional stressors (most notably racism) that exist in American society and are also present in the gay community. Díaz, Peterson, and Choi consider the experiences of racial and ethnic minority MSM in greater detail in Chapter 12.

Urban versus Rural Residence

The prevalence of same-gender contact is considerably higher among men living in large urban areas than among men living in smaller cities or rural areas. This finding is robust and has been reported in a number of large studies.[43,55-57] Using data from the 1998–2002 General Social Surveys, Turner and colleagues found that 11.6% of men residing in the 12 largest metropolitan areas in the United States reported sex with a man during adulthood, compared to 3.6% to 6.6% of men living in smaller urban and suburban communities and rural areas.[56] Consistent with this finding, a 2003 population-based sample of men residing in the largest US metropolitan area, New York City, found higher rates of same-gender sex than national surveys. This study found that 13.6% of men who responded to a question about sexual identity had sex with men only (12.4%) or men and women (1.2%) during the prior 12 months.[64] Similar results have been found with regard to sexual identity, with the highest percentage of homosexually or bisexually identified men residing in large cities, compared to smaller cities, suburbs, and rural areas.[43]

The higher concentration of MSM and gay men in urban areas may be influenced by migration into these areas as well as by environmental influences that affect the opportunity for, and acceptability of, same-gender sexual activity.[43,55] Regardless of the specific mechanisms responsible for the increased presence of MSM within the urban centers of large cities, this concentration creates opportunities for the provision of targeted and culturally appropriate health care services for MSM who reside in these areas. It also creates challenges and stressors that may affect the physical and mental health of MSM who live in these environments, particularly those who live in neighborhoods with a very high concentration of MSM (called "gay ghettos" by some).[74,75] Given the increased prevalence of MSM in urban areas, these stressors have the potential to contribute to health disparities experienced by MSM. The influence of these urban environments on the health and well-being of gay and bisexual men is discussed by Stall, Friedman, and Catania in Chapter 9.

Considering MSM within a Health Disparities Framework

Health disparities are measurable differences in the incidence or prevalence of disease, physical or mental health, quality of life, or longevity between members of one group and those of another. Some disparities are inherent to the human condition, such as those that are biologically determined, and are not inherently unjust.[76] Many more disparities, however, are the result of the marginalization, discrimination, and unequal access to health care experienced by the members of some groups, which directly and indirectly affect their health and well-being. Such disparities are often defined as health inequities, which Whitehead describes as differences in health that are unnecessary, avoidable, unfair and unjust.[77] Braveman and Gruskin assert that health inequities "systematically put groups of people who are already socially disadvantaged (for example, by virtue of being poor, female, and/or members of disenfranchised racial, ethnic or religious groups) at further disadvantage with respect to their health."[76]

Health disparities can result from multiple factors that differentially affect the health and well-being of socially disadvantaged groups. Multiple models and theories have been developed to better understand and predict health disparities by accounting for individual, familial, social, and environmental determinants of health. For example, King and Williams have developed a framework for understanding the relationship between race/ethnicity and health that identifies five key influences: (1) biological factors that predispose individuals to develop or protect them from disease, (2) cultural factors that influence health behavior and coping strategies, (3) socioeconomic factors, such as income and education, that affect living circumstances and ability to access care, (4) racism that creates psychological stressors and limits access to resources including high-quality medical care, and (5) political factors that contribute to policies and laws that directly and indirectly affect health and well-being.[9] These factors affect health and well-being by influencing health practices (e.g., a nutritious diet, exercise, condom use) and risk behaviors (e.g., unsafe sexual behavior, use of tobacco, alcohol and illicit drugs), environmental stressors (e.g., exposure to noise, crime, crowding, toxic chemicals), psychological stressors (e.g., strained family relationships, concern about finances), psychological resources that buffer stress (e.g., strong family ties, supportive social networks, church involvement), and access to, and quality of, medical care.

We argue that sexual orientation should be routinely considered when addressing health disparities and that the models and frameworks that have been used to understand disparities among racial and ethnic minorities provide an important foundation for understanding the health of MSM. A key element of work on health disparities in racial and ethnic groups is the dynamic that occurs between majority groups that systematically deprive marginalized minority groups equal access to economic, social, health-related, and other resources.[4,6,9,23,76] In their review of effects of racial discrimination on the health of African Americans, King and Williams[9] defined a minority group as follows:

. . . a collective that, regardless of size, is distinguishable on the basis of color, language, culture, sex, religion or other recognizable features. Moreover, a minority group exerts less power than the majority group over societal decision-making processes, controls fewer vital social resources, and is unequal in access to opportunity structures, social rewards, and status (economic, political, health status) as a result of discrimination, intentional or unintentional. (p. 94)

This definition is readily applicable to MSM in contemporary American society. All MSM share a defining feature that distinguishes them from their heterosexual peers, namely their sexual relationships with same-gender partners. However, this distinction goes beyond the gender of their sex partners. Many MSM have common developmental experiences that profoundly shape their lives,[48,49] they share and participate in various aspects of the gay community,[78–82] and often live in close proximity to each other in gay-identified areas of major metropolitan areas.[74,75,83,84]

Not only do MSM represent a collective of individuals distinct from the majority, they experience stigma and discrimination as a result of their minority status.[10,85–89] The majority of self-identified homosexual or bisexual persons (76%) participating in a 1995 nationally representative study of men and women 25 to 74 years of age reported having personally experienced discrimination versus 65% of their heterosexual peers.[86] Homosexually and bisexually identified men in this study were more significantly likely than heterosexually identified men to report having been fired from a job (19.5% vs. 5.9%) and to experience multiple types of day-to-day discrimination (e.g., were treated with less respect, received poorer service than others, were called names or insulted). Gay and bisexual adolescents and young men also experience high rates of stigma and discrimination.[48,85,90,91] A 1996–1997 three-city study of young gay and bisexually identified men 18 to 27 years of age found that, in the prior 6 months, 37% had experienced anti-gay verbal harassment, and 11% experienced discrimination.[85] As reviewed by Herek and Sims in Chapter 2, MSM are also at increased risk of physical violence as a result of their sexual orientation. In addition to these personal experiences with discrimination, MSM in the United States also experience stigma and discrimination as a result of organized efforts to prevent same-gender couples from marrying and gaining other equal rights and protections under the law.

Unique Aspects of Minority Group Status among MSM

Although MSM have much in common with other minority groups, they are also unique in a number of ways that merit further consideration. These include: (1) the definition of minority status based on behavior or attraction to same-gender partners, rather than genetic traits or other characteristics that are universally accepted to be immutable, (2) a lack of strong intergenerational influences that perpetuate disparities within families, (3) the acquisition of minority status by MSM later in life, (4) the ability of MSM to selectively hide their minority group status, and (5) historical differences. Each of these distinctions is considered below.

Definition of Minority Group Status

Some have resisted the inclusion of sexual minorities in efforts to address health disparities because they view same-gender sex as a "lifestyle choice" that has inherent consequences that MSM should have to bear. This perspective is inconsistent with the bulk of scientific evidence indicating that sexual orientation is not a choice (i.e., it is determined by biological influences, environmental influences, or both).[45,92–96] Regardless of the basis of sexual orientation, it is important to recognize the negative effects of stigma, prejudice, and discrimination on the health and well-being of MSM and to identify steps that can be taken to ameliorate these disparities. The amount of data regarding the stresses of homophobia and discrimination on the mental and physical health of sexual minorities has grown considerably in recent years and provides an empirical basis for understanding and addressing the effects of discrimination and social marginalization on MSM's health.[10,25,26,86,89,97] A developmental model that links the effects of key stressors experienced by many MSM with negative health outcomes over the life course is presented in Chapter 9.

Lack of Strong Intergenerational Influences

Perhaps most importantly, the minority group status of gay and bisexual men is different from that of some other minorities because of a lack of intergenerational influences and learning. Among racial and ethnic minorities, minority status is passed down within a family from one generation to the next. Gonsiorek describes racial and ethnic groups as being "vertically integrated" and sexual minorities as being "horizontally integrated."[98] In vertically integrated groups, information and norms are passed through families from one generation to the next. In horizontally integrated groups, such as gay and bisexual men, the learning of cultural norms and information occurs largely from peers, not one's family of origin.

In much the same way, the effects of discrimination, unequal socioeconomic status, and health disparities experienced by earlier generations of racial/ethnic minorities are passed on to their children.[7] African Americans have a greater likelihood of being born into poverty in the United States and starting life in a disadvantaged position because of the effects of racism and discrimination experienced by their parents and grandparents. This perpetuates the effects of discrimination long after the formal systems that enforced racial segregation and unequal access to education, safe and well-paying jobs, and good living conditions have been dismantled. Homosexuality, however, is not related to race or the socioeconomic class into which one is born. Thus, male infants who grow up to have sex with men in adulthood have the same probability as do their heterosexual peers of being born into rich, poor, or middle-class families.

Acquisition of Minority Group Status in Later Life

Many minority group members are identifiable as members of a minority group at birth. Sexual minorities acquire their minority status later in life, typically during adolescence or young adulthood. This distinction has important implications. Early disadvantages that are often associated with minority group status are not experienced by many sexual minorities until early adulthood. Thus, all other things being equal, access to high-quality nutrition, medical care, and education during childhood are unlikely to differ for MSM and heterosexual men of the same socioeconomic class. Sexual minorities who begin life with a more-or-less equal standing compared to their peers may not experience some of the negative economic, educational, social, and health outcomes experienced by persons whose minority status is evident at birth. It is important to recognize, however, that some children are non-gender-conforming at an early age or develop traits that are perceived to be associated with sexual minority status (e.g., an effeminate boy being labeled as a "sissy") and as a result do experience stigma and discrimination early in life.[90,91]

Although many sexual minorities may start out life on an equal footing compared to their majority peers, they risk losing this status as they (and others) become aware of their attraction to same-gender partners. The process of acknowledging, acting on, and disclosing one's same-gender sexual attraction ("coming out") can be very stressful for many individuals. Part of this stress is associated with acquisition of minority status (or dual minority status for some, such as racial/ethnic minorities) and the potential losses that come with it, such as disruption of existing relationships and loss of social status and support from friends and family members. Thus, unlike members of other minority groups, sexual minorities risk losing important sources of social, emotional, and financial support that can help buffer the effects of stigma, discrimination, and other stressors.

The loss of these supports can have a substantial impact on mental and physical health. If they lose some or all of these supports, sexual minorities are forced to develop new sources of support, which sometimes creates additional stressors such as moving away from their community of origin and the struggles associated with integrating sexual and other identities (e.g., racial/ethnic identity, professional identity, religious affiliation and participation).

Ability to Hide Minority Group Status

Some minority groups and their members are more recognizable than are others. For example, most women and many members of racial and ethnic minority groups are readily perceived by others as such. Their minority group status is a perceivable characteristic in most aspects of their lives, and the question of whether or not to disclose their status as a member of a minority group is moot. For MSM, however, their minority group status is often not apparent unless it is disclosed to others, and it can be denied if their sexual orientation is questioned. This presents MSM with the opportunity to selectively disclose their sexual orientation in some settings, and to certain individuals, but not others.

The ability to hide minority group status could be hypothesized to have either positive or negative effects on physical and mental health. On one hand, keeping minority group status secret might be protective because the individual would not be a target of stigma and discrimination. On the other hand, failure to disclose might contribute to stress and limit the individual's ability to access social support from other members of the minority group, which could buffer the effects of stigma, discrimination, and other stressors.[9,10,99]

Keeping secrets, including concealing one's own sexual orientation, has been shown to negatively affect health.[100–106] Research with MSM living with HIV has shown that hiding sexual orientation is associated with more rapid progression of HIV-related illness.[102,103,106] Similarly, a study of HIV-seropositive men and women found that disclosure of sexual orientation was associated with improvement in immune function over time.[104] One study has also demonstrated the negative effects of nondisclosure of sexual orientation among HIV-seronegative MSM. In this study, those who concealed their sexual orientation were more likely to develop cancer and infectious diseases at a higher rate than were MSM who were more open about their sexual orientation.[101] Although most studies indicate that concealing sexual orientation has negative health outcomes, disclosure in some settings, such as the workplace, has been associated with increased physiological signs of stress, negative affect, and discrimination.[107–109]

Historical Influences

All minority groups in the United States have their own history that affects the context of their present-day lives. The nature, duration, and magnitude of the oppression experienced by various minority groups differ substantially. Many of these groups have experienced not only social stigma and prejudice, but also horrific exploitation and systematic discrimination in (and exclusion from) key aspects of community life that were codified into laws and institutional policies. Various laws that served to perpetuate discrimination based on race, ethnicity, and gender were struck down decades ago, and new laws that provide safeguards against discrimination based on race, ethnicity, gender, age, religion, and disability have been enacted. These laws have not eliminated prejudice and discrimination in the United States, nor have they erased long-standing disparities; however, they have gone a long way toward establishing a more equitable playing field for members of many minority groups, and they offer an opportunity for legal recourse when overt discrimination occurs in key areas of individuals' lives such as housing and employment.

Until relatively recently, gay, bisexual, and other MSM have largely sought to remain hidden in American society because of the stigma and discrimination associated with homosexuality. Highly visible and well-organized gay communities did not begin to develop on the East and West Coasts of the United States until the 1960s. Efforts to obtain civil rights and to address the health care needs of gay and bisexual men were hampered by the medical profession's classification of homosexuality as a psychological disorder, as well as laws that criminalized homosexuality. It was not until 1973 that the American Psychiatric Association removed homosexuality from its official list of psychiatric disorders. The last of the laws criminalizing same-gender relationships between consenting adults in the United States were struck down in only the last decade. Same-gender sexual relationships were illegal in some states until 2003, when the remaining state laws were invalidated by the U.S. Supreme Court.

The devastation of AIDS has also profoundly influenced the current context of MSM's lives. Before the first cases of AIDS were identified in 1981, the HIV virus had already spread widely among MSM. The staggering numbers of deaths devastated an entire generation of MSM, and AIDS continues to exact a grim toll among MSM in the United States even today. As of 2005, AIDS had claimed the lives of more than 300,000 MSM, more than 16,500 of whom died in that year alone.[110] A five-city study completed in 2005 found that HIV prevalence remains high among MSM.[111] Overall, one in four MSM were infected with HIV. Nearly half (46%) of African American MSM in this study were HIV-seropositive, compared to 21% of non-Hispanic whites and 17% of Hispanics. Alarmingly high rates of HIV infection were found even among the youngest men who participated in the study. Fourteen percent of MSM between the ages of 18 and 24 were infected with HIV, and HIV prevalence rates were more than 30% among men who were 40 years of age or older.

The impact of the HIV epidemic affects the current context of MSM's lives in a number of ways. The loss of partners, friends, and acquaintances has negatively affected the mental health of many MSM.[112–114] HIV-seropositive MSM have the additional stressors of living with HIV, dealing with the stigma still associated with the disease, and meeting the demands on time and financial resources that are associated with having a serious long-term illness. However, the HIV epidemic also brought the gay community together and demonstrated its considerable resilience. The gay community mobilized in response to the AIDS epidemic in an unprecedented way—providing care to the sick and dying, supporting those living with HIV, disseminating information about AIDS and its prevention, and organizing to hasten the government's response to the epidemic, stimulate research leading to new treatments, and ensure that these treatments were available to those who needed them.[115,116] The HIV epidemic and the gay community's response to it has had a lasting impact, including the creation of new organizations that continue to serve the community, greater visibility for sexual minorities, and broader public recognition of the struggles faced by gay, bisexual, and other MSM.

The AIDS epidemic also created an urgent need to learn more about the sexual health-related practices and needs of MSM. As a result, a number of ongoing studies began to collect data about MSM, and many new studies began. These studies provided important information not only about HIV risk and its prevention, but also about a constellation of other health problems that disproportionately affected MSM. It is largely this research, which began in response to the HIV epidemic, that has provided the most extensive evidence of the health disparities described in this volume.

Individual and Social Determinants of Health among MSM

Research on the underlying causes of health disparities among racial and ethnic minorities and other disadvantaged groups have identified a large number of factors that account for these inequities.[3,4,6,9,23] This substantial body of research clearly shows the central role of social, environmental, and structural influences in the creation of disparities in health and access to health care. This research also identifies the role that individual health behaviors play in the health status of disadvantaged groups and the effects that social, environmental, and structural influence have on individuals' ability and motivation to choose healthy behaviors and discontinue unhealthy practices.

Much remains to be learned about the determinants of health disparities among MSM. The chapters that follow this introduction review what is known about the determinants of specific health disparities in this population. In order to set the stage for these chapters, we briefly discuss a number of cross-cutting factors that have the potential to influence a range of health disparities among MSM. These factors are: (1) socioeconomic status, (2) the effects of prejudice and discrimination, (3) laws and policies that affect health, health behavior, and access to health care, and (4) individual behavior and cultural norms within the gay community.

Socioeconomic Status

Employment, income, and educational attainment are among the traditional measures of socioeconomic status that have been shown to affect the health of racial and ethnic minorities, women, and other marginalized groups.[6,7,9,117] One might reasonably expect that the stigma and discrimination experienced by MSM in the United States would negatively affect their socioeconomic status in much the same way that these factors have affected other marginalized groups. It is possible, however, that the nature of homosexuality may have a differential impact on socioeconomic status and its subsequent influence on health. Educational attainment may be less strongly affected by anti-gay bias because same-gender attractions or the development of a gay or bisexual identity may not occur until many gay and bisexual men's education is well under way. Educational attainment and income may be relatively unaffected by anti-gay bias because some gay and bisexual men successfully hide their sexual orientation from teachers, classmates, and employers. Furthermore, as discussed previously, MSM are likely to start life out on an equal footing compared to their heterosexual peers because sexual minority status is not due to the race, ethnicity, or other characteristics of the families into which MSM are born.

Available data indicate that MSM have comparable, or better, levels of education than their heterosexual counterparts. Analyses of GSS data for 1988–1998[62] and 1998–2002[56] found that men reporting same-gender sex during adulthood had educational levels that were comparable to those of other men. Another nationally representative survey conducted in 1991, the National Survey of Men, found that higher education was associated with having had same-gender sex in the prior 10 years, but education was not associated with having only same-gender partners during this period.[59] Other studies have found that MSM have higher levels of education compared to heterosexual men. Using data from the 1990 U.S. Census, Black and colleagues found that, in all age groups, male same-gender partners residing in the same household were better educated than were married men and unmarried men in opposite-gender partnerships.[118] The same pattern of differences in educational attainment was also observed by these researchers using data from the GSS and the NHSLS.[118] Similarly, more highly educated men living in urban areas accounting for the majority of AIDS cases in the United States were more likely than less educated men to report same-gender sex in the prior five years.[55]

Even though MSM have levels of educational attainment that are comparable to or higher than those of other men, most studies indicate that they earn less than their heterosexual peers.[118–122] This finding has been replicated using several nationally representative samples and can be observed within groups that differ in terms of educational attainment. That is, whether they are poorly or highly educated, MSM earn less than their heterosexual peers with comparable educational backgrounds. Some data suggest that income differences may not be driven by differences in hourly wages,[119] but rather by the professions that gay men enter and by differential participation in the workforce.[118,120,121] Tebaldi and Elmslie found that men living with a same-gender partner worked fewer hours and were more likely to work part-time than were married and unmarried heterosexual men.[120] Furthermore, they found that men living with a same-gender partner who became unemployed were more likely to remain unemployed than were their heterosexual peers. Decreased income, part-time work, and unemployment have the potential to not only affect MSM's ability to pay for health care, but also their ability to access health insurance, which many Americans enjoy as a benefit of full-time employment. On the other hand, a greater proportion of MSM (but certainly not all MSM) may be able to afford health care because they are less likely than heterosexual men to have financial responsibility for raising one or more children. Issues related to MSM's ability to obtain health insurance and access appropriate health care services are discussed in more detail by Ramchand and Fox in Chapter 13.

Effects of Prejudice and Discrimination

Like other minority groups, MSM and other sexual minorities also experience stigma and discrimination that can adversely affect mental and physical health.[10,85–89,123] Public attitudes toward homosexuality have become more tolerant in recent decades, but 40% of Americans interviewed in a 2006 poll stated that they thought sex between same-gender partners should not be legal.[124] Although the majority of Americans (89% of those interviewed in 2006) agree in concept that homosexuals should have equal rights in terms of job opportunities, substantial minorities of Americans interviewed in 2005 believed that homosexuals should not be hired as doctors (19%), elementary school teachers (43%), high school teachers (36%), clergy (49%), or even sales clerks (7%).[124] The most extreme manifestations of negative attitudes toward minority group members are physical attacks that are motivated by hostility toward minority group members (i.e., hate crimes). Like racial/ethnic, religious, and other minority group members, MSM are also the target of hate crimes. Herek and Sims review the data on hate crimes experienced by MSM in Chapter 2.

Unlike other minority groups, however, MSM often experience discrimination and rejection from their families of origin. The initial reaction of many family members when they learn that a child or sibling is gay or bisexual is negative.[125–128] Some of these reactions are extremely negative and lead to verbal or physical abuse, lifelong estrangement, or, for some youth, being forced to leave their homes. Rejection by family members not only adds to the stress experienced by sexual minorities, it eliminates key sources of social, emotional, and material support that can affect individuals' coping ability as well as their physical and mental health. These strained relationships can be a lifelong source of stress for some MSM, but for others the initial negative reactions of family members give way to supportive and nurturing relationships, which become beneficial sources of support that enhance the lives of MSM and their family members.

Stigma and discrimination from within and outside MSM's families represent stressors that can negatively affect physical and mental health.[10,25,86,89,129] As discussed previously, even anticipated stigma and discrimination have substantial effects on the health of MSM who conceal their sexual orientation in some or all settings.[101,102,106] Societal disapproval of same-gender relationships is internalized to some degree by many MSM. The internalization of stigmatizing attitudes (termed internalized homophobia, internalized homonegativity, or internalized heterosexism) represents another source of stress that can negatively affect the health of MSM.[10,97] Taken as a whole, the direct effects of discrimination and the stress of rejection and negative attitudes toward homosexuality represent significant threats to the health of MSM.

Laws and Policies

MSM and other sexual minorities do not have equal protection under the law. Under existing federal law and the laws of many states, sexual minorities do not have specific protections against employment discrimination and cannot serve openly in the military. Most do not have the right to enter into civil marriage or to have their long-term relationships formalized through legally recognized alternatives to marriage, such as civil unions or domestic partnerships. This lack of legal protections represents a systematic form of discrimination that can affect MSM's health and their ability to access health care services. For example, the lack of legal recognition of same-gender relationships deprives MSM of the economic advantages afforded married couples by American laws, including the ability to obtain health insurance through a spouse's employer, death benefits, and community property laws.[130–133] Further, same-gender partners may be deprived of other potential health benefits of marriage; being married has been associated with reduced mortality and improved physical health and mental health among heterosexuals.[132,134–136]

Although they do not carry the force of law, policies of public and private institutions can enhance or diminish the health and well-being of MSM and other sexual minorities. Many companies and state and local governments have established policies that address the equal treatment of sexual minority employees in the absence of a federal workplace nondiscrimination law that clearly addresses sexual orientation and extends health care benefits to same-gender partners.[137]

The effects of changing laws and policies to protect the rights of sexual minorities and provide access to health care and other services are not fully understood. However, some evidence suggests that changing laws and policies affecting sexual minorities could have a measurable public health impact. A comparison of data from states with laws protecting sexual minorities to states without these laws found significant differences in suicide rates among male adolescents.[138] This observational study found that states with antidiscrimination laws experienced a differential reduction of 29.1 suicides per million white male adolescents when compared to states without such laws. These findings provide additional support for the public health benefit of efforts to eliminate legal and policy-related barriers to the equal treatment of MSM and other sexual minorities.

Individual Behavior and Community Norms

The choices that individuals make about their own behaviors have a significant effect on physical and mental health. Many serious chronic health problems and diseases are strongly influenced by individual behaviors related to nutrition, exercise, smoking, substance use, and sexual behavior. As will be discussed in later chapters, personal behavior is clearly a factor in many of the health disparities experienced by MSM, and it is important that the contributions of individuals' behavior be studied and addressed in prevention efforts. All people, including MSM, need to be encouraged to take responsibility for their own health, and much can be done to change individual risk behaviors through targeted intervention programs. However, an exclusive focus on the behaviors of individuals that does not recognize the environmental context reinforcing these behaviors is counterproductive and limits the ability to achieve public health goals. Focusing only on personal responsibility prevents the identification of potential underlying causes of these behaviors, will not result in the structural and cultural changes needed to sustain community-wide behavior change, and is tantamount to "blaming the victim."[139,140]

An integrated approach that recognizes the contributions of both individual and external influences, such as those discussed above, is warranted. In recent years, a number of studies and reviews have begun to address these external influences existing within and outside the gay community and their impact on the health of MSM.[10,25,75,89,141,142] These publications provide an important foundation for future research and prevention efforts, but much more remains to be done to further an ecological understanding of the causes of health disparities among MSM and strategies for improving the health of this population.

Public Health Efforts to Address Health Disparities

Public health seeks to prevent disease and promote health among all members of the community—especially those who are at heightened risk. As such, public health has a fundamental concern with the identification and elimination of health disparities that are rooted in social inequities.[23] This concern has led to the development of formal efforts to reduce racial, ethnic, gender, and other disparities in the United States and elsewhere.

The World Health Organization and other governmental organizations have played a leading role in efforts to identify and eliminate health disparities. In the United States, the federal government has established a variety of programs and initiatives to address racial, ethnic, and other health disparities in this country. Many of these efforts do not explicitly address health disparities associated with sexual orientation. The most notable exception is *Healthy People 2010*, which is a comprehensive set of disease prevention and health promotion objectives established by the U. S. Department of Health and Human Services.[24] *Healthy People 2010* established measurable objectives for the United States that address two overarching goals: (1) to help individuals of all ages increase life expectancy and improve their quality of life, and (2) to eliminate health disparities among segments of the population, including differences that occur by gender, race or ethnicity, education or income, disability, geographic location, or sexual orientation. *Healthy People 2010* has a very broad scope—it identifies 467 specific objectives for improving the nation's health, which are clustered in 28 separate focus areas. Sexual orientation is addressed in 29 of the objectives, which cover 10 of the focus areas.[143]

The inclusion of sexual orientation in the *Healthy People 2010* goals and objectives represents a significant milestone in efforts to identify and eliminate health disparities among MSM and other sexual minorities. The importance of the inclusion of sexual orientation cannot be overstated. It represents one of the first times that the federal government has recognized the existence of health disparities associated with sexual orientation and has established formal objectives for reducing these disparities. Despite the importance of this effort, concern has been raised that other objectives related to sexual orientation that were supported by empirical data were not included in the final *Healthy People 2010* conference report and that data for assessing many other potential health disparities associated with sexual orientation were lacking.[143,144] In addition, the ability to monitor *Healthy People 2010* objectives that address disparities related to sexual orientation has been called into serious question because of deficiencies in the information systems used to evaluate progress toward meeting these objectives.[143]

Health Disparities among MSM

In recent years, a growing number of studies has documented the existence of multiple health disparities among MSM in the United States.[20,21,26] Some disparities, such as HIV and other sexually transmitted infections, are associated with the sexual practices of MSM. Others, however, are not a direct result of differences in sexual practices between MSM and heterosexual men and likely result in part from stressors associated with stigma and discrimination experienced by MSM.[10,25,97] These disparities include mental health problems, substance use, violence and victimization, as well as chronic and infectious disease.

In the chapters that follow, experts from a variety of fields systematically review and synthesize evidence of health disparities affecting MSM, identify individual and community factors that contribute to these disparities, and articulate strategies for public health efforts to eliminate these disparities. These chapters review the evidence supporting (or in some cases, not supporting) the existence of disparities among MSM in the following areas: hate crimes and domestic violence; sexual abuse; mental health; alcohol, tobacco, and drug use; HIV and other sexually transmitted diseases; and hepatitis. By bringing together chapters on these issues that are usually studied and discussed in isolation from each other, we hope to further an integrated approach to the examination of these problems, their underlying causes, and potential solutions. In addition to highlighting what is known about health disparities among MSM, this volume also identifies critical gaps in our knowledge about the health of MSM and suggests directions for future research, prevention, and treatment efforts.

In this volume, we have focused on the health issues that have received the most study to date. As this area of research is still young, we recognize that some data on other health issues do exist and that new data will continue to emerge over time. There will be an ongoing need for the critical evaluation and synthesis of new findings as the number of studies in this area grows so that new data can be used to inform future research and public health efforts.

The term *men who have sex with men* describes an incredibly diverse population, which contains numerous subpopulations that have much in common but that also have important differences. Various subpopulations of MSM have unique experiences and circumstances that affect their health and mental health needs as well as their ability to receive high-quality medical, psychosocial, and preventive health services. In this volume, we invited authors to draw attention to the unique needs and experiences of several subpopulations that are particularly vulnerable to health disparities: racial and ethnic minority MSM, younger MSM, and older MSM.

The final chapters of the volume address crosscutting issues that affect MSM as a whole, including underlying mechanisms that may contribute to health disparities among MSM and issues affecting MSM's access to health care and the quality of the care that they receive. In the final chapter, we present a framework for future research on health disparities among MSM and offer suggestions for broad-based efforts to reduce the impact of stigma and discrimination on the health and well-being of MSM. Taken as a whole, we hope that the chapters in this volume provide a useful foundation for stimulating and guiding future research, prevention, and medical care that aims to improve the health and well-being of gay, bisexual, and other MSM in the United States.

Authors' Note

The findings and conclusions in this chapter are those of the authors and do not necessarily represent the views of the US Centers for Disease Control and Prevention or the US Department of Veterans Affairs.

References

1. DeNavas-Walt C, Proctor BD, Lee CH. *Income, Poverty, and Health Insurance Coverage in the United States: 2005*. Washington, DC: US Government Printing Office; 2006. US Census Bureau, Current Population Reports, P60–231.
2. US Census Bureau Housing and Household Economic Statistics Division. *Housing Vacancies and Homeownership (CPS/HVS): Annual Statistics: 2005*. Washington, DC: US Census Bureau; 2006.
3. Institute of Medicine. *Unequal Treatment: Confronting Racial and Ethnic Disparities in Health Care*. Washington, DC: National Academy Press; 2002.
4. Wilkinson R, Marmot M, eds. *Social Determinants of Health: The Solid Facts*. Copenhagen, Denmark: World Health Organization; 2003.

5. Moss N. Socioeconomic disparities in health in the US: An agenda for action. *Soc Sci Med.* 2000;51:1627–1638.

6. House J, Williams D. Understanding and reducing socioeconomic and racial/ethnic disparities in health. In: Smedley BD, Syme LS, eds. *Promoting Health: Intervention Strategies From Social and Behavioral Research.* Washington, DC: National Academy Press; 2000:81–124.

7. Marmot M, Bell R. The socioeconomically disadvantaged. In Levey BS, Sidel VW, eds. *Social Injustice and Public Health.* New York, NY: Oxford University Press; 2006:25–45.

8. Amick BC, Levine S, Tarlov AR, Walsh DC, eds. *Society and Health.* New York, NY: Oxford University Press; 1995.

9. King G, Williams DR. Race and health: a multidimensional approach to African-American health. In: Amick BC, Levine S, Tarlov AR, Walsh DC, eds. *Society and Health.* New York, NY: Oxford University Press; 1995:93–130.

10. Meyer IH. Prejudice, social stress, and mental health in lesbian, gay, and bisexual populations: conceptual issues and research evidence. *Psychol Bull.* 2003;129:674–697.

11. Raphael D. A society in decline: the political, economic, and social determinants of health inequalities in the United States. In: Hofrichter R, ed. *Health and Social Justice: Politics, Ideology, and Inequity in the Distribution of Disease.* San Francisco, CA: Jossey-Bass; 2003:59–88.

12. Williams DR, Neighbors HW, Jackson JS. Racial/ethnic discrimination and health: findings from community studies. *Am J Public Health.* 2003;93:200–208.

13. Brunner EJ. Stress and the biology of inequality. *BMJ.* 1997;314:1472–1476.

14. Centers for Disease Control and Prevention. Health disparities experienced by Hispanics—United States. *MMWR Morb Mortal Wkly Rep.* 2004;53:935–937.

15. Centers for Disease Control and Prevention. Health disparities experienced by Black or African Americans—United States. *MMWR Morb Mortal Wkly Rep.* 2005;54:1–3.

16. National Center for Health Statistics. *Health, United States, 2006.* Hyattsville, MD: Author; 2006.

17. Centers for Disease Control and Prevention. Health status of American Indians compared with other racial/ethnic minority populations—selected states, 2001–2002. *MMWR Morb Mortal Wkly Rep.* 2003;52:1148–1152.

18. Lasser KE, Himmelstein DU, Woolhandler S. Access to care, health status, and health disparities in the United States and Canada: results of a cross-sectional population-based survey. *Am J Public Health.* 2006;96:1300–1307.

19. Trivedi A, Zaslavsky AM, Schneider EC, Ayanian JZ. Trends in quality of care and racial disparities in Medicare managed care. *N Engl J Med.* 2005;353:692–700.

20. Lombardi E, Bettcher T. Lesbian, gay, bisexual, and transgender/transsexual individuals. In: Levey BS, Sidel VW, eds. *Social Injustice and Public Health.* New York, NY: Oxford University Press; 2006:130–144.

21. Dean L, Meyer IH, Robinson K, et al. Lesbian, gay, bisexual, and transgender health: findings and concerns. *J Gay Lesbian Med Assoc.* 2000;4:101–151.

22. Safford L. Building the pillars of diversity in the U.S. health system. *Clin Res Regulatory Affairs.* 2001;19:125–152.

23. Levy BS, Sidel VW, eds. *Social Injustice and Public Health.* New York, NY: Oxford University Press; 2006.

24. US Department of Health and Human Services. *Healthy People 2010: Understanding and Improving Health.* Washington, DC: US Government Printing Office; 2000.

25. Diaz RM, Ayala G. *Social Discrimination and Health: The Case of Latino Gay Men and HIV Risk.* New York, NY: Policy Institute of the National Gay and Lesbian Task Force; 2001.

26. Omoto AM, Kurtzman HS, eds. *Sexual Orientation and Mental Health: Examining Identity and Development in Lesbian, Gay, and Bisexual People.* Washington, DC: American Psychological Association; 2006.

27. Koop CE. Health and health care for the 21st century: for all the people. *Am J Public Health.* 2006;96:2090–2092.

28. Bernhard LA. Lesbian health and health care. *Annu Rev Nurs Res.* 2001;19:145–177.

29. Hutchinson MK, Thompson AC, Cederbaum JA. Multisystem factors contributing to disparities in preventive health care among lesbian women. *J Obstet Gynecol Neonatal Nurs.* 2006;35:393–402.

30. McNair RP. Lesbian health inequalities: a cultural minority issue for health professionals. *Med J Aust.* 2003;178:643–645.

31. O'Hanlan KA, Dibble SL, Hagan HJ, Davids R. Advocacy for women's health should include lesbian health. *J Womens Health.* 2004;13:227–234.

32. Saunders JM. Health problems of lesbian women. *Nurs Clin North Am.* 1999;34:381–391.

33. Solarz AL, ed. *Lesbian Health: Current Assessment and Directions for the Future.* Washington, DC: National Academy Press; 1999.

34. Bradford J, Ryan C, Honnold J, Rothblum E. Expanding the research infrastructure for lesbian health. *Am J Public Health.* 2001;91:1029–1032.

35. Stevens PE. Lesbian health care research: a review of the literature from 1970 to 1990. *Health Care Women Int.* 1992;13:91–120.

36. Abbott LJ. The use of alcohol by lesbians: a review and research agenda. *Subst Use Misuse.* 1998;33:2647–2663.

37. Celments-Nolle K, Marx R, Guzman R, Katz M. HIV prevalence, risk behaviors, health care use, and mental health status of transgender persons: implications for public health interventions. *Am J Public Health.* 2001;91:915–921.

38. Garolfalo R, Deleon J, Osmer E, Doll M, Harper GW. Overlooked, misunderstood and at-risk: Exploring the lives and HIV risk of ethnic minority male-to-female transgender youth. *J Adolesc Health.* 2006;38:230–236.

39. Kenagy GP. Transgender health: findings from two needs assessment studies in Philadelphia. *Health Soc Work.* 2005;30:19–26.

40. Lombardi E. Enhancing transgender health care. *Am J Public Health.* 2001;91:869–872.

41. Nemoto T, Operario D, Keatley J, Han L, Soma T. HIV risk behaviors among male-to-female transgender persons of color in San Francisco. *Am J Public Health.* 2004; 94:1193–1199.

42. Herek GM. Homosexuality. In: Kazdin AE, ed. *Encyclopedia of Psychology.* Vol. 4. Washington, DC: American Psychological Association; 2000:149–153.

43. Laumann EO, Gagnon JH, Michael RT, Michaels S, eds. *The Social Organization of Sexuality: Sexual Practices in the United States.* Chicago, IL: The University of Chicago Press; 1994.

44. Savin-Williams RC. Who's gay? Does it matter? *Curr Dir Pschol Sci.* 15:40–44.

45. Kauth MR, Kalichman SC. Sexual orientation and development: an interactive approach. In: Diamant L, McAnulty RD, eds. *The Psychology of Sexual Orientation, Behavior, and Identity: A Handbook*. Westport, CT: Greenwood Press; 1995:81–103.

46. Rowland DL. The psychobiology of sexual arousal and behavior. In: Diamant L, McAnulty RD, eds. *The Psychology of Sexual Orientation, Behavior, and Identity: A Handbook*. Westport, CT: Greenwood Press; 1995:19–42.

47. Diamond M. Biological aspects of sexual orientation and identity. In: Diamant L, McAnulty RD, eds. *The Psychology of Sexual Orientation, Behavior, and Identity: A Handbook*. Westport, CT: Greenwood Press; 1995:45–80.

48. D'Augelli AR. Developmental and contextual factors and mental health among lesbian, gay, and bisexual youths. In: Omoto AM, Kurzman HS, eds. *Sexual Orientation and Mental Health: Examining Identity Development in Lesbian, Gay, and Bisexual People*. Washington, DC: American Psychological Association; 2006:37–53.

49. D'Augelli AR. Identity development and sexual orientation: toward a model of lesbian, gay, and bisexual development. In: Trickett EJ, Watts RJ, Birman D, eds. *Human Diversity: Perspectives on People in Context*. San Francisco, CA: Jossey-Bass; 1994:312–333.

50. Doll LS, Beeker C. Male bisexual behavior and HIV risk in the United States: synthesis of research with implications for behavioral interventions. *AIDS Educ Prev*. 1996;8:205–208.

51. Garland JT, Morgan RD, Beer AM. Impact of time in prison and security level on inmate's sexual attitude, behavior, and identity. *Psycol Serv*. 2005;2:151–162.

52. Rietmeijer CA, Wolitski RJ, Fishbein M, Corby NH, Cohn DL. Sex hustling, injection drug use, and non-gay identification by men who have sex with men: associations with high-risk sexual behaviors and condom use. *Sex Transm Dis*. 1998; 25:353–360.

53. Lichtenstein B. Secret encounters: black men, bisexuality, and AIDS in Alabama. *Med Anthropol Q*. 2000;14:374–393.

54. Kinsey AC, Pomeroy WB, Martin CE. *Sexual Behavior in the Human Male*. Philadelphia, PA: W. B. Saunders Company; 1948.

55. Binson D, Michaels S, Stall R, Coates TJ, Gagnon JH, Catania JA. Prevalence and social distribution of men who have sex with men: United States and its urban centers. *J Sex Res*. 1995;32:245–254.

56. Turner CF, Villarroel MA, Chromy JR, Eggleston E, Rogers SM. Same-gender sex among U.S. adults: trends across the twentieth century and during the 1990s. *Public Opin Q*. 2005;69:439–462.

57. Rogers SM, Turner CF. Male-male sexual contact in the U.S.A.: findings from five sample surveys, 1970–1990. *J Sex Res*. 1991;28(4):491–519.

58. U.S. Census Bureau. *Statistical Abstract of the United States: 2007*. Washington, DC: Author; 2005.

59. Billy JOG, Tanfer K, Grady WR, Klepinger DH. The sexual behavior of men in the United States. *Fam Plann Perspect*. 1993;25:52–60.

60. Hewitt C. Homosexual demography: implications for the spread of AIDS. *J Sex Res*. 1998;35:390–396.

61. Grov C, Bimbi DS, Nanin JE, Parsons JT. Race, ethnicity, gender, and generational factors associated with the coming-out process among gay, lesbian, and bisexual individuals. *J Sex Res*. 2006:115–121.

62. Butler AC. Trends in same-gender sexual partnering, 1988–1998. *J Sex Res*. 2000; 37:333–343.

63. Goldbaum G, Perdue T, Wolitski R, et al. Differences in risk behavior and sources of AIDS information among gay, bisexual, and straight-identified men who have sex with men. *AIDS Behav.* 1998;2:13–21.

64. Pathela P, Hajat A, Schillinger J, Blank S, Sell R, Mostashari F. Discordance between sexual behavior and self-reported sexual identity: a population-based survey of New York City men. *Ann Intern Med.* 2006;145:416–425.

65. McKirnan DJ, Stokes JP, Doll L, Burzette RG. Bisexually active men: social characteristics and sexual behavior. *J Sex Res.* 1995;32:65–76.

66. Doll LS, Petersen LR, White CR, Johnson ES, Ward JW, the Blood Donor Study Group. Homosexually and nonhomosexually identified men who have sex with men: A behavioral comparison. *J Sex Res.* 1992;29:1–14.

67. Millett G, Peterson JL, Wolitski RJ, Stall R. Greater risk for HIV infection of black men who have sex with men: a critical literature review. *Am J Public Health.* 2006; 96:1007–1019.

68. Barrett DC, Pollack LM. Whose gay community? Social class, sexual self-expression, and gay community involvement. *Sociological Quarterly.* 2005;46:437–456.

69. Millett G, Malebranche D, Mason B, Spikes P. Focusing "down low": bisexual black men, HIV risk and heterosexual transmission. *J Nat Med Assoc.* 2005;97:52S-59S.

70. Beeker C, Kraft JM, Peterson JL, Stokes JP. Influences on sexual risk behavior in young African-American men who have sex with men. *J Gay Lesbain Med Assoc.* 1998;2(2):59–67.

71. Williams JK, Wyatt GE, Resell J, Peterson J, Asuan-O'Brien A. Psychosocial issues among gay- and non-gay-identifying HIV-seropositive African American and Latino MSM. *Cul Diversity Ethnic Minority Psychol.* 2004;10:268–286.

72. Zea MC, Reisen CA, Diaz RM. Methodological issues in research on sexual behavior with Latino gay and bisexual men. *Am J Com Psychol.* 2003;31:281–291.

73. Mays VM, Cochran SD, Zamudio A. HIV prevention research: are we meeting the needs of African American men who have sex with men? *J Black Psychol.* 2004;30: 78–105.

74. Mills TC, Stall R, Pollack L, et al. Health-related characteristics of men who have sex with men: a comparison of those living in "gay ghettos" with those living elsewhere. *Am J Public Health.* 2001;91:980–983.

75. Frye V, Latka MH, Koblin B, et al. The urban environment and sexual risk behavior among men who have sex with men. *J Urban Health.* 2006;83:308–324.

76. Braveman P, Gruskin S. Defining equity in health. *J Epidemiol Community Health.* 2003;57:254–258.

77. Whitehead M. The concepts and principles of equity in health. *Int J Health Serv.* 1992;22:429–445.

78. Woolwine D. Community in gay male experience and moral discourse. *J Homosex.* 2000;38:5–37.

79. Haldeman DC. The village people: identity and development in the gay male community. In: Bieschke KJ, Perez RM, DeBord KA, eds. *Handbook of Counseling and Psychotherapy With Lesbian, Gay, Bisexual, and Transgender Clients.* 2nd ed. Washington, DC: American Psychological Association; 2007:71–89.

80. Peacock B, Eyre SL, Quinn SC, Kegeles S. Delineating differences: sub-communities in the San Francisco gay community. *Cult Health Sex.* 2001;3:183–201.

81. Nardi PM; *Gay Men's Friendships: Invincible Communities.* Chicago, IL: University of Chicago Press; 1999.

82. Ramirez-Valles J, Fergus S, Reisen CA, Poppen PJ, Zea MC. Confronting stigma: community involvement and psychological well-being among HIV-positive Latino gay men. *Hisp J Behav Sci.* 2005;27:101–119.
83. Black D, Gates G, Sanders S, Taylor L. Why do gay men live in San Francisco? *J Urban Econ.* 2002;51:54–76.
84. Anacker KB, Morrow-Jones HA. Neighborhood factors associated with same-sex households in U. S. cities. *Urban Geogr.* 2005;26:385–409.
85. Huebner DM, Rebchook GM, Kegeles SM. Experiences of harassment, discrimination, and physical violence among young gay and bisexual men. *Am J Public Health.* 2004;94:1200–1203.
86. Mays VM, Cochran SD. Mental health correlates of perceived discrimination among lesbian, gay, and bisexual adults in the United States. *Am J Public Health.* 2001;91:1869–1876.
87. Rose SM, Mechanic MB. Psychological distress, crime features, and help-seeking behaviors related to homophobic bias incidents. *Am Behav Sci.* 2002;46:14–26.
88. Herek GM, Gillis JR, Cogan JC. Psychological sequelae of hate-crime victimization among lesbian, gay, and bisexual adults. *J Consult Clin Psychol.* 1999;67:945–951.
89. Diaz RM, Ayala G, Bein E, Henne J, Marin BV. The impact of homophobia, poverty, and racism on the mental health of gay and bisexual Latino men: findings from 3 US cities. *Am J Public Health.* 2001;91:927–932.
90. D'Augelli AR, Pilkington NW, Hershberger SL. Incidence and mental health impact of sexual orientation victimization of lesbian, gay, and bisexual youths in high school. *School Psychol Q.* 2002;17:148–167.
91. Pilkington N, D'Augelli AR. Victimization of lesbian, gay, and bisexual youth in community settings. *J Community Psychol.* 1995;23:34–56.
92. Bailey JM, Pillard RC. A genetic study of male sexual orientation. *Arch Gen Psychiatry.* 1991;48:1089–1096.
93. Bailey JM, Pillard RC. Genetics of human sexual orientation. *Annu Rev Sex Res.* 1996;6:126–150.
94. Mustanski BS, Chivers ML, Bailey JM. A critical review of recent biological research on human sexual orientation. *Annu Rev Sex Res.* 2002;13:89–140.
95. Pillard RC, Bailey JM. Human sexual orientation has a heritable component. *Hum Biol.* 1998;70:347–365.
96. Kendler KS, Thornton LM, Gilman SE, Kessler RC. Sexual orientation in a US national sample of twin and nontwin sibling pairs. *Am J Psychiatry.* 2000;157:1843–1846.
97. Meyer IH. Minority stress and mental health in gay men. *J Health Soc Behav.* 1995;36(1):35–56.
98. Gonsiorek JC. Gay male identities: concepts and issues. In: D'Augellis AR, Patterson CJ, eds. *Lesbian, Gay, and Bisexual Identities Over the Lifespan.* New York, NY: Oxford University Press; 1995:24–47.
99. House JS, Landis KR, Umberson D. Social relationships and health. *Science.* 1988;241:540–545.
100. Pennebaker JW, Ed; *Emotion, Disclosure, and Health.* Washington DC: American Psychological Association; 1995.
101. Cole SW, Kemeny ME, Taylor SE, Visscher BR. Elevated physical health risk among gay men who conceal their homosexual identity. *Health Psychol.* 1996;15:243–251.

102. Cole SW, Kemeny ME, Taylor SE, Visscher BR, Fahey JL. Accelerated course of human immunodeficiency virus infection in gay men who conceal their homosexual identity. *Psychosom Med.* 1996;58:219–231.

103. Ullrich PM, Lutgendorf SK, Stapleton JT. Concealment of homosexual identity, social support and CD4 cell count among HIV-seropositive gay men. *J Psychosom Res.* 2003;54:205–212.

104. Strachan ED, Bennett WRM, Russo J, Roy-Byrne PP. Disclosure of HIV status and sexual orientation independently predicts increased absolute CD4 cell counts over time for psychiatric patients. *Psychosom Med.* 2007;69:74–80.

105. Morris JF, Waldo CR, Rothblum ED. A model of predictors and outcomes of outness among lesbian and bisexual women. *Am J Orthopsychiatry.* 2001;71:61–71.

106. Cole SW, Kemeny ME, Taylor SE. Social identity and physical health: accelerated HIV progression in rejection-sensitive gay men. *J Pers Soc Psychol.* 1997;72:320–335.

107. Huebner DM, Davis MC. Gay and bisexual men who disclose their sexual orientation in the workplace have higher workday levels of salivary cortisol and negative affect. *Ann Behav Med.* 2005;30:260–267.

108. Waldo CR. Working in a majority context: a structural model of heterosexism as minority stress in the workplace. *J Counseling Psychol.* 1999;46:218–232.

109. Croteau JM. Research on the work experiences of lesbian, gay, and bisexual people: an integrative review of methodology and findings. *J Vocat Behav.* 1996;48:195–209.

110. Centers for Disease Control and Prevention. *HIV/AIDS Surveillance Report.* Atlanta, GA: Department of Health and Human Services; 2006;11.

111. Centers for Disease Control and Prevention. HIV prevalence, unrecognized infection, and HIV testing among men who have sex with men—five U.S. cities, June 2004-April 2005. *MMWR Morb Mortal Wkly Rep.* 2005;54:597–601.

112. Gluhoski VL, Fishman B, Perry SW. The impact of multiple bereavement in a gay male sample. *AIDS Educa Prev.* 1997;9:521–531.

113. Martin JL. Psychological consequences of AIDS-related bereavement among gay men. *J Consult Clin Psychol.* 1988;56:856–862.

114. Martin JL, Dean L. Effects of AIDS-related bereavement and HIV-related illness on psychological distress among gay men—A 7-year longitudinal-study, 1985–1991. *J Consult Clin Psychol.* 1993;61:94–103.

115. Valdiserri RO. HIV/AIDS in historical profile. In: Valdiserri RO, ed. *Dawning Answers: How the HIV/AIDS Epidemic Has Helped to Strengthen Public Health.* New York, NY: Oxford University Press; 2003:3–32.

116. Shilts R. *And the Band Played on: Politics, People, and the AIDS Epidemic.* New York, NY: St. Martin's Press; 1987.

117. Adler NE, Boyce T, Chesney MA, et al. Socioeconomic status and health: the challenge of the gradient. *Am Psychol.* 49:15–24.

118. Black D, Gates G, Sanders S, Taylor L. Demographics of the gay and lesbian population in the United States: evidence from the available systematic data sources. *Demography.* 2000;37:137–154.

119. Carpenter CS. Self-reported sexual orientation and earnings: evidence from California. *Ind Labor Relations Rev.* 2005;58:258–273.

120. Tebaldi E, Elmslie B. Sexual orientation and labour supply. *Appl Econ.* 2006;38:549–562.

121. Allegretto S, Arthur MM. An empirical analysis of homosexual/heterosexual male earnings differentials: unmarried and unequal? *Ind Labour Relations Rev.* 2001;54:631–646.

122. Badgett MV. The wage effects of sexual orientation discrimination. *Ind Labour Relations Rev.* 1995;48:726–729.

123. Harper GW, Schneider M. Oppression and discrimination among lesbian, gay, bisexual, and transgender people and communities: a challenge for community psychology. *Am J Community Psychol.* 2003;31:243–252.

124. The Gallup Organization. *The Gallup Poll: Homosexual Relations;* 2007. http://www.galluppoll.com/content/default.aspx?ci=1651&pg=1. Accessed January 14, 2007.

125. Damien MA, Hetrick ES. The stigmatization of the gay and lesbian adolescent. *J Homosexuality.* 1988;15:163–183.

126. Hetrick ES, Damien MA. Developmental issues and their resolution for gay and lesbian adolescents. *J Homosexuality.* 1987;14:25–43.

127. Strommen EF. "You're a what?": family member reactions to the disclosure of homosexuality. *J Homosexuality.* 1989;18:37–58.

128. D'Augelli AR, Hershberger SL. Lesbian, gay, and bisexual youth in community settings: personal challenges and mental health problems. *Am J Community Psychol.* 1993;21:421–448.

129. Meyer IH, Dean L. Patterns of sexual behavior and risk taking among young New York City gay men. *AIDS Educ Prev.* 1995;7(Suppl.):13–23.

130. Herek GM. Legal recognition of same-sex relationships in the United States. *Am Psychol.* 2006;61:607–621.

131. Riggle EDB, Thomas JD, Rostosky SS. The marriage debate and minority stress. *PS: Political Sci Polit.* 2005;April:221–224.

132. King M, Bartlett A. What same sex civil partnerships may mean for health. *J Epidemiol Community Health.* 2006;60:188–191.

133. Ash MA, Badgett MVL. Separate and unequal: the effect of unequal access to employment-based health insurance on same-sex and unmarried different-sex couples. *Contemporary Economics Policy.* 2006;24:582–599.

134. Kiecolt-Glaser JK, Newton TL. Marriage and health: his and hers. *Psychol Bull.* 2001;127:472–503.

135. Gordon HS, Rosenthal GE. Impact of marital status on outcomes in hospitalized patients: evidence from an academic medical center. *Arch Int Med.* 1995;155:2465–2471.

136. Johnson NL, Backlund E, Sorlie PD, Loveless CA. Marital status and mortality: The National Longitudinal Mortality Study. *Ann Epidemiol.* 2000;10:224–238.

137. Human Rights Campaign Foundation. The State of the Workplace; 2007. Available at http://hrc.org/workplace. Accessed August 22, 2007.

138. Jesdale BM, Zierler, S. Enactment of gay rights laws in U.S. states and trends in adolescent suicide: an investigation of non-Hispanic white boys. *J Gay Lesbian Med Assoc.* 2002;6:61–69.

139. Ryan W. *Blaming the Victim.* New York, NY: Random House; 1971.

140. Sumartojo E. Structural factors in HIV prevention: concepts, examples, and implications for research. *AIDS.* 2000;14(Suppl 1):S3-S10.

141. Stall R, Mills T, Williamson J, et al. Co-occurring psychosocial health problems among urban men who have sex with men are associated with increased vulnerability to the HIV/AIDS epidemic. *Am J Public Health.* 2003;93:939–942.

142. Rotello G. *Sexual Ecology: AIDS and the Destiny of Gay Men.* New York, NY: Dutton; 1997.

143. Sell RL, Becker JB. Sexual orientation data collection and progress toward Healthy People 2010. *Am J Public Health.* 2001;91:876–882.

144. Sell RL, Bradford J. *Elimination of Health Disparities Based on Sexual Orientation: Inclusion of Sexual Orientation as a Demographic Variable in Healthy People 2010 Objectives.* San Francisco, CA: Gay and Lesbian Medical Association; 2000.

PART II

EVIDENCE OF HEALTH DISPARITIES
AFFECTING GAY AND BISEXUAL MEN

2

Sexual Orientation and Violent Victimization: Hate Crimes and Intimate Partner Violence among Gay and Bisexual Males in the United States

Gregory M. Herek and Charles Sims

On February 2, 2006, an 18-year old man entered the Puzzles Lounge in New Bedford (MA). After ordering a drink, he asked the bartender if it was a gay bar and, when the bartender confirmed it was, the teenager pulled out a hatchet and struck a customer with it, then shot two other customers and fled the scene. Two of the victims were hospitalized in critical condition.[1]

> My partner, who I have been living with for a number of years, has been abusive on and off for much of that time. Most recently, he stabbed me several times. I dialed 911 and was hospitalized. He was arrested and is in jail and I have an automatic restraining order against him, which is good. But now, I am homeless because we were on a month-to-month lease and have now been kicked out. I have a congenital lung condition and so I receive SSI benefits but I cannot pull together deposit and first month's rent from it. Even though I am a victim of partner abuse, I can't get into any of the local domestic violence shelters because I am male. I will be able to get some motel vouchers but I am not sure if it will be enough time for me to save up my SSI.
>
> —*"William," age 28, p. 15* [2]

These events illustrate two kinds of violent victimization that men experience as a result of being gay or bisexual: criminal violence based on their sexual minority status (hereafter referred to as *hate crimes* or *bias crimes*) and violence from a male intimate partner (hereafter referred to as *domestic violence* or *intimate partner violence*). Consistent with the present volume's theme of health-related disparities, gay and bisexual men are disproportionately at risk for hate crime victimization because nearly all hate crimes based on the victim's sexual orientation target sexual minorities. In the case of intimate partner violence, currently available data do not permit conclusions to be drawn about disparities among men across sexual orientation groups. Nevertheless, such violence can have especially negative consequences for men in a same-sex relationship.

The present chapter summarizes current knowledge about hate crimes and intimate partner violence as they affect gay and bisexual men. We begin by describing the forms that anti-gay bias crimes take and discuss current data on their incidence and prevalence. We also consider the limitations of these data, as well as the challenges faced by researchers studying anti-gay violence and by providers attempting to address the problem. After discussing the correlates of anti-gay victimization, we briefly discuss community and societal responses to such victimization. Then we address similar topics for intimate partner violence. The chapter concludes with suggestions for future research directions.

Before discussing these phenomena, it is important to acknowledge the broader cultural context in which violence against sexual minority men occurs. Homosexual behavior and sexual minority identities remain widely stigmatized in the United States,[3] a fact with important implications for the continuing enactment of anti-gay violence as well as for individual, community, and societal responses to it. This is perhaps clearest in the case of anti-gay hate crimes, which can be understood as an extreme expression of society's sexual stigma,[4,5] but stigma and prejudice also play important roles in exacerbating the problem of intimate partner violence. As this chapter goes to press, same-sex marital relationships are recognized only in Massachusetts, with a handful of additional states according same-sex couples limited legal rights through institutions such as civil unions or domestic partnerships. Most states have enacted legislation expressly forbidding such recognition. Whereas legal recognition does not eliminate intimate partner violence (as attested by the widespread problem of abuse in heterosexual married couples), the lack of social legitimation and its accompanying benefits (including financial benefits[6] and social support[7]) imposes added stress on same-sex partners.[8] Such stress may foster relationship conflict and abuse in some cases. Reflecting negative societal attitudes toward sexual minorities and gender stereotypes, gay male victims of intimate partner violence may be viewed more negatively than heterosexual victims,[9] and male-male partner violence may be regarded as less serious than male-female abuse.[10,11]

Hate Crime Violence Targeting Gay and Bisexual Men

Regardless of one's sexual orientation or the perpetrator's motivation, being a victim of violent crime typically has negative psychological consequences. These can include acute anxiety disorder, depression, and post-traumatic stress disorder.[12,13] Such experiences also challenge victims' beliefs about their own safety, their self-worth, and their perception of the world as meaningful.[14] In addition to the negative psychosocial consequences of violent crime in general, victims of anti-gay violence are at heightened risk for psychological distress.[15,16] Hate crimes may have especially negative psychological sequelae because they attack a core aspect of the victim's personal identity and community membership, components of the self that are particularly important to sexual minority individuals because of the stresses created by sexual stigma.[3,15,17]

Anti-gay hate crimes take many forms. In documented victimizations, public settings are the most frequent locales for attacks, and the perpetrators most often are strangers to their victims. About 45% of the attacks reported to community-based anti-violence organizations and compiled by the National Coalition of Anti-Violence Programs (NCAVP)[18] occurred in public settings, such as on a street or in another public area, on public transportation, at a public accommodation, or in a gay-identified venue. In NCAVP annual reports between 1995 and 2004, strangers perpetrated between roughly one-third and one-half of the attacks, depending on the year (median across years = 43.5%). The most common scenario for hate crimes is the street attack, in which a group of perpetrators descends upon one or two gay or bisexual men in a public place, often in proximity to a gay neighborhood, gay bar, or other gay-identified venue. The perpetrators of such attacks typically are groups of male adolescents or young adults with no prior acquaintance with the victim.[19,20]

Although the streets are common settings, anti-gay attacks can occur virtually anywhere, and perpetrators evidence a variety of relationships to their victims. For example, interviews conducted with a convenience sample of 450 lesbian, gay, and bisexual adults in the greater Sacramento, California, area revealed that 27% of simple, aggravated, and sexual assaults, as well as robberies (hereafter referred to as *person crimes*) based on sexual orientation occurred in an indoor private setting (e.g., a home or office) and 30% were perpetrated by someone known to the victim.[20]

Anti-gay Violence: Incidence and Prevalence

Four main sources of data are available for estimating the incidence and prevalence of anti-gay violence: (1) reports by victims to advocacy and social service organizations, (2) reports by victims to law enforcement authorities, (3) the National Crime Victimization Survey, and (4) surveys of victim populations. We consider each in turn.

Historically, the earliest source of data about the prevalence of anti-gay violence was the gay community itself. As visible gay communities began to flourish in the 1960s and 1970s, first in large cities and later in smaller urban areas, community-based groups organized to respond to anti-gay attacks.[21,22] The first action of many groups was to develop procedures for documenting the frequency and characteristics of such incidents. In the mid-1980s, the National Gay Task Force (later the National Gay and Lesbian Task Force, or NGLTF) Anti-Violence Project, under the leadership of Kevin Berrill, began compiling data from individuals and community groups into annual reports on anti-gay victimization.[23]

As NGLTF and the local organizations acquired more resources and became more sophisticated in their approach to documentation, their reporting procedures evolved through three distinct stages. Between 1985 and 1990, the NGLTF compiled annual reports of anti-gay harassment, crimes, and victimization in the United States, based on whatever data were submitted to them by individuals and community-based organizations. Beginning in 1991, the NGLTF shifted to a more selective strategy, limiting the annual reports to data obtained from a small number of local anti-violence projects with professional staffs. This change represented an attempt to increase the quality of the data, to standardize data-collection procedures across cities, and to facilitate accurate tracking of trends. In 1994, responsibility for the annual reports shifted from NGLTF to an umbrella organization of community groups, the National Coalition of Anti-Violence Programs (NCAVP). Under the leadership of the New York City Anti-Violence Project, the NCAVP continues to compile and coordinate annual releases of tracking data. Table 2-1 summarizes the data compiled by the NCAVP since 1994, broken down by year, victim characteristics, and severity of injuries.

National data about hate crimes were not compiled by law enforcement agencies until the federal Hate Crime Statistics Act was passed in 1990. In 1991, the first year in which figures were tallied, the FBI recorded 422 anti-homosexual or anti-bisexual crimes (comprising 99% of the 425 reported crimes based on sexual orientation).[24] Through 2004, a total of 14,823 incidents based on sexual orientation were reported to the FBI, representing roughly 17,000 victims.* In any given year, sexual orientation incidents have comprised roughly 11–17% of all bias crimes recorded by the FBI. Tables 2-2, 2-3, and 2-4 report the characteristics of the crimes recorded in the annual statistics, including the number of incidents, victims, and criminal offenses for each category of sexual orientation used by the FBI (Table 2-2), the types of offenses reported (Table 2-3), and the crime settings (Table 2-4).

Since July 2000, questions about hate crime victimization have been included in the National Crime Victimization Survey (NCVS). The NCVS is conducted annually by the U.S. Bureau of Justice Statistics (BJS) with a sample of approximately 42,000 households comprising nearly 76,000 persons.[25] Data are collected by the US Census Bureau. As of this writing, only limited analyses of the NCVS hate crime data have been published.[26] Based on these analyses, the BJS estimated an annual average of 210,430 hate crime victimizations in 190,840 separate incidents from July 2000 through December 2003. Nearly one-fifth (17.9%) of the victimizations—more than 37,800—were motivated

---

*In contrast to subsequent years, the FBI did not release figures that separated the number of victims or offenses by target group in 1991. Consequently, these figures do not include 1991 crimes.

Table 2-1. Characteristics of victims of anti-gay violence, based on data compiled annually by community anti-violence programs

Victim characteristics	1994	1995	1996	1997	1998	1999	2000	2001	2002	2003	2004
Victim's gender											
Male	61	61	61	63	64	62	64	60	58	59	54
Female	30	27	29	27	24	25	23	25	26	25	26
Transgender	n/a	2	4	3	6	8	9	9	11	10	11
Unknown	0	0	0	3	4	3	3	3	3	4	6
Not applicable (organization/institution)	8	10	6	3	3	3	2	3	2	2	3
Total N	2,739	3,153	3,105	3,213	2,901	2,231	2,475	2,232	2,254	2,384	2,131
Victim's age											
Under 18	2	4	5	6	3	4	4	3	8	n/a	n/a
18–22	27	11	9	10	10	8	8	9	9	n/a	n/a
23–29	0	19	20	18	17	15	16	19	16	n/a	n/a
30–44	35	32	36	34	35	37	37	34	35	n/a	n/a
45–64	7	9	11	10	13	12	14	16	14	n/a	n/a
65 and over	0	0	1	1	1	1	1	2	1	n/a	n/a
Unknown				17	18	20	18	14	15	n/a	n/a
Not applicable (organization/institution)	28	25	19	3	3	3	2	3	2	n/a	n/a
Total N	2,162	3,153	3,105	3,213	2,901	2,234	2,475	2,232	2,254	n/a	n/a
Victim's sexual orientation											
Lesbian/gay	n/a	82	75	74	70	76	77	75	70	70	66
Bisexual	n/a	5	7	5	4	3	3	3	5	3	3
Heterosexual	n/a	2	3	4	3	5	6	8	10	9	9
Unsure	n/a	1	1	1	2	1	1	1	2	1	1

(*continued*)

Table 2-1. (*continued*)

Victim characteristics	1994	1995	1996	1997	1998	1999	2000	2001	2002	2003	2004
Unknown	n/a	n/a	n/a	13	18	13	11	10	12	16	18
Not applicable (organization/institution)	n/a	10	14	3	3	2	2	3	2	2	3
Total *N*	n/a	3,153	3,105	3,213	2,901	2,234	2,475	2,232	2,254	2,384	2,131
Victim's injuries											
None	38	66	64	68	62	63	64	66	56	65	65
Minor	27	15	18	16	18	16	18	16	16	13	13
Serious	32	8	9	8	10	11	9	10	10	9	11
Death	3	1	1	<1	1	1	1	<1	1	1	1
Unknown/not applicable (organization/institution)	n/a	9	8	8	9	9	8	8	17	12	10
Total *N*	632	3,153	3,105	3,196	2,896	2,235	2,475	2,209	2,254	2,291	2,136

Except for Total *N*, all entries in the table are percentages rounded to the nearest whole number. NCAVP made a transition to new age categories in 2003–2004 but these categories were adopted at different times by different participating agencies. Consequently, data for ages of victims were not uniformly categorized in 2003 and 2004 and thus are not displayed in the table. "Institution" refers to crimes against community organizations and institutions (e.g., vandalism).

n/a = Data not available

Source: Tabular data in annual reports from the National Coalition of Anti-Violence Programs (http://www.ncavp.org)

Table 2-2. FBI data on reported incidents, victims, and offenses in crimes based on sexual orientation 1991–2004, compiled by FBI

Target	1991	1992	1993	1994	1995	1996	1997	1998	1999	2000	2001	2002	2003	2004
Total incidents (N)	*425*	*767*	*860*	*685*	*1,019*	*1,016*	*1,102*	*1,260*	*1,317*	*1,299*	*1,393*	*1,244*	*1,239*	*1,197*
Anti-male homosexual	n/a	73%	72%	73%	72%	75%	69%	67%	69%	69%	70%	66%	63%	62%
Anti-lesbian	n/a	12%	14%	15%	14%	15%	17%	18%	14%	14%	15%	14%	15%	14%
Anti-homosexual	99%	13%	11%	9%	10%	8%	12%	13%	14%	14%	12%	18%	20%	20%
Anti-bisexual	<1%	<1%	<1%	1%	2%	1%	1%	1%	2%	2%	1%	1%	1%	1%
Anti-heterosexual	<1%	2%	3%	2%	2%	1%	1%	1%	1%	2%	1%	1%	1%	3%
Total victims (N)	n/a	*972*	*1,043*	*809*	*1,347*	*1,281*	*1,401*	*1,488*	*1,558*	*1,558*	*1,664*	*1,513*	*1,479*	*1,482*
Anti-male homosexual	n/a	70%	69%	72%	70%	73%	66%	68%	69%	68%	69%	65%	62%	61%
Anti-lesbian	n/a	14%	15%	15%	14%	15%	17%	18%	15%	15%	15%	15%	16%	14%
Anti-homosexual	n/a	14%	14%	10%	14%	8%	15%	12%	14%	15%	13%	18%	21%	21%
Anti-bisexual	n/a	<1%	<1%	1%	1%	1%	1%	1%	2%	1%	1%	1%	1%	1%
Anti-heterosexual	n/a	2%	3%	2%	1%	3%	1%	1%	1%	2%	1%	2%	1%	2%
Total offenses (N)	n/a	*949*	*998*	*793*	*1,266*	*1,256*	*1,375*	*1,439*	*1,487*	*1,486*	*1,592*	*1,464*	*1,430*	*1,406*
Anti-male homosexual	n/a	70%	70%	72%	72%	74%	66%	68%	69%	69%	69%	65%	62%	61%
Anti-lesbian	n/a	14%	15%	15%	15%	15%	17%	18%	15%	14%	15%	14%	15%	14%
Anti-homosexual	n/a	14%	12%	10%	10%	7%	15%	12%	14%	14%	13%	18%	21%	21%
Anti-bisexual	n/a	<1%	<1%	1%	1%	1%	1%	1%	2%	1%	1%	1%	1%	1%
Anti-heterosexual	n/a	2%	3%	2%	2%	3%	1%	1%	1%	1%	1%	2%	1%	2%

A single crime incident can target numerous victims and involve multiple criminal offenses

n/a = Data not available in category for that year.

All percentages are rounded to the nearest whole number.

Source: FBI annual hate crime reports (http://www.fbi.gov/ucr/ucr.htm)

Table 2-3. Types of offenses in crimes based on sexual orientation 1992–2004, compiled by FBI

Offense type	1992	1993	1994	1995	1996	1997	1998	1999	2000	2001	2002	2003	2004
Murder	<1%	1%	1%	<1%	<1%	<1%	<1%	<1%	<1%	<1%	<1%	<1%	<1%
Forcible rape	<1%	<1%	<1%	<1%	0%	<1%	<1%	<1%	0%	<1%	<1%	<1%	0%
Aggravated assault	20%	20%	17%	15%	18%	15%	14%	12%	15%	13%	14%	11%	15%
Simple assault	26%	25%	25%	24%	23%	25%	26%	26%	27%	29%	28%	31%	27%
Intimidation	35%	33%	37%	37%	36%	35%	34%	32%	29%	29%	30%	30%	28%
Other person crime	n/a	n/a	1%	<1%	0%	0%	0%	<1%	<1%	1%	<1%	0%	1%
Robbery	4%	4%	3%	4%	3%	3%	3%	3%	3%	3%	3%	3%	3%
Burglary/larceny/theft	1%	1%	2%	2%	1%	2%	2%	3%	2%	2%	2%	3%	2%
Arson	<1%	0%	1%	<1%	1%	<1%	1%	<1%	1%	1%	<1%	<1%	<1%
Vandalism	12%	16%	14%	17%	17%	19%	20%	23%	22%	23%	20%	21%	25%
Crimes against society	n/a	n/a	0%	0%	<1%	<1%	<1%	<1%	<1%	<1%	<1%	<1%	<1%
Other	n/a	<1%	n/a	<1%	<1%	<1%	<1%	<1%	<1%	<1%	<1%	0%	<1%
Total N	932	970	777	1,247	1,218	1,361	1,426	1,471	1,464	1,572	1,438	1,415	1,371

Incidents categorized as "anti-heterosexual" are not included in the table.
n/a = Data not available in category for that year.
All percentages are rounded to the nearest whole number.

Source: FBI annual hate crime reports (http://www.fbi.gov/ucr/ucr.htm)

Table 2-4. Locations of incidents in crimes based on sexual orientation 1992–2004, compiled by FBI

Location of incidents	1992	1993	1994	1995	1996	1997	1998	1999	2000	2001	2002	2003	2004
Street/alley/highway	28%	30%	27%	28%	26%	28%	24%	23%	21%	23%	25%	25%	25%
Parking lot/garage	7%	5%	6%	6%	6%	5%	7%	7%	6%	7%	5%	6%	5%
Bar/nightclub	5%	4%	5%	5%	5%	5%	4%	4%	5%	3%	3%	4%	3%
School/college	9%	6%	7%	7%	8%	11%	9%	10%	11%	12%	13%	12%	13%
Church/temple	<1%	2%	1%	<1%	1%	0%	<1%	1%	1%	1%	<1%	1%	1%
Other public setting	8%	11%	8%	10%	12%	11%	12%	10%	11%	12%	11%	10%	12%
Field/woods/waterway	2%	1%	1%	1%	2%	2%	2%	1%	2%	2%	1%	2%	<1%
Jail/prison	0%	<1%	0%	<1%	<1%	<1%	<1%	<1%	<1%	1%	<1%	1%	<1%
Home/residence	17%	26%	27%	26%	31%	28%	27%	31%	35%	33%	31%	30%	34%
Other/unknown	24%	15%	19%	16%	10%	10%	14%	15%	9%	7%	10%	10%	6%
Multiple locations	n/a	n/a	<1%	0%	<1%	<1%	0%	<1%	<1%	0%	0%	0%	<1%
Total N	767	860	685	1,019	1,016	1,102	1,260	1,317	1,299	1,393	1,244	1,239	1,197

All percentages are rounded to the nearest whole number.
n/a=Data not available in category for that year.

Source: FBI annual hate crime reports (http://www.fbi.gov/ucr/ucr.htm)

by the victim's sexual orientation. Approximately 42% of the incidents were reported to police authorities.

A fourth source of data on anti-gay victimization consists of surveys and questionnaire studies conducted by academics and community-based advocates with samples of sexual minority respondents. Such studies query participants about their experiences with criminal victimization and harassment due to their sexual orientation. Because they sample the community at large, they have the advantage of detecting anti-gay crimes that were never reported to law enforcement agencies or a gay community organization. Thus, they provide a basis for tentatively estimating the prevalence of sexual minority victimization.

The earliest such surveys were not designed specifically to assess hate crime victimization but rather inquired about violence as one component of the experience of homosexuals.[27,28] In the 1980s, when anti-gay violence came to be seen as a problem in its own right, individual researchers and community groups began to conduct community surveys designed specifically to document its prevalence.[29] The quality of community-based surveys has varied widely. Some have been methodologically sophisticated—designed and implemented by researchers with extensive training in survey methods, often in collaboration with community-based organizations—whereas others have yielded results with limited value because of flaws in question construction, sampling, methodology, data analysis, or reporting procedures.[30] Nevertheless, substantial proportions of respondents to victimization surveys have consistently reported experiencing criminal victimization because of their sexual orientation.

Berrill[19] compiled the data from 24 such studies conducted with convenience samples of gay men, lesbians, and bisexuals between 1977 and 1991. Most of them did not report data separately by respondents' gender or sexual orientation. Across the studies, a median of 9% of respondents reported aggravated assault (i.e., assault with a weapon) because of their sexual orientation; 17% reported simple physical assault (i.e., without a weapon); 19% reported vandalism of personal property; 44% had been threatened with violence; 33% had been chased or followed; 25% reported having objects thrown at them; 13% had been spat upon; and 80% had been verbally harassed.[19]

More recent academic research has provided additional data. The previously mentioned interview study[20] was conducted with a subset of respondents from a larger survey project in which 2,259 respondents completed a lengthy questionnaire concerning their experiences with violence.[15] In that larger group, 13% of gay men (total $n = 898$) and 11% of bisexual men (total $n = 191$) had experienced a simple or aggravated assault based on their sexual orientation, and 4% of gay men and 7% of bisexual men had experienced sexual assault. Overall, more than one-fourth of the male respondents (28% of gay men, 27% of bisexual men) had experienced some type of criminal victimization since age 16 because of their sexual orientation.

Other studies have focused on particular age groups in sexual minority communities. Huebner and colleagues reported data from a sample of 1,248 young gay and bisexual men ($M = 23$ years, range $= 18–27$ years) recruited in three southwestern U.S. cities. Five percent reported that they had experienced physical violence during the previous 6 months because of their sexual orientation.[31] In another study, conducted with a convenience sample of 194 lesbian, gay, and bisexual youths (age range $= 15–21$ yrs), 9% reported at least one aggravated assault (i.e., assault with a weapon) based on their sexual orientation, 18% had experienced a simple assault, 22% had been sexually assaulted, and 44% had been threatened with attack.[32] At the other end of the age continuum, D'Augelli and Grossman[33] documented the lifetime occurrence of hate crime victimization among older (over 59 years) lesbian, gay, and bisexual adults, using a convenience sample ($n = 416$) recruited from across the United States. In that sample, 16% had been physically attacked at some time in their life, 11% reported having had objects thrown at them, 12% had been threatened with weapons, 7% had been sexually assaulted, and 29% had been threatened with violence.

It is difficult to estimate the prevalence of hate crime victimization from these studies because of variations in the categorization of crimes, time frames in which victimization was assessed, and differences in reporting (e.g., some studies reported findings separately for men and women, or for homosexuals and bisexuals, whereas others did not). Across studies, roughly 11–18% of male respondents report having experienced a hate crime assault. Because the surveys all used convenience samples, the extent to which their results describe the entire U.S. gay and bisexual male population cannot be determined.

Data collected in three studies with probability samples confirm that hate crime victimization is widespread. In a 1989 *San Francisco Examiner* telephone survey with a national probability sample that included 287 gay men, 5% reported having been physically abused or assaulted in the previous year because they were gay.[34] In a 2000 Kaiser Family Foundation survey of 405 lesbian, gay, and bisexual adults residing in major US population centers, 32% of the respondents said they had ever been targeted for violence against their person or property because of their sexual orientation. When asked how worried they were that they someday "might be physically assaulted or beaten by someone who dislikes gay people," 39% were "very worried" or "somewhat worried."[35] In a probability sample of 912 Latino men who have sex with men (MSM)—recruited from social venues in the cities of New York, Miami, and Los Angeles—10% had experienced violence as an adult because of their sexual orientation or femininity.[36]

Limitations of Existing Data

Each of the existing sources of data described above has limitations. The organizations contributing to the NGLTF and NCAVP compilations have varied from year to year. In its 1989 report, for example, the NGLTF noted that "more than half of the groups reporting to NGLTF in 1988 did not do so in 1989 because of a lack of resources to continue data collection, inability to meet NGLTF reporting deadlines, or dissolution of the group. Meanwhile, other groups provided documentation to NGLTF for the first time in 1989" (p. 7).[37] These discontinuities in reporting made it problematic to compare data from one year to the next. The shift to collecting data only from cities with ongoing anti-violence projects—which was subsequently continued by the NCAVP—addressed this problem and made the figures more comparable from one year to the next. Even so, because statistics were collected locally and then reported to a central clearinghouse, there were probably variations across sites in how incidents were classified. A related consideration is that, as is often the case in community service organizations operating on limited budgets, personnel turnover occurs frequently in many local anti-violence projects. Staff changes can adversely affect the consistency of their data collection and reporting from year to year. In addition, the decision whether or not to categorize any incident as anti-gay was made locally. Although the compilers of the NGLTF and NCAVP provided explicit guidelines for classifying incidents as anti-gay, some incidents may have been inappropriately included in or excluded from the count.

Data collected by law enforcement agencies may not have the same limitations, but they almost certainly underestimate the true number of anti-gay crimes for several reasons. First, reporting of such crimes by law enforcement agencies is voluntary. Many localities are not consistently represented in the statistics in Tables 2-2, 2-3, and 2-4. Fewer than 3,000 law enforcement agencies contributed to the 1991 data (by contrast, more than 16,000 agencies provided data for the FBI Uniform Crime Reports that year).[24] Since 1991, ever larger proportions of U.S. law enforcement agencies have participated in hate crime reporting each year. By 2004, the number had climbed to more than 12,000 agencies, representing jurisdictions covering approximately 87% of the US population.[38] Consequently, hate crime statistics for recent years can be considered more reliable than for earlier years.

A second problem is that the quality of the data submitted to the FBI varies from one local jurisdiction to another. In contrast to the community anti-violence agencies, high levels of bureaucratization in local law enforcement agencies may increase the consistency of reporting from one year to the next. However, inter-agency differences exist. Some police departments—especially in larger cities—have staff assigned to deal with crimes that might be bias-motivated, and all members of the force receive training for identifying and reporting hate crimes. Those departments are in the minority, however; most others devote no special resources to hate crimes. In a 1999 national survey of police chiefs in large and medium-sized cities, for example, Haider-Markel found that slightly more than one-third of the responding departments had a special officer, task force, or unit to investigate and track such crimes. Nearly 40% of responding departments did not require any training of officers for identifying hate crimes.[39] Without training or resources, officers on the scene often may not know which questions to ask or how best to ask them to ensure accurate responses. Consequently, many anti-gay crimes probably go undetected.

A third important reason why criminal justice agencies undercount hate crimes is that many victims never report their experience to police authorities. Underreporting of all crime is a problem in the United States, and victims decide not to report for many reasons. These include believing the incident was not serious enough to report; uncertainty about whether it was actually a crime; doubts about whether reporting will accomplish anything because the police are unlikely to catch the perpetrator; and a desire to put the experience behind them and move on with their lives. In addition to these reasons, victims of anti-gay crimes often do not report a crime because they fear harassment by law enforcement personnel as a result of their sexual minority status or because they do not want their sexual orientation to become a matter of public record. Still others do not believe the police will seriously attempt to apprehend the perpetrators of a crime when the victim is gay.[20,40]

Community-based gay and lesbian organizations are likely to receive reports of crimes not reported to the police because many gay people are more willing to volunteer information to a gay-identified agency than to law enforcement personnel. Their experiences indicate that a substantial number of incidents reported to them would qualify for inclusion in police data but are never reported to police. For example, the 2005 NCAVP report[18] noted that in 2003,

> only 1,239 bias-related incidents based on sexual orientation (including 14 based on anti-heterosexual sentiment) were contained in the FBI's data representing 82.8% of the nation's population, whereas NCAVP captured 1,792 incidents in areas representing only 27.2% of the nation's population. Of the incidents for which NCAVP collected data, there were at least 758 'arrest-able' offenses such as murder, assault or rape that if reported to local law enforcement should have been documented as hate incidents and submitted to the FBI under Uniform Crime Reporting. Additionally, the FBI identified just 6 anti-LGTB murders in 2003, while in the same year, NCAVP documented 23. (p. 21, footnotes omitted)

How extensive is police undercounting of anti-gay crimes? The NCVS data indicate that only 42.3% of hate crime incidents between July 2000 and December 2003 were reported to law enforcement authorities, accounting for 43.5% of all hate crime victimizations during that period (a single incident can include multiple victims).[26] Of the hate crimes not reported to police, 15.6% were based on the victim's sexual orientation (compared to 21.4% of those reported to police). Another study found that the reporting of hate crimes by sexual minority individuals varies according to their gender and sexual orientation (bisexual versus homosexual), and that hate crimes are considerably less likely to be reported to law enforcement officials than crimes unrelated to sexual minority status ("routine" crimes).[15] In that study, gay men had reported 72% of their routine victimizations to police, but only 46% of their hate crime victimizations; bisexual men were even less likely to report hate crime victimizations (24%, compared to 61% of routine crimes).[15] Follow-up interviews with a subsample of the survey respondents revealed that concerns about police prejudice influenced the decision not to report for more than two-thirds of the victims of anti-gay assaults, robberies, and rapes, but for fewer than one-fifth of the gay and bisexual victims of otherwise comparable routine crimes. Among victims of anti-gay property crimes, almost half (44%) said that such concerns affected their decision, compared to only 6% of routine property crime victims.[20] These data indicate that nonreporting affects police statistics and leads to underestimation of the full extent of anti-gay victimization.

Despite their limitations, community-based organization data and law enforcement agency reports complement each other. Green and colleagues mapped anti-gay attacks reported to the New York City police and those reported to a community anti-violence group.[41] Although considerably more incidents were reported to the community group than to the police, the attacks reported to both entities tended to manifest the same geographic distribution, with the greatest likelihood of occurrence in gay neighborhoods such as Greenwich Village. The link between gay population density and prevalence of attacks was stronger for gay men than for lesbians, perhaps because gay men tended to be more geographically concentrated in gay neighborhoods.[41]

Challenges in Documenting the Incidence and Prevalence of Anti-gay Violence

In addition to the data limitations already noted, the task of obtaining incidence and prevalence data on anti-gay violence poses several special challenges. First, because all data in this area are based on some form of self-report (whether survey responses or reports to agencies), assessing their validity requires an understanding of the decision criteria used by gay and bisexual people for labeling a particular experience as an instance of anti-gay violence. Two studies[20,42] have examined the strategies that sexual minority respondents use to determine whether or not a victimization experience was based on their sexual orientation. Four variables appeared to play a central role in victims' assessments: (1) whether or not the perpetrator(s) made explicit anti-gay statements during the incident; (2) whether or not the incident occurred in a gay-identified location or situation; (3) whether or not it occurred immediately after they (or others with them) had behaved in a way that made their gay or lesbian identity apparent to others (e.g., the victim was holding hands with a same-sex partner or had affixed a gay bumper sticker to his car); and (4) the timing of the incident (e.g., whether it occurred simultaneously with an event such as a local gay pride march). Overall, the patterns observed in these two studies suggest that the motivations for a majority of anti-gay crimes are frequently unambiguous. Either the perpetrators make explicit statements, or the attack occurs in a gay-identified location or is closely associated with behaviors by the victim that identify her or him as gay.

A second important question about data quality is whether self-reports of anti-gay violence are reliable, that is, whether respondents are consistent over time in recalling and categorizing their experiences. To address this question, Herek and colleagues[42] assessed consistency in reports of victimization experiences between self-administered questionnaires and face-to-face interviews. From a convenience sample of 150 individuals who completed an initial questionnaire, 45 were recontacted for a follow-up interview between 1 and 7 months later. Of these, 39 respondents provided complete data that permitted comparisons across data collection modes. Roughly half (51%) of them were consistent in their self-reports of bias crimes across data-collection modes: 11 reported a bias incident in both their questionnaire and interview, whereas 9 reported no bias incidents in either mode. Another 28% reported a crime in the interview that they had not previously reported in the self-administered questionnaire, a pattern that the researchers attributed to the greater number of memory cues and prompts available in an interview setting compared to a self-administered questionnaire. The remaining 21% reported a crime in the questionnaire but did not subsequently report it in the interview.[42] The researchers noted that the time lag between completion of the questionnaire and the interview could have induced memory problems (e.g., an incident that was relatively recent at the time of questionnaire completion might have faded in memory by the time the interview was conducted) and might also have created confusion about the time frame for incidents (e.g., events that were appropriately reported as having happened "in the past year" on the questionnaire might have been appropriately reported as happening more than one year ago in the interview). To the best of our knowledge, this is the only published study to systematically examine consistency in the recall and reporting of anti-gay victimization. The results suggest that, for some victims, accurate and complete recall of incidents may be affected by memory factors (e.g., elapsed time since the incident) and by the mode of data collection (self-administered questionnaire versus personal interview). Further research is needed to better understand how to increase the accuracy and completeness of victim self-reports.

Correlates of Victimization

Three major correlates of victimization have been observed in the studies described above: gender, age, and visibility. Data from the National Crime Victimization Surveys[43] show that men are considerably more likely than women to be victims of violent crime, especially crimes perpetrated by strangers. Consistent with this pattern, most empirical studies of anti-gay crimes, including compilations of reports to law enforcement agencies and community organizations, show that men are more frequent targets than women in all violent crime categories other than sexual assault. In reports compiled by NCAVP between 1994 and 2004, for example, the number of incidents with male victims outnumbered those with female victims by a ratio of roughly 2:1 (see Table 2-1). Males were victims in 54% to 64% of incidents, depending on the year, compared to 23% to 30% for females. Gender disparities are even greater in the FBI data: Crimes classified as "anti-male homosexual" outnumber those classified as "anti-lesbian" by roughly 4:1 (see Table 2-2).

Berrill found that gay men experienced higher rates than women of most forms of physical violence and intimidation.[19] More recent studies have noted similar patterns. In D'Augelli and Grossman's[33] study of sexual minority adults over 60, significantly more men than women reported having been threatened: respectively, 34% versus 16%. In addition, more men than women were physically attacked because of their sexual orientation: about 20% compared to 4%. Men were also threatened more often with weapons: 15% of the men were threatened with a weapon compared to 4% of the women. In Herek and colleagues' study,[15] gay and bisexual men were almost twice as likely as lesbian and bisexual women to have been victimized. However, women were more likely than men to experience a crime they did not attribute to their sexual orientation, especially an assault. It is possible that lesbians and bisexual women, in contrast to gay and bisexual men, tend to interpret victimizations as misogynistic rather than anti-lesbian.[44] This is an area in which further research is needed.

Age is another correlate of anti-gay victimization.[15] Federal crime statistics show that, in general, younger people are more likely than older people to experience a violent crime.[43] Consistent with this pattern, young people account for a substantial portion of crimes documented in the NCAVP reports (see Table 2-1). Between 1994 and 2003, the percentage of victims under 30 years of age ranged from 27% (in 1999) to 34% (in 1995, 1996, and 1997). Evidence for younger gay and bisexual males' risk for violent victimization is also found in studies with probability samples of adolescents, which further suggest that victimization is correlated with increased risk for a variety of social and psychological problems, including alcohol and drug use and suicide attempts.[45,46,47] However, interpretation of the findings from these studies is complicated by differing operational definitions of sexual orientation across studies and the relatively small numbers of sexual minority respondents in the samples.

Although age is correlated with victimization, older sexual minority men are nevertheless at risk for anti-gay violence. In the NCAVP reports between 1994 and 2003 (Table 2-1), the proportion of victims in the 30–44 year age group was about as high as in younger age groups, ranging from 32% (in 1995) to 37% (in 1999 and 2000). Thus, the age range for targets of anti-gay violence may be considerably wider than is the case for other types of crime, with many victims in their thirties and forties.

A third important correlate of victimization is visibility and the extent to which individuals have publicly disclosed their sexual orientation (i.e., are publicly "out of the closet," or "out"). D'Augelli and colleagues[48,49] found that victimization[†] in their sexual minority youth samples was predicted by greater visibility (indicated by gender nonconformity and disclosure of sexual orientation to others). Tewksbury and colleagues[50] also found that anti-gay victimization was predicted by visibility, operationally defined as being out in one's workplace. Herek and colleagues similarly found that, controlling for other relevant factors, the extent to which one was publicly out was a significant correlate of anti-gay victimization.[15]

The linkage between visibility and risk for victimization has probably changed over the past half century as opportunities for being publicly out have increased for most sexual minority adults. With the rise of gay culture after World War II, gay neighborhoods and communities became more visible in most cities and towns in the United States.[51] Although the existence of gay-identified spaces has had many positive consequences, it also has made their inhabitants more visible targets for attack. Similarly, the greater willingness of gay people to make their sexual orientation known in spaces not defined as gay—including workplaces, schools, homes, and neighborhoods—has created new freedom for them but also has increased their vulnerability.[52]

The factors of visibility and age probably interact to increase risk for sexual minority youth. Although comparison data from probability samples are not available, data from convenience samples suggest that the average age at which sexual minority youth recognize their same-sex attractions, act on them, and come out as lesbian, gay, or bisexual has declined over the past several decades.[53,54] This is consistent with an overall trend among American youth to have sexual experiences at a younger age than in the past.[55] Adolescents and young adults are especially vulnerable to bullying in school and college settings, and violence and harassment appear to be more likely the earlier that youth publicly identify as gay or lesbians.[32]

Trends

Given the uneven quality of data in this area, tracking time trends in victim reports is problematic. The FBI data have included more police agencies with each passing year since 1991. The cities and organizations reflected in NGLTF and NCAVP reports have changed over time. With both sets of data, nonreporting by victims is an ongoing problem. Despite the lack of adequate data, the perception that anti-gay violence is increasing is widespread. When asked whether they believed "there is more violence or less violence directed against gays and lesbians in this country today" compared to "a few years ago," 41% of

---

[†]In this study, the researchers did not report predictors of violence per se; rather, victimization was operationalized as an ordinal variable that included verbal harassment and threats of violence as well as actual assault.

the gay, lesbian, and bisexual respondents to the Kaiser Family Foundation's 2001 survey believed there was more violence today than in the past. When the question was posed to a sample drawn from the general population, the result was essentially the same—39% believed that violence had increased.[35]

Violence may well be on the rise because sexual stigma has become increasingly overt in recent decades. Even as gay and bisexual people have become more visible and have made significant social and legal gains, messages of anti-gay bigotry, intolerance, and resentment have increasingly become a part of daily discourse in the United States.[56] When sexual minorities are blamed for society's ills, some members of society are likely to interpret such messages as legitimizing anti-gay violence and to act accordingly.

At the same time, the popular belief that anti-gay crimes have become more common might reflect shifts in perception more than an actual increase in the number of violent attacks. Until relatively recently, anti-gay violence was widely perceived to be simply the price one paid for being a sexual minority. This seemingly "natural" state of affairs was rarely questioned, and the frequency with which lesbians, gay men, and bisexuals were attacked went undocumented. The upsurge in the number of crimes reported throughout the 1980s and 1990s undoubtedly reflected a gradual change in how the gay and lesbian community regarded such incidents. The community stopped accepting harassment and attacks as inevitable, and began to define them as crimes warranting a response from law enforcement and other government entities. This shift reflected a growing sense among gay and bisexual people that they deserve to be fully participating members of society, entitled to pursue their day-to-day lives without being attacked. Thus, anti-gay crimes may seem more common today than in the past because gay communities have organized and, in the process, have become less willing to accept victimization as their lot.

In addition, community standards for reporting probably evolved at different rates in different parts of the country and in different kinds of settings. In the wake of the 1998 murder of Matthew Shepard, for example, anti-violence projects in larger cities noted a decline in reports of anti-gay harassment, whereas observers in smaller towns and rural areas noted an increase. The 2000 NCAVP report speculated that the widely publicized Shepard murder may have had different effects in the two types of settings. Urban gay men and lesbians may have become less likely to report experiences such as verbal harassment, regarding them as relatively trivial in comparison to Shepard's murder, whereas gay men and lesbians in less populated areas were inspired to report every incident to honor Shepard's memory.[57]

Responses to Anti-gay Violence

As noted above, many victims of anti-gay violence are reluctant to report their experiences to local police, even today. Historically, this pattern effectively made the problem of anti-gay violence invisible to law enforcement personnel, government authorities, and the general public. It is not surprising, therefore, that early efforts to document the nature and prevalence of anti-gay violence were initiated within gay communities. Indeed, the felt need for documentation—and the credibility it conveys—provided the main impetus for establishing many community antiviolence groups. Of the 32 community-based US anti-violence projects analyzed by Jenness and Broad,[58] approximately two-thirds had established programs to document local incidents of anti-gay violence, and more than half focused on incident documentation as their primary activity.

In addition to documenting violence, community groups also have developed programs for crisis intervention and victim assistance. In many cases, the latter activities grew out of initial documentation efforts through, for example, telephone hot lines.[58] The history of the New York City Anti-Violence Project (AVP) illustrates this pattern. The AVP has its roots in community organizing by residents of Manhattan's Chelsea neighborhood in 1980, when neighborhood residents were becoming aware of what appeared to be an increasing number of street attacks by groups of young white males coming to Chelsea specifically to harass and assault gay men. As Wertheimer[22] described,

> Members of the Chelsea Gay Association, a local lesbian and gay community organization, began to address the problem by sponsoring a number of well-attended town meetings. Numerous assault victims came forward publicly for the first time to report precisely what had happened to them. As a result of these meetings, two members of the Chelsea Gay Association placed a special telephone hotline in their own home to take reports from individuals who had been gay-bashed. Volunteers from the group were recruited and trained to respond to messages left on an answering machine, document incidents of violence, and provide basic crisis intervention services to callers. The group decided to provide volunteers who could accompany crime victims who wished to make police reports to the local precinct, and to monitor the progress of any cases that resulted in arrests and entered into the criminal court system. Palm cards with the new hotline number were distributed throughout the community. As word spread, calls came in to the hotline from all over the City. The project organizers quickly realized that anti-gay and anti-lesbian violence was not limited to any one neighborhood, but was in fact present throughout every part of the region. (p. 230)

Whereas the Chelsea Gay Association began to offer victim services soon after its initial establishment of a phone reporting hotline, many other community groups took longer to develop service provision programs, and still others have lacked the resources to do so.[58]

Yet another response by community organizations has been to conduct educational campaigns. Some campaigns have been designed to alert gay men, lesbians, and bisexuals about the dangers of violence, ways to avoid it, tactics for self-defense, and resources for victims. Others have tried to make the general public aware of the problem of anti-gay violence and to prevent it by influencing community attitudes and norms, often through speakers' bureaus, training sessions for employers and law enforcement personnel, and public media campaigns.[58]

One consequence of community-based activism and the general public's increasing awareness of anti-gay hate crimes has been the passage of state and federal laws that explicitly address violence based on the victim's actual or perceived sexual orientation. Such laws were initially enacted at the state level, beginning with a 1978 California statute, and focused mainly on crimes that targeted victims because of their race, national origin, or religion.[59] Throughout the 1980s and 1990s, more states passed hate crime statutes and began to include sexual orientation within the purview of those laws.[60] By early 2006, 32 states and the District of Columbia had enacted hate crime statutes that included sexual orientation. Another 14 states had enacted hate crime laws that did not include sexual orientation.[61,62] Most of these statutes enhance the penalties for existing crimes when the victim was selected because of her or his status.[60]

Currently, only two federal laws address hate crimes based on sexual orientation. The Hate Crimes Statistics Act, signed into law by President George H.W. Bush in 1990, mandates the attorney general to collect and compile hate crimes data from local jurisdictions. The Hate Crimes Sentencing Enhancement Act of 1994 directs the U.S. Sentencing Commission to provide a sentencing enhancement (i.e., a more severe penalty than would otherwise be imposed) for bias crimes, including those based on the victim's sexual orientation. This law's impact is limited because it applies only to existing federal crimes, which, for those involving sexual orientation, include only crimes committed in national parks and on other federal property. Since 1998, new legislation has been introduced repeatedly in Congress to expand federal definitions and enforcement of hate crimes, including those based on sexual orientation. Labeled variously as the "Hate Crimes Expansion Act" and the "Local Law Enforcement Enhancement Act," somewhat different versions of the bill have been passed by the House of Representatives and the Senate, but not by both houses in the same session.

Intimate Partner Violence in Male Same-Sex Couples

When community anti-violence projects established hot lines for reporting victimization, agency staffs soon discovered that some acts of violence were being committed by gay people against other gay people. In particular, the problem of violence perpetrated by lovers and intimate partners emerged, and it became apparent that domestic violence was a problem in same-sex relationships just as in heterosexual couples. As with hate crime violence, community organizations responded by attempting to document the extent of intimate partner violence as well as by creating victim services programs and public education campaigns.[58]

Intimate partner violence (IPV) refers to "physical, sexual, or psychological harm by a current or former partner or spouse."[63] This term is increasingly used instead of the once common *domestic violence* because it better differentiates the phenomenon from other forms of family violence (e.g., child and elder abuse) and carries fewer presumptions about the genders of the individuals involved.[64] The rubric of IPV can encompass physical violence, sexual violence, threats of physical or sexual violence, and psychological or emotional violence but, as noted below, operational definitions of IPV have varied widely.

Regardless of the participants' sexual orientation, victimization through IPV has negative consequences, including psychological trauma (e.g., depression, anxiety, lowered self-esteem), self-destructive behaviors (including substance abuse and suicide), economic instability, physical injury, and even death.[65,66] Violence in intimate relationships creates additional stressors for gay and bisexual men, in part because society stigmatizes sexual minorities and in part because gay communities and society at large have been slow to recognize and address the problem. Most existing social services and resources for IPV victims are designed for women in heterosexual relationships. Consequently, male victims of IPV from a same-sex partner often are unable to find appropriate assistance. Because most states do not accord legal recognition to same-sex relationships, IPV between two people of the same gender often is not even acknowledged as such, and victims lack the legal safeguards offered to heterosexual victims, such as protection orders in family courts.[67] Ignorance and misinformation about male-male IPV can have direct negative consequences. For example, law enforcement personnel who are summoned to intervene in a violent incident may incorrectly assume that male-male violence must be mutual and thus arrest both the abuser and the victim.[68,69] Similarly, courts may issue restraining orders against both parties.[67,68] This overall lack of support and accurate information make it difficult for gay and bisexual male IPV victims to seek help, receive treatment, and leave abusive relationships, thereby exacerbating the extent and severity of their abuse and complicating their recovery from it.[70,71,72]

These deficiencies in services for the victims of violence are closely related to the stigmatization associated with being gay or bisexual, which deters victims not only from seeking help but also from openly acknowledging that a problem exists. Victims may justifiably feel that law enforcement personnel, social service workers, and other potential resources for help are unknowledgeable, unsympathetic, and perhaps even hostile toward them. Fearing secondary victimization,[40] they may avoid official agencies entirely. Furthermore, the belief that the existence of IPV will be used to justify and promote anti-gay prejudice may make victims even more reluctant to attempt to obtain assistance. Such concerns have a basis in fact. For example, the Web site of one anti-gay activist group[73] cites studies of same-sex domestic violence in an effort to support its claims that same-sex marriage is "a health hazard" and to argue that "rather than being a 'shelter against the storms of life,' as traditional marriage is sometimes characterized, being homosexually partnered actually increases the physical dangers associated with homosexuality."‡

Given the largely hidden nature of same-sex IPV, it is perhaps not surprising that the empirical research literature in this area is limited, especially for male couples. This dearth of empirical studies hampers attempts to understand its prevalence, correlates, consequences, and treatment. Before reviewing the available studies, we briefly consider some important conceptual and methodological issues that affect the interpretation of data.

Definition, Measurement, and Sampling

Accurate estimates of the prevalence of intimate partner violence among gay and bisexual men are hampered by definitional, measurement, and sampling problems. We consider each of these in turn. First, empirical studies have used differing conceptual and operational definitions of IPV. Prevalence estimates are strongly affected by how broadly or narrowly researchers define IPV. For example, prevalence estimates are inevitably higher when the scope of IPV includes verbal behavior than when it is restricted to physical aggression. Unfortunately, studies have often failed to distinguish among physical, sexual, and psychological forms of abuse.[74] This problem is not exclusive to research on same-sex IPV. In the area of heterosexual partner violence, dramatically different views of IPV have emerged, depending on how partner violence was operationalized. Studies using crime victimization data have focused on severe forms of violence, whereas studies that operationalized IPV in terms of responses to measures of family conflicts (e.g., the Conflict Tactics Scale, or CTS[75]) have often identified behaviors of relatively minor severity as IPV. Crime victim studies "typically find that domestic violence is rare, serious, escalates over time, and primarily perpetrated by men" (p. 466),[76] whereas family conflict studies tend to show "higher rates of domestic violence, stable

---

‡The FRI Web page buttresses its claims about domestic violence by citing only two published research studies of same-sex IPV.[83,105] Our examination of those papers revealed that the FRI site's assertions substantially inflated the prevalence figures reported in both. The FRI page also cites two unpublished dissertations on IPV in same-sex couples; we could not check the accuracy of the FRI's statements about those studies. As noted below, even when they are accurately characterized, the data from unpublished theses and dissertations are of limited value because they have not been subjected to the same level of peer review as studies published in academic journals. Although the quality of peer review varies across journals and flawed studies sometimes survive the process, unpublished research has not been subjected to even this level of scrutiny.

levels of severity, and low rates of injury and find it perpetrated equally by women and men" (p. 1341).[77]

Another definitional problem that arises in studies of same-sex IPV is determining what constitutes an intimate relationship. Whereas studies of heterosexual couples often use marriage as a marker, the vast majority of gay and bisexual men in the United States are legally barred from claiming this status. Even limited societal recognition of same-sex relationships, such as that accorded to civil unions and domestic partnerships, is available in only a few states. This ambiguity in defining relationship boundaries can make it difficult to determine when a violent act should be classified as occurring in the context of an intimate relationship, making comparisons between heterosexual and same-sex couples highly problematic. Whereas most studies operationally define IPV in heterosexual relationships as occurring between legal spouses or cohabiting partners, studies of same-sex IPV typically ask respondents to define whether or not they were in a relationship when a violent incident occurred. Consequently, unlike much of the data from heterosexuals, self-reports obtained from gay and bisexual men may include violence that occurred in the context of dating or a noncohabiting relationship. This may result in overestimates of the prevalence of IPV in male couples relative to heterosexual couples.

Second, studies have differed widely in how they operationalized IPV. Many studies of IPV in same-sex relationships have employed a version of the Conflict Tactics Scale[75] but some have used original checklists or questionnaires created specifically for the study, often without evaluation of their psychometric properties. Because only summary scores were often reported (rather than responses to individual items), comparisons across studies are problematic. Even among studies that used the CTS, results may not be directly comparable. Categorization of respondents is affected by the specific CTS subscales that were used to operationally define IPV. Some studies have reported overall abuse; others have distinguished among physical, psychological, and sexual abuse; others have separated actual from threatened abuse; and still others have differentiated severe from mild violence. Studies also vary in the time frame they use for asking about violence, ranging from the previous six months to the respondent's entire lifetime. In addition, because the CTS was originally developed for heterosexual respondents,[78] most studies with gay and bisexual males have used modified forms of the scale. However, the scale modifications have not been consistent across studies, and the validity of the modified versions with gay and bisexual male samples has not been established. Yet another measurement problem is that the gender of abusive partners has not always been assessed. Because the relationship histories of some gay and bisexual men include one or more female partners, it cannot be assumed that all of their reports of IPV involved a male perpetrator. Consequently, questions about past experiences of IPV yield data of dubious quality if they do not ascertain the gender of the partner who perpetrated it.

Third, as with research on hate crimes, most studies of IPV have relied on convenience samples recruited through friendship networks, community venues, organization lists, and similar sources. The generalizability of findings from these samples cannot be known.

Incidence and Prevalence of IPV

Incidence data on IPV in same-sex relationships has been collected both through federal surveys and by community organizations. Based on responses to the National Crime Victimization Survey (NCVS), the Bureau of Justice Statistics estimated that an average of 13,740 male-male partner victimizations occurred annually in the years 1993–1999. These incidents represented 9.7% of the estimated average of 142,290 intimate partner victimizations committed annually against males during that period.[79] Incidence data compiled by the National Coalition of Anti-Violence Programs (NCAVP) are less extensive but nevertheless highlight the seriousness of the problem. In 2003, the NCAVP's member organizations and affiliated programs documented 6,523 domestic violence incidents in 11 US cities and regions and in Toronto, Canada. This total represented an increase of 13% over the 5,718 cases reported by the same agencies the previous year.[2]

Although IPV clearly occurs in male-male couples, relatively few published studies have reported prevalence rates. Perhaps as a consequence of the dearth of empirical research in this area, past reviews of the male–male IPV literature have cited unpublished masters theses, doctoral dissertations, and conference papers. Because such reports are not widely available and typically have not been subjected to rigorous peer review, we omit them from the present discussion. We also limit our review to studies of men in the United States (including Puerto Rico) to avoid problems of noncomparability of data across cultures.

Seven published papers have reported data from US convenience samples that included men in same-sex relationships. They reported rates of male-male IPV ranging from 11%[80] to 44%.[81] Only one of these studies[82] included a comparison group of heterosexuals, and it did not reveal disparities in IPV among men in same- versus different-sex relationships. Because these studies utilized nonprobability samples—some of them quite small—they cannot be used as the basis for estimating the population prevalence of IPV among men in same-sex relationships. Nevertheless, owing to the paucity of relevant data, the results of each study are briefly summarized here in ascending order of IPV prevalence.

- In a study of 560 gay male couples recruited through organizations and community publications, Bryant and Demian[80] found that 11% reported their relationship had suffered from the presence of physical abuse. As Burke and Follingstad[74] observed, the wording of this question required respondents to simultaneously report the presence of abuse and their judgment of how it had affected the relationship. This makes comparisons to other prevalence estimates difficult.

- Waterman, Dawson, and Bologna[83] obtained questionnaire data from 34 male students, of whom 7 (approximately 20%) reported violence from their partner on the CTS; of these, four men (12% of the sample) also reported that a partner had forced them to have sex against their will.
- Toro-Alfonso and Rodriguez-Madera[84] administered an original questionnaire to 199 Puerto Rican men and found that 26% reported physical violence from a partner and 25% reported sexual violence.
- Burke, Jordan, and Owen[85] administered an original questionnaire via the Internet to a snowball U.S. sample of 11 lesbians and 24 gay men and found that 28.6% reported having been "hit, slapped, kicked or otherwise physically harmed" (p. 243). The researchers did not report responses separately by gender.
- Waldner-Hagrud, Gratch, and Magruder[86] administered a modified version of the CTS to 165 gay men and found that 29.7% reported some type of partner violence, including verbal abuse.
- Balsam and colleagues[82] recruited 226 gay and 38 bisexual men through advertisements in publications. In addition, they recruited 185 heterosexual siblings of the respondents as a comparison group. Based on responses to the Physical and Injury subscales of the CTS, they found that 47.1% of the bisexual men and 38.8% of the gay men reported being physically assaulted by a partner since age 18, compared to 43% of the heterosexual men. According to Balsam et al.'s Table 2–3, of the men who experienced physical abuse, 80.8% of the gay men and 56.3% of the bisexual men said it was perpetrated by a male partner, whereas 94.4% of the heterosexual men said it was perpetrated by a female partner. Extrapolating from the data in Balsam et al.'s Tables 1 and 3, we estimate that approximately 31.4% of the gay men (38.8%×80.8%) and 26.5% of the bisexual men (47.1%× 56.3%) were physically abused by a male partner, and that 40.6% of heterosexual men (43.0%×94.4%) were abused by a female partner.
- Turell[81] administered an original questionnaire to 227 men in the Houston, Texas, area and found that 44% reported ever experiencing physical abuse from a partner or lover in a current or past relationship, whereas 12% reported sexual abuse. The high prevalence rate in this sample may be due in part to the broad range of behaviors counted as physical abuse. Although the published report is not explicit about how it was operationalized, the summary measure of physical abuse appears to have included items such as "called you and hung up repeatedly" and "hurt you in anger *or in play*" (emphasis added).

Whereas the aforementioned studies were based on convenience samples, two studies have examined IPV in probability samples of individuals in same-sex intimate relationships. Tjaden and colleagues[87] used data from the National Violence Against Women (NVAW) Survey to examine lifetime intimate partner violence in same- and different-sex cohabiting relationships, measured by a revised version of the CTS. The NVAW was a national telephone survey conducted in 1995 and 1996 with a probability sample of 8,000 men and 8,000 women. About 1% of the respondents (65 men and 79 women) reported involvement in a current or past same-sex cohabiting relationship. Their rates of physical and sexual assault by a same-sex partner were 15.4% (men) and 11.4% (women). For comparison purposes, Tjaden et al. reported rates for randomly selected subsamples of 300 men and 300 women in current or past cohabiting relationships with a person of the other sex, but no same-sex intimate cohabitation. Those rates were 7.7% (men) and 20.3% (women).

Although the authors did not report standard errors or confidence intervals (CI) for their point estimates, our own calculations (based on data reported by Tjaden et al. in their Table 2–5) suggest that same-sex and different-sex male cohabitors differed significantly in self-reports of abuse. For male same-sex cohabitors, we estimate the 95% CI = 10.9%–19.9%; for male different-sex cohabitors, estimated CI = 6.2%–9.2%. However, the amount of abuse reported by male same-sex cohabitors did not differ significantly from that reported by female different-sex cohabitors (estimated CI = 18%–22.6%). Thus, men and women with a male partner did not differ significantly in their rates of physical abuse, but both reported significantly more abuse than men with a female partner.[87]

This study's strength lies in its use of a probability sample and the fact that IPV was measured uniformly for all participants, making possible direct comparisons of lifetime rates. Nevertheless, the results are limited by the small number of respondents in a same-sex couple and by the fact that respondents' sexual orientation was not assessed, which precludes separate assessments of IPV among bisexual, gay, and heterosexual respondents. In addition, the same-sex and different-sex cohabitors differed on potentially relevant characteristics, including income, employment status, and educational level.

Greenwood and colleagues[88] used data from the Urban Men's Health Study (UMHS) to assess battering victimization in intimate relationships in a probability sample of men who have had sex with men. The UMHS sample was recruited in San Francisco, Los Angeles, Chicago, and New York through random-digit dialing with a multistage design that focused on census tracts inhabited by high concentrations of men who have sex with men. Greenwood et al. reported data from 2,881 participants who completed a modified version of the CTS that measured IPV over a 5-year period. The researchers found that 22% of respondents reported physical violence (CI = 20.1%–24%), 5.1%

reported sexual violence (CI = 4.1%–6.4%), and 34% reported psychological violence (CI = 31.8%–36.2%). In all, 39.2% reported at least one form of abuse (CI = 37%–41.5%), with 18.2% (CI = 16.5%–20.1%) reporting two or more forms. Greenwood et al. compared their findings to data on physical abuse from other published studies of IPV among heterosexuals and concluded that the UMHS estimates were "substantially higher than those reported for heterosexual men and higher than or comparable to those reported for heterosexual women" (p. 1967). There were several important limitations to this comparison, however, including that somewhat different measures and time frames were used in the survey questions, and that the comparison samples were not matched demographically to the UMHS four-city sample.

Greenwood et al. also examined correlates of IPV among gay and bisexual men. In their sample, IPV experiences were not correlated with race or ethnicity, income, or city of residence. However, partner violence was more likely to be experienced by men to the extent that they were younger, less well-educated, employed full-time, and HIV-positive.[88] These patterns are somewhat different from those reported for different-sex IPV, which indicate greater risk among Blacks and Hispanics. In addition, whereas the correlates of different-sex IPV may differ across racial and ethnic groups, low income and other indicators of lower socioeconomic status appear to be consistent predictors.[89,90]

In the UMHS, 28.7% of HIV-infected respondents reported experiencing physical abuse from a partner in the previous 5 years (95% CI = 23.7%–34.2%).[88] Two additional studies have also examined experiences of violence among HIV-infected gay and bisexual men. In one study, a convenience sample of 51 HIV-infected men who were currently or recently in an intimate relationship with a male partner reported their IPV experiences, using a modified version of the CTS.[91] Nearly half (45.1%) of the men reported that they were the victim of physical abuse during the previous year, and 33.3% reported being the victim of sexual coercion. About one-fourth reported that they suffered physical injury as a result of the abuse. By contrast, in the HIV Costs and Service Utilization Study, which employed a national probability sample of HIV-positive individuals who sought treatment for HIV disease in 1996 (N = 2,864), only 11.5% of gay and bisexual men reported they had been "physically hurt by your partner or someone important to you" since their HIV diagnosis.[92] Because of the differing measurement and sampling strategies, direct comparison of the results across these three studies is difficult. The differing prevalence estimates derived from the UMHS and the HIV Costs and Service Utilization Study may be due to the fact that the UMHS sample was limited to four large urban centers whereas the HIV Costs and Service Utilization Study included data from throughout the US. It appears that the convenience sample[91] may have overrepresented HIV-infected men who experienced IPV.

In summary, data from probability samples suggest that roughly 15% to 22% of gay and bisexual men may have experienced physical abuse from a male intimate partner at some time in their adult life. This range is lower than the median estimate (26.5%) across the seven previously cited studies conducted with convenience samples.[§] Data from the sole study based on a probability sample that included heterosexual comparison groups suggest that men may experience violence from a male partner at a rate similar to that of women with a male partner, but more frequently than men or women with a female partner.[87] However, any attempt to derive a single prevalence estimate from the published research is extremely risky and necessarily tentative, given the conceptual and methodological differences across studies, the paucity of research with probability samples, and the many other limitations of data in this area, as described above.

Responses to Intimate Partner Violence

As noted earlier, community responses to IPV grew out of existing anti-violence programs that were originally designed in response to hate crimes. Because this has been a fairly recent occurrence, resources for the victims of same-sex IPV—especially male victims—are still lacking in most parts of the United States. Thus, there is a basic need to recognize the existence of male-male IPV and to make emergency services, treatment, and social services available to male victims. As illustrated in the case of "William," described at the beginning of this chapter, male IPV victims who need emergency financial assistance and shelter typically lack access to the community resources available to female IPV victims.[69]

Public education programs are also needed to teach sexual minority communities to recognize and respond to IPV, thereby fostering earlier help-seeking by victims and greater community support for them. In addition, it is important to teach criminal justice personnel, health care workers, mental health providers, and social workers about the needs of gay and bisexual victims of IPV.[69] Such interventions, for example, might protect IPV victims from the threat of dual arrest and thus foster reporting of IPV to police authorities.[68] All of these responses will be facilitated to the extent that statutes related to IPV are modified so that they unambiguously include victims of IPV in all 50 states.[67]

[§]To calculate this figure, we used our estimates of the percentages of gay and bisexual men who were physically abused by a male partner in the Balsam et al.[82] study (31.4% and 26.5%, respectively). If the figures in this study's Table 1 (which included victimizations by female partners) are used instead, the median rate across studies is 28.6%.

Recommendations for Research

Whether or not gay and bisexual men experience more IPV than heterosexual men, the fact that practically all hate crimes based on sexual orientation target sexual minority individuals and institutions makes it is reasonable to hypothesize that sexual minority men are at generally greater risk for violent victimization than their heterosexual counterparts. This hypothesis of disparities in risk for violence is even more plausible when other demographic correlates of sexual orientation are considered. For example, sexual minority men may be disproportionately likely to live in large urban centers.[93] This residential pattern affords gay and bisexual men greater tolerance and increased opportunities for establishing committed relationships and community ties, but it also locates them in settings where the risk for routine criminal violence is higher than in less densely populated areas.[25]

Thus, research is needed with large probability samples of sexual minorities to permit accurate assessment of the incidence and prevalence of hate crimes, intimate partner violence, and violent victimization of all kinds. Perhaps the most feasible way to conduct such research would be to routinely include measures of sexual orientation in ongoing government surveys. As noted above, for example, the NCVS, which is conducted annually with a sample of 42,000 households comprising nearly 76,000 persons,[25] includes questions about hate crime victimizations (including those based on sexual orientation) and the gender of perpetrators of intimate partner violence. If the sexual orientation of adult household members were directly assessed, the resultant sample would yield prevalence estimates of violence and victimization among sexual minority individuals that would be substantially better than those currently available.

In addition to seeking probability samples, future research should utilize standardized assessment techniques with demonstrated reliability. In the area of hate crime victimization, data are likely to be of higher quality if respondents are asked to relate their personal history of victimization in both hate crimes and routine crimes on an incident-by-incident basis.[15] As in other survey research, self-reports of violent incidents, especially those of low or moderate severity that occurred in the distant past, are likely to be more accurate and reliable if researchers provide respondents with multiple memory aids and prompts.[94] In the area of intimate partner violence, the need for separate assessment and reporting of physical, sexual, and psychological abuse has already been noted.[74] In addition, we have argued for the need to assess respondents' sexual orientation and the gender of their partner in order to permit valid comparisons among gay, bisexual, and heterosexual respondents. We have also noted the need for more rigorous operational definitions of intimate relationships (e.g., restricting the definition to include only cohabiting relationships) to make comparisons between same-sex and different-sex couples more valid.

Still another definitional issue concerns the motivation for aggressive acts against an intimate partner. As Renzetti[95] noted, "there are important differences between initiating violence, using violence in self-defense, and retaliating against a violent partner. This is more than simply an issue of who hits first, since individuals may be motivated to strike first because they believe violence against them is imminent" (pp. 107–108). Applying this observation to male-male IPV, Letellier suggested that gay men, by virtue of their gender socialization experiences, are more likely than women to respond with violence when they are attacked by an intimate partner.[96] The knowledge that they aggressed against their partner, albeit in self-defense, may lead some battered males to believe that they themselves are perpetrators of IPV and that they share culpability with their partner.[71,96]

Moving beyond methodological issues, a host of substantive questions should be addressed in empirical research on the violent victimization of gay and bisexual men. We briefly note five of them. First, data are needed on the psychological consequences of victimization. Only a few studies have addressed this question for male victims of anti-gay hate crimes.[15,42,97] They suggest that by linking violent victimization with one's identity as a gay or bisexual man, hate crimes have the potential for inflicting substantial psychological harm.[15,98] For male-male IPV, a few studies have reported qualitative data about victims,[69,71,72] but large-scale studies employing standardized psychological measures are needed. In addition to systematically assessing psychological symptoms, such research should investigate how violent victimization interacts with preexisting minority stress and internalized stigma.[3,96,99]

Empirical research is also needed to identify the major predictors of victimization. As noted above, the available data on anti-gay attacks indicate that gender, public visibility, and age are important correlates.[15,33,50] However, further research is needed with an eye to developing interventions for reducing gay and bisexual men's individual risk for hate crime victimization. Even fewer studies have examined the correlates of male-male IPV. The available data, along with findings from studies of IPV in female and heterosexual couples, suggest that relationship quality, power differentials and control issues, alcohol and drug use, and experience of childhood abuse are likely to be important correlates.[71,74,100] (For a discussion of child sexual abuse, see Chapter 3 by Purcell et al. in this volume.) In addition, men's HIV status may play an important role in IPV and its aftermath. As noted earlier, HIV-infected gay and bisexual men may be at greater risk for IPV than their uninfected counterparts.[88] HIV-positive men, possibly fearing that they will be left without assistance or support when ill, may be more likely than other men to remain in an abusive relationship.[69] HIV also introduces an added risk dimension to sexual coercion if an HIV-infected man forces his uninfected partner to engage in unprotected anal sex.[91]

A third substantive area that warrants empirical inquiry concerns the variables that influence gay and bisexual men to report their victimization to law enforcement authorities and to seek assistance in recovering from violence. A variety of factors have been found to affect reporting of hate crime victimization, including concerns about having one's sexual orientation publicly disclosed and fears of secondary victimization at the hands of law enforcement personnel. [20,40] Some preliminary research has described factors that motivate victims of male-male IPV to seek assistance or leave an abusive relationship.[69,71,72] More research is needed, however, to ascertain how barriers to reporting can best be overcome, both through changing the institutions in which secondary victimization is perpetrated and educating gay and bisexual men about the availability of assistance and advocacy.

A fourth substantive question to be addressed concerns the perpetrators of violence. Although some research suggests that the perpetrators of criminal violence display somewhat predictable psychological profiles or patterns of personality traits,[101] Franklin's research[5,102] highlights the important roles played by peer groups, social norms, and situational variables in fostering anti-gay attacks. Systematic data about the perpetrators of male-male IPV are not available in the published scientific literature. Thus, research is needed to identify the individual and situational characteristics that promote the perpetration of anti-gay hate crimes and intimate partner violence.

Fifth, more research is needed on the social structural factors that perpetuate the violent victimization of sexual minority men and interfere with their recovery from its negative effects. We have already noted the importance of recognizing the cultural context of sexual stigma and prejudice in which anti-gay hate crimes and IPV occur.[3] In addition, the negative psychological and social impact of laws and political campaigns that are perceived by sexual minority individuals as promoting stigma and prejudice are not well understood, but may be substantial.[103] For example, laws that prohibit same-sex couples from marrying not only deny such couples the protective benefits of marriage,[8] but also could conceivably be used to prevent victims of intimate partner violence from obtaining government funded services if provision of such services is equated with state recognition of same-sex relationships. Similarly, hate crimes—especially crimes that inflict severe injury or death—may have traumatic consequences for the entire sexual minority community.[104] Indeed, part of the rationale underlying hate crime legislation is that such crimes target not only individual victims but entire classes of people.

Conclusion

Whereas clear disparities between heterosexual and sexual minority men are evident in risk for hate crime victimization, data are not currently adequate for assessing differential risks for intimate partner violence. Nevertheless, both types of violence significantly affect the lives of gay and bisexual men. Carefully designed research with large probability samples is needed to understand their prevalence, causes, and consequences. Such research should be designed with the ultimate goal of developing effective interventions to prevent hate crimes and intimate partner violence.

References

1. Zezima K. Teenager attacks three men at gay bar in Massachusetts. *New York Times.* February 3, 2006;A17.
2. National Coalition of Anti-Violence Programs. *Lesbian, gay, bisexual, and transgender domestic violence: 2003 supplement.* 2004. http://www.ncavp.org. Accessed February 1, 2006.
3. Herek GM, Chopp R, Strohl D. Sexual stigma: putting sexual minority health issues in context. In: Meyer I, Northridge M, eds. *The Health of Sexual Minorities: Public Health Perspectives on Lesbian, Gay, Bisexual, and Transgender Populations.* New York, NY: Springer; 2006.
4. Herek GM. Psychological heterosexism and anti-gay violence: The social psychology of bigotry and bashing. In: Herek GM, Berrill KT, eds. *Hate Crimes: Confronting Violence Against Lesbians and Gay Men.* Thousand Oaks, CA: Sage; 1992: 149–169.
5. Franklin K. Antigay behaviors among young adults: Prevalence, patterns and motivators in a noncriminal population. *J Interpersonal Violence.* 2000;15:339–362.
6. Congressional Budget Office. The potential budgetary impact of recognizing same-sex marriages. 2004. http://www.cbo.gov. Accessed June 22, 2004.
7. Kurdek LA. What do we know about gay and lesbian couples? *Curr Dir Psychological Science.* 2005;14:251–254.
8. Herek GM. Legal recognition of same-sex relationships in the United States: a social science perspective. *Am Psychol.* 2006;61:607–621.
9. Harris RJ, Cook CA. Attributions about spouse abuse: it matters who the batterers and victims are. *Sex Roles.* 1994;30:553–568.
10. Seelau EP, Seelau SM, Poorman PB. Gender and role-based perceptions of domestic abuse: does sexual orientation matter? *Behav Sci Law.* 2003;21:199–214.
11. Seelau SM, Seelau EP. Gender-role stereotypes and perceptions of heterosexual, gay and lesbian domestic violence. *J Fam Violence.* 2005;20:363–371.
12. Bisson JI, Shepherd JP. Psychological reactions of victims of violent crime. *Br J Psychiatry.* 1995;167:718–720.
13. Weaver TL, Clum GA. Psychological distress associated with interpersonal violence: a meta-analysis. *Clin Psychol Rev.* 1995;15:115–140.
14. Janoff-Bulman R. *Shattered Assumptions: Towards a New Psychology of Trauma.* New York, NY: Free Press; 1992.
15. Herek GM, Gillis JR, Cogan JC. Psychological sequelae of hate crime victimization among lesbian, gay, and bisexual adults. *J Consult Clin Psychol.* 1999;67:945–951.
16. Mills TC, Paul J, Stall R, et al. Distress and depression in men who have sex with men: The Urban Men's Health Study. *Am J Psychiatry.* 2004;161:278–285.
17. Garnets L, Herek GM, Levy B. Violence and victimization of lesbians and gay men: mental health consequences. *J Interpersonal Violence.* 1990;5:366–383.
18. National Coalition of Anti-Violence Programs. Anti-lesbian, gay, bisexual, and transgender violence in 2004. 2005. http://www.ncavp.org. Accessed February 1, 2006.
19. Berrill KT. Antigay violence and victimization in the United States: an overview. In: Herek GM, Berrill KT, eds. *Hate Crimes: Confronting Violence Against Lesbians and Gay Men.* Thousand Oaks, CA: Sage Publications; 1992:19–45.

20. Herek GM, Cogan JC, Gillis JR. Victim experiences in hate crimes based on sexual orientation. *J Social Issues.* 2002;58:319–339.
21. Herek GM. The community response to violence in San Francisco: an interview with Wenny Kusuma, Lester Olmstead-Rose, and Jill Tregor. In: Herek GM, Berrill KT, eds. *Hate Crimes: Confronting Violence Against Lesbians and Gay Men.* Thousand Oaks, CA: Sage; 1992:241–258.
22. Wertheimer DM. Treatment and service interventions for lesbian and gay male crime victims. In: Herek GM, Berrill KT, eds. *Hate Crimes: Confronting Violence Against Lesbians and Gay Men.* Newbury Park, CA: Sage Publications, Inc; 1992: 227–240.
23. National Gay Task Force. *Anti-Gay/Lesbian Victimization.* Washington, DC: Author; 1984.
24. Federal Bureau of Investigation. *Press Release.* Washington, DC: US Department of Justice; 1992.
25. Bureau of Justice Statistics. Crime and victims statistics. 2006. http://www.ojp .usdoj.gov/bjs/cvict.htm. Accessed February 19, 2006.
26. Harlow, CW. Hate Crime Reported by Victims and Police. 2005. http://www.ojp .usdoj.gov/bjs/pub/pdf/hcrvp.pdf. Accessed July 4, 2006.
27. Bell AP, Weinberg TS. *Homosexualities: A Study of Diversity Among Men and Women.* New York, NY: Simon & Schuster; 1978.
28. Saghir MT, Robins E. *Male and Female Homosexuality: A Comprehensive Investigation.* Baltimore, MD: Williams and Wilkins; 1973.
29. Aurand SK, Addessa R, Bush C. *Violence and Discrimination Against Philadelphia Lesbian and Gay People.* Philadelphia, PA: Philadelphia Lesbian and Gay Task Force; 1985.
30. Herek GM, Berrill KT. Documenting the victimization of lesbians and gay men: methodological issues. In: Herek GM, Berrill KT, eds. *Hate Crimes: Confronting Violence Against Lesbians and Gay Men.* Thousand Oaks, CA: Sage; 1992:270–286.
31. Huebner DM, Rebchook GM, Kegeles SM. Experiences of harassment, discrimination, and physical violence among young gay and bisexual men. *Am J Public Health.* 2004;94:1200–1203.
32. Pilkington NW, D'Augelli AR. Victimization of lesbian, gay, and bisexual youth in community settings. *J Community Psychol.* 1995;23:34–56.
33. D'Augelli AR, Grossman AH. Disclosure of sexual orientation, victimization, and mental health among lesbian, gay, and bisexual older adults. *J Interpersonal Violence.* 2001;16:1008–1027.
34. Results of poll. *San Francisco Examiner.* June 6, 1989;A-19.
35. Kaiser Family Foundation. *Inside-Out: A Report on the Experiences of Lesbians, Gays, and Bisexuals in America and the Public's View on Issues and Politics Related to Sexual Orientation.* Menlo Park, CA: Author. http://www.kff.org. Accessed November 14, 2001.
36. Díaz RM, Ayala G, Bein E, Henne J, Marín BV. The impact of homophobia, poverty, and racism on the mental health of gay and bisexual Latino men: findings from 3 US cities. *Am J Public Health.* 2001;91:927–932.
37. National Gay and Lesbian Task Force. *Anti-Gay Violence, Victimization and Defamation in 1988.* Washington, DC: Author; 1989.
38. Federal Bureau of Investigation. *Hate Crime Statistics 2004.* Washington, DC: US Department of Justice; 2005.

39. Haider-Markel DP. Implementing controversial policy: results from a national survey of law enforcement activity on hate crime. *Justice Research and Policy.* 2001; 3:29–61.

40. Berrill KT, Herek GM. Primary and secondary victimization in anti-gay hate crimes: Official response and public policy. In: Herek GM, Berrill KT, eds. *Hate Crimes: Confronting Violence Against Lesbians and Gay Men.* Thousand Oaks, CA: Sage Publications; 1992:289–305.

41. Green DP, Strolovitch DZ, Wong JS, Bailey RW. Measuring gay populations and anti-gay hate crime. *Soc Sci Quarterly.* 2001;82:281–296.

42. Herek GM, Gillis JR, Cogan JC, Glunt EK. Hate crime victimization among lesbian, gay, and bisexual adults: prevalence, psychological correlates, and methodological issues. *J Interpersonal Violence.* 1997;12:195–215.

43. Catalano S, Bureau of Justice Statistics. Criminal victimization, 2004. 2005. http://www.ojp.usdoj.gov/bjs/abstract/cv04.htm. Accessed February 19, 2006.

44. Von Schulthess B. Violence in the streets: anti-lesbian assault and harassment in San Francisco. In: Herek GM, Berrill KT, eds. *Hate Crimes: Confronting Violence Against Lesbians and Gay Men.* Thousand Oaks, CA: Sage Publications; 1992: 65–75.

45. DuRant RH, Krowchuk DP, Sinal SH. Victimization, use of violence, and drug use at school among male adolescents who engage in same-sex sexual behavior. *J Pediatr.* 1998;133:113–118.

46. Faulkner AH, Cranston K. Correlates of same-sex sexual behavior in a random sample of Massachusetts high school students. *Am J Public Health.* 1998;88:262–266.

47. Russell ST, Franz BT, Driscoll AK. Same-sex romantic attraction and experiences of violence in adolescence. *Am J Public Health.* 2001;91:903–906.

48. Hershberger SL, D'Augelli AR. The impact of victimization on the mental health and suicidality of lesbian, gay, and bisexual youths. *Dev Psychol.* 1995;31:65–74.

49. Waldo CR, Hesson-McInnis MS, D'Augelli AR. Antecedents and consequences of victimization of lesbian, gay, and bisexual young people: a structural model comparing rural university and urban samples. *Am J Community Psychol.* 1998;26: 307–334.

50. Tewksbury R, Grossi EL, Suresh G, Helms J. Hate crimes against gay men and lesbian women: a routine activity approach for predicting victimization risk. *Humanity and Society.* 1999;23:125–142.

51. D'Emilio J. *Sexual Politics, Sexual Communities: The Making of a Homosexual Minority in the United States 1940–1970.* Chicago, IL: University of Chicago Press; 1983.

52. Herek GM. Why tell if you're not asked? Self-disclosure, intergroup contact, and heterosexuals' attitudes toward lesbians and gay men. In: Herek GM, Jobe J, Carney R, eds. *Out in Force: Sexual Orientation and the Military.* Chicago, IL: University of Chicago Press; 1996:197–225.

53. Herdt GH, Boxer A. *Children of Horizons: How Gay and Lesbian Teens Are Leading a New Way Out of the Closet.* Boston, MA: Beacon; 1993.

54. Savin-Williams RC, Cohen KM. Homoerotic development during childhood and adolescence. *Child Adolesc Psychiatr Clin N Am.* 2004;13:529–549.

55. Cooksey EC, Rindfuss RR, Guilkey DK. The initiation of adolescent sexual and contraceptive behavior during changing times. *J Health Soc Behav.* 1996;37:59–74.

56. Herman D. *The Antigay Agenda: Orthodox Vision and the Christian Right.* Chicago, IL: University of Chicago Press; 1997.

57. National Coalition of Anti-Violence Programs. Anti-lesbian, gay, bisexual, and transgender violence in 1999. http://www.ncavp.org. Accessed October 11, 2000.
58. Jenness V, Broad K. *Hate Crimes: New Social Movements and the Politics of Violence.* New York, NY: Aldine de Gruyter; 1997.
59. Grattet R, Jenness V, Curry TR. The homogenization and differentiation of hate crime laws in the United States, 1978 to 1995: innovation and diffusion in the criminalization of bigotry. *Am Sociol Rev.* 1998;63:286–307.
60. Jenness V, Grattet R. *Making Hate a Crime: From Social Movement to Law Enforcement.* New York, NY: Russell Sage; 2001.
61. Anti-Defamation League. Combating Hate. 2006. http://www.adl.org/combating_ hate. Accessed February 21, 2006.
62. National Gay and Lesbian Task Force. Hate crime laws in the U.S. 2005. http:// www.thetaskforce.org/downloads/hatecrimesmap.pdf. Accessed February 21, 2006.
63. Centers for Disease Control and Prevention. Intimate partner violence: Overview. 2006. http://www.cdc.gov/ncipc/factsheets/ipvoverview.htm. Accessed June 28, 2006.
64. McClennen JC. Domestic violence between same-gender partners: Recent findings and future research. *J Interpersonal Violence.* 2005;20:149–154.
65. Robinson GE. Current concepts in domestic violence. *Primary Psychiatry.* 2003;10: 48–52.
66. Tjaden P, Thoennes N. Prevalence and consequences of male-to-female and female-to-male intimate partner violence as measured by the National Violence Against Women Survey. *Violence Against Women.* 2000;6:142–161.
67. Aulivola M. Outing domestic violence: affording appropriate protections to gay and lesbian victims. *Family Court Review.* 2004;42:162–177.
68. Hirschel D, Buzawa E. Understanding the context of dual arrest with directions for future research. *Violence Against Women.* 2002;8:1449–1473.
69. Merrill GS, Wolfe VA. Battered gay men: an exploration of abuse, help seeking and why they stay. *J Homosex.* 2000;39:1–30.
70. Merrill GS. Ruling the exceptions: same-sex battering and domestic violence theory. *J Gay and Lesbian Social Services.* 1996;4:9–22.
71. Cruz JM, Firestone JM. Exploring violence and abuse in gay male relationships. *Violence Vict.* 1998;13:159–173.
72. Cruz JM. "Why doesn't he just leave?": gay male domestic violence and the reasons victims stay. *J Men's Studies.* 2003;11:309–320.
73. Family Research Institute. Getting the facts: Same-sex marriage. 2005. http://www .familyresearchinst.org/Default.aspx?tabid=80. Accessed February 25, 2006.
74. Burke LK, Follingstad DR. Violence in lesbian and gay relationships: theory, prevalence, and correlational factors. *Clin Psychol Rev.* 1999;19:487–512.
75. Straus MA. Measuring intrafamily conflict and violence: the Conflict Tactics (CT) Scales. *J Marriage and the Family.* 1979;41:75–88.
76. Field CA, Caetano R. Intimate partner violence in the US general population: progress and future directions. *J Interpersonal Violence.* 2005;20:463–469.
77. Kimmel MS. "Gender symmetry" in domestic violence: a substantive and methodological research review. *Violence Against Women.* 2002;8:1332–1363.
78. Regan KV, Bartholomew K, Oram D, Landolt MA. Measuring physical violence in male same-sex relationships: an item response theory analysis of the Conflict Tactics Scales. *J Interpersonal Violence.* 2002;17:235–252.

79. Rennison, CM. Intimate partner violence and age of victim, 1993–99. 2001. http://www.ojp.usdoj.gov/bjs/pub/pdf/ipva99.pdf. Accessed July 4, 2006.
80. Bryant AS, Demian. Relationship characteristics of American gay and lesbian couples: findings from a national survey. *J Gay and Lesbian Social Services.* 1994;1: 101–117.
81. Turell SC. A descriptive analysis of same-sex relationship violence for a diverse sample. *J Family Violence.* 2000;15:281–293.
82. Balsam KF, Rothblum ED, Beauchaine TP. Victimization over the life span: a comparison of lesbian, gay, bisexual, and heterosexual siblings. *J Consult Clin Psychol.* 2005;73:477–487.
83. Waterman CK, Dawson LJ, Bologna MJ. Sexual coercion in gay male and lesbian relationships: predictors and implications for support services. *J Sex Res.* 1989; 26:118–124.
84. Toro-Alfonso J, Rodríguez-Madera S. Domestic violence in Puerto Rican gay male couples: perceived prevalence, intergenerational violence, addictive behaviors, and conflict resolution skills. *J Interpersonal Violence.* 2004;19:639–654.
85. Burke TW, Jordan ML, Owen SS. Cross-national comparison of gay and lesbian domestic violence. *J Contemp Criminal Justice.* 2002;18:231–257.
86. Waldner-Haugrud LK, Gratch LV, Magruder B. Victimization and perpetration rates of violence in gay and lesbian relationships: gender issues explored. *Violence Vict.* 1997; 12:173–184.
87. Tjaden P, Thoennes N, Allison CJ. Comparing violence over the life span in samples of same-sex and opposite-sex cohabitants. *Violence Vict.* 1999;14:413–425.
88. Greenwood GL, Relf MV, Huang B, Pollack LM, Canchola JA, Catania JA. Battering victimization among a probability-based sample of men who have sex with men. *Am J Public Health.* 2002;92:1964–1969.
89. Field CA, Caetano R. Longitudinal model predicting partner violence among White, Black, and Hispanic couples in the United States. *Alcohol Clin Exp Res.* 2003;27:1451–1458.
90. Field CA, Caetano R. Ethnic differences in intimate partner violence in the US general population: the role of alcohol use and socioeconomic status. *Trauma, Violence, & Abuse.* 2004;5:303–317.
91. Craft SM, Serovich JM. Family-of-origin factors and partner violence in the intimate relationships of gay men who are HIV positive. *J Interpersonal Violence.* 2005;20:777–791.
92. Zierler S, Cunningham WE, Andersen R, et al. Violence victimization after HIV infection in a US probability sample of adult patients in primary care. *Am J Public Health.* 2000;90:208–215.
93. Laumann EO, Gagnon JH, Michael RT, Michaels S. *The Social Organization of Sexuality: Sexual Practices in the United States.* Chicago, IL: University of Chicago Press; 1994.
94. Tourangeau R, Rips LJ, Rasinski KA. *The Psychology of Survey Response.* Cambridge, England: Cambridge University Press; 2000.
95. Renzetti CM. *Violent Betrayal: Partner Abuse in Lesbian Relationships.* Newbury Park, CA: Sage; 1992.
96. Letellier P. Gay and bisexual male domestic violence victimization: challenges to feminist theory and responses to violence. *Violence Vict.* 1994;9:95–106.
97. McDevitt J, Balboni J, Garcia L, Gu J. Consequences for victims: a comparison of bias- and non-bias-motivated assaults. *Am Behav Sci.* 2001;45:697–713.

98. Garnets L, Herek GM, Levy B. Violence and victimization of lesbians and gay men: mental health consequences. In: Herek GM, Berrill KT, eds. *Hate Crimes: Confronting Violence Against Lesbians and Gay Men.* Thousand Oaks, CA: Sage; 1992: 207–226.

99. Meyer IH. Prejudice, social stress, and mental health in lesbian, gay, and bisexual populations: conceptual issues and research evidence. *Psychol Bull.* 2003;129: 674–697.

100. Cruz JM, Peralta RL. Family violence and substance use: the perceived effects of substance use within gay male relationships. *Violence Vict.* 2001;16:161–172.

101. Heide KM. *Young Killers: The Challenge of Juvenile Homicide.* Thousand Oaks, CA: Sage; 1999.

102. Franklin K. Unassuming motivations: contextualizing the narratives of anti-gay assailants. In: Herek GM, ed. *Stigma and Sexual Orientation: Understanding Prejudice Against Lesbians, Gay Men, and Bisexuals.* Thousand Oaks, CA: Sage; 1998:1–23.

103. Russell GM, *Voted Out: The Psychological Consequences of Anti-Gay Politics.* New York, NY: NYU Press; 2000.

104. Noelle M. The ripple effect on the Matthew Shepard murder: impact on the assumptive worlds of members of the targeted group. *Am Behav Sci.* 2002;46: 27–50.

105. Lockhart LL, White BW, Causby V, Isaac A. Letting out the secret: violence in lesbian relationships. *J Interpersonal Violence.* 1994;9:469–492.

3

Childhood Sexual Abuse Experienced by Gay and Bisexual Men: Understanding the Disparities and Interventions to Help Eliminate Them

David W. Purcell, Jocelyn D. Patterson, and Pilgrim S. Spikes, Jr.

Childhood sexual abuse (CSA) is a complex, often misunderstood, and highly charged area for scientific inquiry, and these challenges are particularly acute when examining CSA among males.[1–6] Despite widely acknowledged methodological weaknesses, evidence indicates that CSA of males is more common than originally believed, and that there appear to be important gender differences in understanding the effects of CSA[3,7–9] and in providing appropriate treatment.[10] It is also clear that CSA can be associated with immediate as well as delayed negative effects across a number of social and emotional domains[3,11,12]; although negative effects are not always reported or observed, they may be mitigated by a variety of contextual factors, and they may vary depending on the definition used for abuse.[2]

Recovery from CSA for men may be difficult because their abuse experience runs counter to gender role expectations of male self-reliance/self-protection, and because the experience of CSA conflicts with the standard stereotypes about abuse that females are helpless victims while men are powerful abusers.[1,13] Among men, CSA may be even more challenging for gay and bisexual men (or men who have sex with men, MSM) for a number of intertwining personal, social, and psychological reasons. First, it is a particularly sensitive subject because of the myths that MSM are more likely to seduce male children, that they seek out boys to "recruit" to be gay, and that they are gay because they were abused.[15] In fact, sexual abuse of males by men is often perceived as indicating that the victim, the perpetrator, or both, are homosexually oriented, which may not be the case, and CSA can disrupt development of sexual identity.[1,13] In addition, gender roles and expectations regarding what it means to be a man are challenging for male victims of CSA, particularly those who, as adults, are attracted to men. MSM are particularly vulnerable to self-blame, even if they were not aware of same-sex attractions when the abuse occurred.[1] Boys who are abused by older males and subsequently grow up to experience same-sex attractions often feel that they were responsible for the abuse because of their own actions or attractions. MSM also may feel guilty or responsible because sexual behavior that is legally defined as "abuse" may not have been perceived by them as abusive, particularly if they were older adolescents when they sought out the sexual experience.[6,15,16]

CSA among MSM is important for health care practitioners and public health because of the elevated rates of abuse among MSM (discussed below), the potential negative sequelae of CSA for men, and the potential reverberations among their partners, families, and communities. CSA among MSM is different from the disparities described in other chapters in this volume because the actual trigger event occurs during childhood or adolescence (sometimes before sexual orientation is consolidated), and the ranges of possible outcomes are broad and can occur over the lifespan. In addition, some of the disparities discussed in other chapters, such as elevated rates of substance abuse and HIV infection, are potential secondary outcomes of CSA; in other words, a childhood disparity regarding CSA could be part of the genesis for some of the other disparities among MSM described in this volume.

In this chapter, first we will examine prevalence of CSA among MSM, and then compare it to prevalence among heterosexual men. Because the same methodological issues apply regardless of sexual orientation, we next briefly cover methodological issues for interpreting prevalence studies. Then, we will examine the outcomes of CSA and the ramifications of elevated rates of CSA among MSM. Finally, we will discuss interventions for addressing this health disparity and directions for future research.

How Prevalent Is CSA among MSM?

Relatively high rates of CSA have been reported in every sample of MSM that has been reported, with rates being similar to rates of abuse for women.[7] Table 3–1 lists data from 17 different samples from the past 15 years that have reported CSA prevalence among MSM. The range of prevalence rates is from 11.8% to 37.0%. We calculated 95% confidence intervals for each estimate (shown in the fourth column of Table 3–1) and report the rates for heterosexual men in the few studies that included both samples. Also, we report the citation or Web site for the study, the geographic location(s) of data collection, the definition of CSA used in the study, the sampling method and average age of the sample, and any demographic differences between MSM reporting CSA versus those not reporting CSA. Studies are presented starting with the most recently published, except that publications using the same study sample are presented serially. Definitions of abuse in most studies required coercion or force and sexual behavior before a certain age (somewhere from 13 to 18), although some used very broad definitions of abuse (e.g., including non-contact incidents as abuse), and some studies also asked reporters of CSA about perceptions of harm and willingness to engage in the behavior.

Many studies used convenience or clinic samples in which elevated risk for CSA might be expected (e.g., STD clinic patients, homeless youth, or those seeking an HIV test). However, some of the studies used stronger sampling methods, and their point prevalence estimates were similar to those using convenience samples. For example, Paul and colleagues,[17] using a larger and more representative sample of urban MSM, found 20.6% prevalence of coercive CSA with physical contact before age 18. When they used two different methods to make their definition of coercive more restrictive (by adding various measures of age differences between partners), they found only slightly reduced prevalence rates (16.7% and 17.3%). Jinich and colleagues[4] also used stronger sampling methods and found 27.4% prevalence of CSA. A national probability sample of almost 5000 men ages 15 to 44 collected in 2002 for the National Survey of Family Growth (NSFG) found that 14.9% of MSM reported coercive CSA before age 18.[18] Thus, the best-designed studies tend to converge on CSA prevalence of 15% to 25%, which is at the lower range for all studies.

The last column of Table 3-1 summarizes the data regarding demographic differences found between MSM who reported and did not report CSA. Some of these characteristics are the same in childhood and adulthood (e.g., race), and some of them can change between the time of abuse and the time of assessment (e.g., socioeconomic status). Unfortunately, with research on this topic still in its early stages, a majority of studies did not evaluate or report demographic differences between abused and non-abused MSM. Among the convenience samples, there is one study that found the prevalence of CSA for gay men of color in general is higher than among white men,[19] while others found no racial/ethnic differences.[20] In a study of CSA and adult sexual victimization, African American men were more likely to be sexually abused as adults than other racial/ethnic groups,[21] but the authors did not analyze the CSA data by race. Two of the studies in Table 3-1 focused on one ethnic group (Latinos), and in both convenience samples, rates of abuse were above 30%,[16,22] although about half of the sexual behavior reported by participants was described as not having been forced.

Data from the three methodologically stronger studies all point to racial/ethnic differences. With one data set, the authors reported higher rates of abuse for Latinos before age 13 (but no ethnic differences between ages 13 to 16)[23] and lower rates for white and Asian Pacific Islanders (API) men.[17] In another study, higher rates were reported for Latinos, API, and Native American men.[4] Data from the NSFG[18] indicate that there is a trend for a racial/ethnic difference in CSA among MSM. Overall, rates of CSA were 3.3% for African Americans and 1.9% each for Hispanics and for white men (p<.01). Among MSM, rates were about double for African Americans (22.2%) compared to 11.8% for Hispanics and 11.4% for whites (p = 0.09).

Table 3-1. Studies on the prevalence of childhood sexual abuse (CSA) among men who have sex with men (MSM)

Reference and Study Location	Sample Size and Description	Definition of CSA	Prevalence of CSA among MSM (95% CI)	Demographic Differences between MSM Reporting CSA and Those Not
National Survey of Family Growth–Cycle 6* (unpublished data collected in 2002)[18]	National probability sample of 4928 men ages 15 to 44 collected by face-to-face and self-administered computer methods (CSA questions only for ages 18–44)	Coercive anal or vaginal sex before age 18, assessed separately for male and female perpetrators	CSA by males: 14.9% (CI = 10.3, 19.5) (compared to 1.7% of heterosexual men; CI = 1.3, 2.1) CSA by females: 3.4% of MSM versus 3.3% of heterosexual men	Overall abuse rates by men: African American = 3.3% Hispanic = 1.9% White = 1.9% Rates of abuse of MSM by men: African American = 22.2% Hispanic = 11.8% White = 11.4%
Arreola et al., 2005 Chicago, IL; Los Angeles, CA; New York, NY; San Francisco, CA[23]	Telephone probability sample of 2692 urban adult MSM. Median age upper 30s.	Coercive CSA with contact and age of first incident less than 17	20.6% (CI = 18.8, 22.5) <13 – (13.0%) 13–17 – (7.6%)	Significantly higher proportion of Latino MSM reported sex abuse before age 13 (22%) than non-Latino MSM (12%). No differences at ages 13–17.
Paul et al., 2001* (same sample as Arreola et al., above)[17]	See above	See above	See above	Compared to non-abused MSM, abused MSM were younger, less likely to be white or Asian Pacific Islander (API), and reported less gay identification, education, and income, and more unemployment. Abused men were also more likely to be HIV-positive (24% vs. 14%).

(continued)

Table 3-1. (*continued*)

Reference and Study Location	Sample Size and Description	Definition of CSA	Prevalence of CSA among MSM (95% CI)	Demographic Differences between MSM Reporting CSA and Those Not
Parsons et al., 2005 New York, NY[19]	Convenience sample of 46 male escorts recruited through emails collected from Internet profiles. Mean age 31.8 years.	Pressured, forced, or intimidated into doing something sexual prior to age 16.	28.3% (CI = 15.2, 41.3)	Abused men more likely to be: ethnic minority, have a primary male partner, identify as bisexual. Less likely to be receptive partner with paying and non-paying partners.
Kalichman et al., 2004 Atlanta, GA[20]	Convenience sample of 608 men attending gay pride festival. Mean age 34.8 years.	At age 16 or younger forced or pressured to have sex with a man 5 or more years older.	15.3% (CI = 12.4, 18.2)	No difference between abused and non-abused men for age, education level, income, ethnic group, or relationship status. Abused men are more-likely to be HIV-positive (40% vs. 19%).
Stanley et al., 2004 Vancouver, Canada[46]	From a random digit dial sample of MSM, a subsample (64%, n = 192) who chose to participate in a qualitative interview and quantitative survey. Mean age 39 years.	Sexual contact with someone at least 5 years older before age 17.	26.0% (CI = 19.8, 32.2) 51% of CSA men reported being willing	Not reported.

Finlinson et al., 2003* New York, NY; Puerto Rico[32]	38 IDU and crack-smoking Latinos. Mean age 36 years.	Forced sexual encounter at 18 years of age or younger.	26.3% (CI = 12.3, 40.3) (compared to 1.2% of heterosexual men)	Not reported.
O'Leary et al., 2003 New York, NY; San Francisco, CA[48]	456 HIV-positive gay and bisexual men recruited from AIDS service organizations, gay outreach venues. Mean age 37 years.	Pressured, forced or intimidated into doing something sexually that you did not want to do when under 16 years old.	14.9% (CI = 11.6, 18.2)	Not reported.
Ratner et al., 2003 Vancouver, Canada[49]	358 young HIV-negative MSM recruited from medical clinics, doctor's offices, and community outreach. Mean age 28.6 years.	Forced or coerced into sexual activity before age 14 (Canadian criminal definition).	14.0% (CI = 10.4, 17.6)	Not reported.
Dolezal et al., 2002 New York, NY[22]	307 Latino MSM primarily recruited from gay and service venues. Mean age 31 years.	Sexual contact before age 13 with partner 4 or more years older.	32.6% (CI = 27.3, 37.8) 41% of CSA men reported being willing	All Latino sample. Other difference not reported.
Rind, 2001 Ithaca, NY[15]	129 MSM college students. Mean age 21 years.	Age-discrepant sexual relationship. Sexual activity with adult male when participant 12–17 years of age.	20.1% (CI = 13.2, 27.1) 92% of CSA men reported being willing	No differences.

(continued)

Table 3-1. (*continued*)

Reference and Study Location	Sample Size and Description	Definition of CSA	Prevalence of CSA among MSM (95% CI)	Demographic Differences between MSM Reporting CSA and Those Not
Kalichman et al. 2001 Atlanta, GA[21]	595 men recruited at a large gay pride event. Median age 33 years.	Sexual coercion at age 16 or younger.	21.7% (CI = 18.4, 25.0)	Not reported.
Tjaden et al., 1999* United States[33]	National telephone probability sample of 65 men with a lifetime history of same sex cohabitation. Mean age early 40s.	Forced anal or oral sex before age 18.	15.4% (CI = 6.6, 24.2) (compared to <2% of heterosexual men)	Not reported within MSM.
Jinich et al., 1998 Portland, OR, Tucson, AZ[4]	1941 MSM recruited using time-space sampling at gay venues and household telephone sampling. Mean age upper 30s.	CSA: - if <13 years, sex with someone 5+ years older - if 13–15 years, sex with someone 10+ years older - if 13–15, sex with someone 5–9 years older and "physically forced" or "strongly coerced"	27.4% (CI = 25.7, 29.7) No coercion for: 44% events at 13–15 years. 16% of events at <13 years old	Latinos, API, and Native American appear more likely to be abused; abused were less educated, lower income, and were more likely to be HIV-positive (20.5% vs. 15.9%).

Study, Location	Sample	Definition	Results	Comparison
Lenderking et al., 1997 Boston, MA[47]	Cohort study of 327 MSM examining risk factors related to HIV at community health center. Mean age 39.5 years.	CSA: if <13 years, sexual experience with person 5+ years older if 13–16 yrs, sexual experiences with person 10 years older with or without contact whether sex wanted or not.	35.5% (CI = 30.2, 40.7) 63% of CSA occurred before age 13, and 27% between 13–16 65% of CSA involved no bodily contact	Not reported.
Carballo-Dieguez et al., 1995 New York, NY[16]	Community recruited sample of 182 Spanish-and non-Spanish speaking Latino MSM or MSMW. Avoided use of terms *gay* and *bisexual.* Mean age 29.4 years.	Sexual contact before age 13 with person 4 or more years older.	35.7% (CI = 28.8, 42.7) 50% of CSA men reported being willing and unharmed.	All Latino sample. Other difference not reported.
Bartholow et al., 1994 & Doll et al., 1992 Chicago, IL, Denver, CO, San Francisco, CA[13, 14]	1001 STD clinic patients who reported a male sex partner in past 5 years or self-identified as gay or bisexual. Mean age 32.5 years.	Encouraged or forced by older or more powerful person to engage in sexual contact during childhood or adolescence.	37.0% (CI = 34.0, 40.0)	Not reported.
*Duncan, 1990** Illinois[34]	34 MSM and 184 hetero-sexual university undergraduates.	Forced to have sex against their will in their lifetime.	11.8% (CI = 0.01, 22.6) (compared to 3.6% of heterosexual men; (CI = 0.01, 6.4))	Not reported.

* Researchers either included a heterosexual comparison group or compared their data to an appropriate heterosexual comparison group.

Other demographic or health differences between abused and non-abused MSM have only been examined in a handful of studies. Characteristics associated with abuse among MSM include more non-gay identification,[17,19] HIV seropositivity,[4,17,20] less education and income,[4,17] and more unemployment.[17] A methodological challenge to examining demographic differences is that unmeasured family environment factors and socioeconomic factors may be confounded with race. Given the small sample sizes of men of color in most studies, firm conclusions are not possible, but the preliminary differences suggest that men of color and men of less means may require particular attention and treatment resources to address CSA and its effects.[24]

Comparing Prevalence Rates between MSM and Heterosexual Men

Comparing rates of prevalence of CSA between studies of MSM and separate studies of the general male population (which includes MSM) is problematic due to definitional and sampling differences as well as the fact that MSM, although a small segment of the population, are included within general samples.[3,17] For this chapter, it is important to get a sense of the general CSA prevalence rates among men and then to look at studies that examined MSM in comparison to a suitable heterosexual comparison group. In studies that stratify by sexual orientation, MSM are not included in the heterosexual rates, thus making comparisons less problematic.

In their large review of over 150 existing studies of CSA among males, Holmes and Slap[3] reported a wide range of prevalence rates (from 4% to 76%), although in studies with larger, more representative samples, the range was narrower (from 4% to 16%). Other recognized experts have provided prevalence estimates between 5% and 10% for men in general.[25,26] By excluding non-contact abuse from their definition, Gorey and Leslie[27] estimated prevalence of CSA among the general male population at 5% to 8%. Similarly, in a recent population-based study, 6.8% of men reported contact CSA.[28] Another study using a national male sample reported rates of abuse of 7.3%.[29] Two recent large studies found rates of abuse among men of 14.2% among a nationally representative sample[30] and 16.0% among a cohort of 7970 men recruited from an HMO,[11] although both studies used relatively broad definitions of abuse. In general, rates of CSA among general samples of men are less than 10%, although higher rates are reported with broader definitions. These rates are almost all less than the lowest prevalence rate in the studies of MSM reported in Table 3-1.

Five studies either recruited men of all sexual orientations or found an appropriate comparison group for their MSM sample. In these cases, investigators stratified by sexual orientation and compared CSA rates between heterosexual men and MSM. Studies in Table 3–1 that included both MSM and heterosexual men or that looked at a heterosexual comparison sample are noted by an asterisk after the study name. Given an estimate of MSM at approximately 5% of the population,[31] and given the knowledge that CSA is not experienced by most men, it takes large general samples of men to find enough MSM to make a valid comparison of CSA rates. In each of these five studies, MSM were at least three times more likely to report CSA, however defined, than were heterosexual men. Although most studies did not distinguish between CSA by males versus females, those that did found that the difference across sexual orientations only applied for CSA perpetrated by males, not by females.

Two of the research studies[17,18] used probability samples, while the other three used more typical convenience samples. Paul and colleagues[17] used secondary data from a probability sample to try to corroborate their CSA rate of 20.6% among MSM. They examined unpublished data from the National Sexual Health Survey (NSHS), a national general population survey collected in a manner similar to their own (by telephone) and using a similar CSA definition.[17] There were 3746 males in the NSHS survey sample, and MSM were 6 times more likely to report CSA (17.1%; 95% CI = 11.5% to 24.8%) than heterosexual men (2.8%; 95% CI = 2.3% to 3.5%). This study provided both a replication of Paul's data regarding CSA prevalence among MSM as well as a comparison showing a wide disparity in self-reported CSA between MSM and heterosexual men.

Data from the 2002 NSFG[18] found that, of almost 5000 men aged 15 to 44, 5.2% (n = 250) self-identified as gay or bisexual. Men in the sample who were at least 18 years old were asked whether they had ever been forced by a man or a woman to have intercourse and, if yes, at what age. Looking at forced sex for the overall sample (without stratifying by sexual orientation of the victim), 3.5% of men reported abuse by a woman before the age of 18 years and 2.5% reported abuse by a man before the age of 18. There was a difference in the age of the forced sex by female versus male abusers. Of the 306 participants ever abused by a woman, 25% reported abuse that occurred before age 15, 25% occurred between ages 15 to 17, and 50% occurred at age 18 or older. In contrast, most of the forced sex with males (n = 120) occurred before the age of 15 (76% before age 15, 11% between ages 15 to 17, and 13% at age 18 or older). When looking at prevalence of abuse before age 18 by sexual orientation, there was a significant difference for those abused by males and no difference for those abused by females. Specifically, 14.9% of MSM reported CSA by a man compared to 1.7% of heterosexual men, while the rates for abuse by females were nearly identical (3.4% compared to 3.3%).[18]

In the three studies using convenience samples,[32–34] the results are similar. In the first, which investigated 881 injection-drug-using Latinos, 38 (4.3%) identified as gay or bisexual.[32] Rates of CSA were 1.8% for heterosexual men, 25.0% for bisexual men, and 27.3% for gay men, a highly significant difference. Similarly, in a study of men cohabitating with men or with women, the prevalence of CSA among the 65 men living with men was 15.4%.[33] Using information provided by Tjaden and colleagues,[33] we calculated that less than

2% of the 300 men cohabitating with women reported CSA, at least seven times less than the men living with a male partner. Finally, a study of college students found that MSM reported CSA rates three times higher (11.8%) than their heterosexual peers (3.6%).[34]

In sum, regardless of the rigor of the sample selection, when comparing MSM samples to general male population samples, and when comparing MSM and heterosexual men within one sample, MSM consistently report more CSA overall and more CSA with males than heterosexual men do; and no differences are observed for reported abuse by females. A strength of single-study comparisons is that men were recruited in the same manner and the same definition of CSA was applied, regardless of sexual orientation. These studies bolster our conclusion that a disparity exists between gay/bisexual men and heterosexual men when it comes to CSA by males. While it is possible that these differences may be an artifact of reporting biases (e.g., heterosexual men being less willing to report being victimized by a man or to report that early heterosexual contact is abuse as opposed to initiation), it seems unlikely that reporting bias would account for a difference of this consistency and magnitude across a wide range of samples.

Methodological and Theoretical Issues Regarding Prevalence of CSA

Although the data are strong and consistent in showing a disparity regarding CSA between MSM and heterosexual men, there are some methodological and theoretical issues regarding CSA, particularly how CSA is defined, that need to be considered.[2,3,35,36] These differences in definitions have led to heated disagreements about the study of CSA.[37–39] Moreover, these definitional differences make it challenging to compare and generalize research findings, to determine the general prevalence of CSA, and to examine childhood and adult correlates of abuse. Traditionally, CSA definitions consider some combination of; (1) the ages of the youth and abuser, (2) the behaviors of both partners (sometimes assessing contact, force, or coercion), and (3) the perception of the abused person, either immediately or retrospectively, that he was abused.[5,40]

Factors Affecting Estimates of Prevalence Rates of CSA

How researchers define CSA can have a marked effect on prevalence rates. In most cases, researchers ask a series of questions and then determine *post hoc* what experiences to label as CSA. Generally, it is important to distinguish CSA from child sexual behavior, although this can be difficult.[41] In general, CSA has been defined as coercive or manipulative sexual contact with a "child" (as legally defined) by an adult, although some researchers have included non-contact experiences as well (e.g., exhibitionism). A general principle for CSA data is that the prevalence rate in a given sample of men decreases by about 50% when the definition requires contact or physical touch,[3,42] and estimates of the long-term effects of CSA decrease as the definition of abuse is broadened to include non-contact.[43]

Some researchers have used a more legalistic or age-based definition of CSA that does not require coercion. An age-based definition fits with the US legal system, which in most states declares that children under a certain age (often between 14 and 17 years old, depending on the state) cannot legally consent to engage in sexual behaviors, particularly with older adolescents or adults, even if the "child" expresses willingness. Statutes that set a minimum age for sexual consent are the product of the last century; in earlier generations, it was commonly accepted for people to be married and sexually active in their teenage years.[6,44] An age-based definition is based on the premise of inferred power inequities between the partners, that children cannot consent to certain activities, and that child sexual contact is inherently harmful and traumatic.[17] State laws sometimes set an older age of consent for sex between males than between males and females, further stigmatizing and criminalizing same-sex behavior, although the validity of this legal distinction was recently struck down in a high-profile court case,[45] and this may serve to move definitions of CSA toward uniformity regardless of the sexes of the parties.

There is some concern that research definitions for CSA focusing on age differences alone may be overly broad and problematic because they combine very distinct experiences into a single category (e.g., aggregating long-standing sexual abuse of a 9-year-old by his uncle with a one-time consensual sexual liaison between a 16-year-old adolescent male and a 21-year-old unrelated male). The context of the sexual activity is ignored when research definitions treat both of these experiences as equivalent, that is, both as CSA.[45] Such definitions also make it harder to draw conclusions about potential effects of CSA—because the antecedents and outcomes are likely be very different between these two hypothetical situations.[5] In the studies reported in Table 3–1, four required only an age difference between the parties,[15,16,46,47] ten required force or coercion,[3,17,18,21,23,32–34,48,49] and three required force or a specified age difference.[4,20,22]

How Perceptions Affect the Prevalence of CSA among MSM

Because the context in which CSA occurs may be particularly important, some researchers have focused on the perception of the sexual activity from the perspective of the person who is or was a youth when it occurred. In this situation, researchers often ask some combination of three related questions: (1) whether the participant now reports that he willingly engaged in the sexual activity, (2) whether there was coercion or not, and (3) whether the sexual contact was upsetting at the time or is upsetting in the present.[16,17,46] In a perception-based definition of CSA, self-reported lack of harm or willingness to engage in sex are used to argue that such an event should not be included in overall prevalence estimates of CSA.[15] However, at a certain undetermined age, most would agree that consent or willingness is not an appropriate indicator and that the power and relationship dynamics indicate that sexual contact is *per se* abusive. Some researchers have simply measured perception to better describe sexual behaviors that are legally defined as CSA.

Seven of the studies in Table 3-1 assessed perceptions of abuse such as willingness and distress.[4,15–17,21,46,48] In the two studies that asked about distress, most men who had experienced coercion reported past or current distress.[17,48] Among HIV-positive MSM in the first study, 88% of the men reported that the forced sexual activity before age 16 was upsetting.[48] Similarly, 66% of Paul and colleagues' sample[17] reported that the event was moderately or extremely distressing at the time, and 48% felt that way presently. However, in both cases, even with relatively severe definitions of CSA, not all participants reported distress. Other studies indicate that a substantial number of early sexual behaviors, particularly ones reported as noncoercive, were agreed to or sought out by the younger party. For example, of men retrospectively reporting sexual contact with someone at least four years older when they were less than 13 years old, 50% reported that they willingly engaged in the behavior.[16] Thus, the 36% CSA prevalence reported in this sample is made up of 18% willing and 18% unwilling. Other studies found that 51%[46] or 59%[22] of men defined by the researchers as sexually abused reported that they did not feel that the events were negative, coerced, or abusive. Similarly, Jinich and colleagues[4] found that 44% of men who reported sexual behavior when they were 13 to 15 years old reported no coercion, and 26% of those reporting sexual behavior before age 13 reported no coercion. Despite the frequent occurrence of adult men reporting childhood willingness to behavior defined as CSA, it is possible that these experiences were reframed as positive to manage a potentially overwhelming negative experience or that these experiences had harmful effects that the men did not recognize.[4] In a qualitative study using a select sample of young gay men, the participants discussed their sexual experiences with men that had occurred when the participants were 12 to 17 years old.[15] Over 20% of participants reported such an experience, and no differences were found in self-esteem and positive sexual identity between those who engaged in early sexual experiences and those who did not. In addition, 92% of the sexual interactions were reportedly sought out by the youth.

In sum, prevalence rates of CSA are high among MSM in most of the studies, even when removing events for which participants report that they willingly sought sexual activity and did not feel forced. Careful consideration of CSA definitions is important for understanding the phenomena being examined. Various sensitivities and value judgments about sexuality and youth, particularly gay youth, hamper research and our understanding of these complex developmental phenomena and their intersection with CSA.[26]

Characteristics and Outcomes of CSA

A cohesive theoretical framework is lacking for understanding the effects of CSA, although various models (e.g., trauma, attachment, developmental, and evolutionary models) have been proposed.[41] It is challenging to build a model to explain how heterogeneous childhood events such as CSA affect adult functioning. Due to the passage of time between abuse and adulthood, researchers need to account for the role of the number of experiences that precede and follow abuse, including individual and family factors.[2,5,26] Thus, a pervasive pattern of violent abuse is likely to have greater immediate and long-term effects than an isolated incident. The most common research design has been a cross-sectional assessment of childhood experiences and current adult functioning, but these designs are inadequate for understanding phenomena over time.[5,9,50] Longitudinal research is needed in order to separate the effects of CSA from family or other difficulties that precede it or continue after it.[51] Recent data from large national samples and from studies of twin brothers indicate that both family environment and sexual abuse status contribute separately and additively to adult outcomes.[8,52] In addition, attempts to understand the effects of CSA are hampered by a dearth of information regarding the general development of sexuality, regardless of sexual orientation.

Despite these issues, a key principle that emerges from CSA research is that the effects are highly variable and that no single symptom or syndrome characterizes sexually abused children.[51] Thus, even severe CSA does not fully explain adult functioning, and even apparent willingness to engage in sexual activity on the part of the youth does not ensure lack of harm. Two important corollaries to this key principle are that: (1) some children show no effects during or after abuse while others show severe distress,[50] and (2) CSA is a risk factor for adult problems in numerous domains, although not all adults experiencing CSA develop abuse-related problems.[51] Thus, the long-term effects of CSA represent potential vulnerability to negative outcomes, not destiny. Among the important goals for researchers are to understand, first and foremost, how to prevent CSA. Then, if CSA is not prevented, it is important to understand the full context of CSA, how contextual characteristics are related to outcomes, what the general long-term developmental sequelae of CSA are, and how to best prevent some of the negative public health outcomes that occur among some men who experience CSA. In addition, it is important to help elucidate the impact of elevated rates of CSA among MSM and their communities, as well as ways to minimize these public health impacts.

Adult Outcomes of CSA among MSM

There are a number of important adult behavioral correlates of CSA among MSM, most of them emerging from research in the context of the HIV epidemic. Studies have found that MSM who report CSA, compared to those who do not, are more likely to report adult behaviors such as sexual risk behavior,[4,13,17,19,20,48] sexual victimization by non-intimate partners,[53] trading sex for money or drugs,[20] substance use or mental health problems,[13,20,49] nonsexual relationship violence,[20] and HIV or other STDs.[4,13,17,20] It is important to note that these various problems do not happen in isolation, but instead appear to be related. For example, Stall and colleagues[54] found that psychosocial problems among MSM such as CSA, depression, partner violence, and polydrug use were highly related and had an additive effect, such that men reporting more of these experiences also had more sexual risk behavior and higher prevalence of HIV infection. In addition, CSA was related to increased risk for depression and partner violence, but not polydrug use.

While the outcomes of CSA are generally non-specific, sexual issues (sexual orientation, sexuality, gender role, and comfort with intimacy) do seem to be a hallmark of CSA for all men, regardless of sexual orientation, when compared to the effects of other negative childhood events such as physical abuse.[3,30,36] CSA can be considered a form of sexual learning, even if that learning is involuntary and the results dysfunctional.[55] Sexual orientation and gender identity can be particularly confusing for men who experienced arousal during the abuse,[3] and MSM who experienced abuse may continue to be aroused by circumstances that mirror the abusive situation.[56] Some abused men may avoid friendship with other men or may engage in anti-gay activities in an attempt to reassert their masculinity or to manage fears that they are gay or that their femininity contributed to their abuse.[13,16,22,57] Not only heterosexual men but also gay men who have been sexually abused by other men have been found to be more homophobic (some heterosexual men doubt their sexuality, and some gay men are repulsed by various same-sex behaviors).[13,58]

The clinical literature is full of rich descriptions of the potentially harmful effects of CSA among heterosexual men and MSM.[10] Some of the persistent emotional struggles reported by men who experienced CSA include anger and rage, betrayal and loss, intense fear, helplessness and loss of control, sexual identity confusion and struggle with masculinity, isolation and alienation, lack of belief in the legitimacy of both the abuse and the aftereffects, enduring negative beliefs about self and others, repressed or compulsive sexuality, shame, and humiliation.[10,57] An analysis of qualitative data by Dorais identified three risky patterns of sexual behavior among MSM who reported CSA.[55] The first pattern, which posed the most risk for HIV acquisition or transmission, was marked by sexual compulsivity, the perception that sexual urges were strong and impossible to ignore, and the lack of an attempt to control sexual urges. A second pattern was identified by shame, guilt, and a long-standing uncertainty about sexual orientation, leading to sex with male and female partners. Risk for this group was due to the hidden, uncomfortable, and underground nature of their liaisons with men. The third pattern was described as that of the "rebel," marked by knowledge about HIV risks but conscious resistance to institutions and authority figures who deliver safer sex messages.

The typologies described above are important because they synthesize patterns of effects for this complex phenomenon and make clear the implications for individual and community health. To the extent that MSM are more likely to experience CSA and then develop one of these patterns, the more likely these individuals and the MSM community are at risk to miss important public health messages and to have difficulty protecting themselves and others from HIV and other STDs. In other words, higher rates of CSA might be related to higher rates of maladaptive sexual patterns among MSM, and these patterns could negatively affect community norms and the sexual health of the community. This is particularly problematic in the MSM community with its high incidence and prevalence of HIV. In addition, to the extent that African American or Latino MSM do have higher rates of CSA, this may be a factor in their higher rates of HIV. It is also interesting that the second pattern identified above sounds similar to the "down-low" phenomenon (e.g., men being secretive about their male liaisons), which has been the focus of recent media attention.[59] Thus, one might speculate that men who are abused and later not clear about their sexual orientation have both male and female partners and put both at risk for STDs and HIV due to their confusion and secrecy.

Characterizing CSA among MSM and Relationship to Outcomes

Researchers must carefully characterize CSA to develop a better understanding of contextual factors that may affect childhood and adulthood correlates of CSA. In their extensive review, Holmes and Slap[3] found that studies using larger samples reported some common characteristics among those who were abused. First, the average age at abuse was about 10 years, a finding confirmed among MSM.[17] Research is inconsistent about whether the age of abuse is related to worse outcomes,[3] possibly due to differences in CSA definitions and outcomes. However, more recent data among men in general does indicate that abuse before age 10 is related to increased rates of STDs and more lifetime sexual partners,[60] and there is some recent evidence among MSM that earlier abuse is a risk factor for worse outcomes.[46] In general, most abusers are men (53% to 94%),[3] although a recent study of 17,000 heterosexual and homosexual HMO participants found that, among the 16% reporting CSA, 40% of perpetrators were women.[11] However, in studies focusing on MSM, the perpetrators are always at least 90% male.[4,17,22,18,47] Men who were abused only by women have been found to have better adult functioning,[12] although this finding may differ by adult sexual orientation.

The fact that most childhood abusers of MSM were males suggests either an etiological link between CSA and adult sexual orientation, or the existence of childhood characteristics that are related to adult sexual orientation in men that increase vulnerability, or both. For all boys, gender nonconformity (e.g, behaving in ways more traditionally accepted for girls, such as playing with dolls), which is much more prevalent in the childhood recall of MSM, may be an antecedent to abuse.[61] Longitudinal studies have reliably related gender nonconformity in boys to being gay or bisexual in adulthood (without examining or accounting for abuse).[61] Same-sex attractions may precede abuse, be affected by abuse, or both. Gender nonconformity may lead to boys self-labeling themselves as gay or to them being targeted for abuse. Given that almost all abusers of MSM are men, there may be some interaction between the youth's personal desires and the abuser's ability to target boys who may be more likely to be interested. Unfortunately, no longitudinal studies have examined the relationship between CSA and the development of gender role and sexual orientation. Male youth who recognize their same-sex attractions or who are gender nonconforming may seek partners at a young age and may initiate sexual behavior that is labeled CSA.[16] These youth may also place themselves in situations in which they are more likely to be unexpectedly abused. In a recent study, almost none of the men who reported a sexual relationship with a man during adolescence believed that these experiences had a role in creating their same-sex interest, instead reporting that the same-sex interest already existed.[15] Clearly, some early sexual relationships are voluntary or initiated by the youth (particularly adolescents) as part of exploring emerging sexual feelings, even though these experiences may be illegal, exploitive, and may have harmful effects later in life.[16,22]

Other factors such as duration or frequency of abuse, use of force, the sexual behavior involved in the experience, and family response may affect outcomes.[5] Paul and colleagues[17] found that, among measures of severity, increased frequency of abuse was the most powerful correlate of worse adult outcomes for MSM. Physical force is more often used on boys than girls,[36] although in most studies, physical force was used in less than 25% of abusive acts.[3] Force and coercion were used more often if the boy was older and if the abuser was a man (which is more likely for MSM). Those who experienced force or coercion consistently reported greater distress.[4,36,62] Overall, more negative reactions and outcomes were related to the use of force or penetration, longer duration of abuse, a male perpetrator, greater age difference between the two persons, being younger than 12, the abuser being related to the child, and less supportive or more blaming family reactions.[3,12,17,22,43,46,62,63]

While some have argued that one's perception of harm (or lack thereof) should be the defining feature of whether a behavior should be labeled as CSA,[6,44,64] there is also some evidence that there may be unrealized harm, such as increased sexual risk behavior, even among those who perceive their early sexual behavior as positive or willing.[4,13,16] For example, in a study of Latino gay men who did and did not experience CSA before age 13, the researchers divided the abused sample into those who reported that they were willing participants in the sexual activity and those who were unwilling.[16] Among this sample, adult sexual risk behavior was highest among participants who said they were unwillingly abused as a youth, at a medium level among willing abuse participants, and at lowest levels among those who had not had sexual experiences before age 13. Thus, participants who perceived their early sexual experiences as willing were still potentially affected by the experience in that they exhibited higher levels of sexual risk behavior than did men who had not experienced CSA. Another study also found highest rates of sexual risk with casual partners among men who were strongly coerced or forced into sex, medium rates of risk among men mildly coerced or not coerced at all, and lowest rates of risk among those not abused.[4] In contrast, another study found that men who reported CSA that was noncoercive were very similar in psychological adjustment to those who had not been abused,[46] but they confirmed the finding that men who reported coercion had the worst adjustment. In summary, men who perceive early sexual experience as voluntary may have fewer or no psychological symptoms and feel less injured, but deleterious effects may still be evident when examining sexual risk behavior. In a study in South Africa that did not ask about perceptions of abuse, sexual debut before age 15 was significantly associated with a greater number of recent partners and greater sexual risk at sexual debut.[65] Assessing personal perceptions of CSA may help to characterize the experience and to better link context to outcomes, but perceptions should not be the only definitional aspect of CSA.

Interventions for CSA among MSM

The most effective interventions for CSA are those that prevent it from ever happening. Next most desirable would be early intervention shortly after CSA occurs. However, vast numbers of sexually abused men and women are not identified or treated in childhood or adolescence,[26] or if they are identified, they do not feel that they need treatment. For adult MSM affected by CSA, effective interventions would be designed to address a host of potentially interrelated psychological and sexual sequelae. Because of the potential to overlap with other chapters, we will examine specific interventions focused on CSA among MSM, and not on the more generic interventions for some of the other potential sequelae of CSA.

Primary and Early Secondary Prevention

The most effective way to address the disparities of increased CSA and related sequelae among MSM is through the development of primary prevention programs (e.g., treating sex offenders, policing untreated offenders living in the community, raising community awareness about the potential damage from CSA of boys, teaching children appropriate boundaries). Better prosecution and rehabilitation for perpetrators of abuse is an important component of CSA prevention. If a boy's sexual orientation could be identified when he is a youth, then extra efforts might be taken to protect boys who would grow up to be gay so as to help eliminate the CSA disparity. To the extent that child abusers use gender nonconformity in boys as a means of identifying victims who might be easier to target, parents can help protect all of their children by talking about sexuality, self-protection, and boundaries.

Early identification of CSA (i.e., during childhood) is the next line of defense for preventing subsequent abuse and facilitating quick introduction into treatment. Family reactions to CSA are important moderators of adult outcomes.[5,26] For example, communicating acceptance of the child and not blaming the child may decrease or minimize the harm from CSA. However, family reactions are not always helpful, as relatives who want to "save the family honor" by preventing further disclosure sometimes silence boys who had disclosed CSA to a family member.[16] By turning a blind eye to abuse, some parents allow the abuse to continue and potentially to be perpetuated in later generations. In contrast, an exaggerated parental response in front of the child might traumatize him or leave him feeling blamed. Addressing feelings of self-blame may decrease common feelings such as enduring negative self-attributes.[50] Research has found that self-blame among those experiencing CSA is more likely if: (1) the abuser or family members blame them, (2) they became aroused by the experiences or received side benefits, favors, or special treatment, (3) they believe they should have been able to protect themselves, or (4) they believe that men should always be ready for sex, regardless of the circumstances.[12,36]

Health care professionals also play an important role in prevention and early identification of CSA, although average disclosure rates to providers during childhood are poor, ranging from 10% to 33% of cases.[3] Even among cases discovered in childhood, only about half of the male victims are referred for mental health care, and only half of those referred actually seek treatment.[3] CSA victims who have a helpful mental health provider as adults were found to have higher self-esteem and better family functioning in adulthood.[66] Doctors accustomed to working with children and properly trained on detecting CSA are on the frontlines of detection,[67] and their sensitivity may make it easier for children to disclose abuse to them. In order to prevent CSA and stop the further abuse of boys, health professionals need to be aware and ready to discuss CSA with boys and their families. In some cases, this may involve discussion about non-gender-conforming behavior, concerns about the child's sexual orientation, and ways to support the child to avoid re-victimization and vulnerability.

The following efforts are essential to the early identification of CSA: revising socially constructed ideas about male gender roles, tackling stigma against same-sex relations, and employing comprehensive screening strategies. Social expectations that males be self empowered leave little room for boys to report a victimizing event. Research with male college students found that they attributed less blame for CSA to abusers when the victim was a boy rather than a girl,[68] indicating the pervasive impact of social norms. To protect boys, we must acknowledge the violation of boys as abuse and establish an environment in which boys can report their victimization in safe settings. Destigmatizing homosexuality would also help the early identification of CSA, as some failure to report CSA comes from general discomfort with homosexuality and the belief that same-sex abuse necessarily indicates a homosexual orientation. Enabling boys and their parents to view this type of sexual violation as abuse is the first step in freeing the boys from assuming responsibility for the actions of their perpetrators and internalizing self-blame.

Secondary Prevention among Adult MSM

Because there are a number of negative outcomes from CSA, there are likewise a number of interventions that may be relevant to adult men who experienced CSA. However, we will focus our discussion first on holistic interventions that treat men who have been sexually abused and will try to address the effects of CSA on men's lives. As previously stated, it may be difficult for abused men to be identified for treatment, because stigma and shame can keep these histories hidden. Health care providers who treat MSM can play an important role in detection of CSA by asking men about a history of abuse. However, health care providers do not ask adult male patients about a history of CSA about three-quarters of the time,[69] and mental health professionals often lack specific knowledge and training for treating CSA among MSM. Thus, it is crucial to educate providers, particularly those who work with MSM, about the existence of this health disparity and the need for attention to it.

There have been no published randomized controlled trials of treatment for CSA among MSM, and given the heterogeneity of effects, such a trial would be a challenge. Common treatment strategies discussed in the literature include individual and group psychotherapy. More recently, some careful and detailed individual treatment manuals have been developed based on research with abused men.[10] This type of individual work may be particularly important because persons who experienced CSA may be less responsive to broad public health messages.[55,70,71] In terms of the focus in CSA treatment, the following goals were recently suggested by Briere[71]: (1) alter enduring cognitive distortions about helplessness and self-blame and improve self esteem; (2) reduce the need for external tension reduction and substance abuse by reducing post-traumatic stress and increasing skills to regulate emotions; (3) address dysfunctional relationship schemas, including unwanted isolation, desperate need for love, and fear of intimacy and abandonment; (4) increase assertiveness and sexual boundaries; and (5) target HIV-related issues. Providing these more expensive individual services to MSM who experienced CSA may provide both personal and community benefits and may be worth the extra resources if it leads to decreases in substance abuse, mental health problems, and sexual risk.

Conclusions and Future Directions for Research

There is a clear disparity in the frequency of CSA between MSM and heterosexual men. Rates for MSM are 15% to 25% in the best designed studies,[4,17,18] which is at least triple the rates reported among heterosexual men. While CSA research is widely acknowledged to be challenged with methodological issues, those issues do not undermine this particular conclusion. Despite this large disparity, it is actually difficult to explain, and the list of potential or partial explanations includes: gender nonconforming behavior being a cue that men use to abuse certain boys; less shame about recall of same-sex CSA among MSM; teenage sexual exploration by young MSM being captured in the abuse definition; and same-sex CSA being related to the development of a homosexual orientation in adulthood. There is some support for each of these explanations, but further research is needed to better understand the various interrelationships. CSA is associated with a number of negative adult outcomes that also disproportionately affect MSM, including substance use, mental health issues, and sexual risk. Untangling the links between these disparities is a challenge that researcher must address head on.

In terms of improving our general knowledge base to respond to CSA, a thorough research program on sexual development of all people, regardless of adult sexual orientation, would be most illuminating. In addition, a consistent definition of CSA would greatly facilitate accurate reporting and understanding. To bring light to the subject of CSA among MSM, assessing important contextual variables surrounding incidents that are defined as abuse is crucial to move the field beyond dichotomous measures of abuse, and to better capture how the contextual aspects of CSA affect adult outcomes. Once abuse has occurred, early and focused treatment is important, if indicated. Better understanding of how to intervene with children and adults can help to minimize the individual and societal impact of CSA. It also is important to conduct research on the sexual experiences of older gay teens, as their experiences might be labeled as abuse under some state laws and research definitions. Finally, it should be noted that cultural sensitivities surrounding homosexuality and youth sexuality make it likely that social forces will continue to have a large impact on the field and on attempts to understand the effects of abuse and boundaries between normal and abusive sexual behavior.

Authors' Note

The findings and conclusions in this chapter are those of the authors and do not necessarily represent the views of the Centers for Disease Control and Prevention.

References

1. Gartner RB. Sexual victimization of boys by men: meanings and consequences. *J Gay Lesbian Psychother.* 1999;3:1–33.
2. Haugaard J. The challenge of defining child sexual abuse. *Am Psychol.* 2000;55: 1036–1039.
3. Holmes WC, Slap GB. Sexual abuse of boys: definition, prevalence, correlates, sequelae, and management. *J Am Med Assoc.* 1998;280(21):1855–1862.
4. Jinich S, Paul JP, Stall R, et al. Childhood sexual abuse and HIV risk-taking behavior among gay and bisexual men. *AIDS Behav.* 1998;2(1):41–51.
5. Purcell D, Malow RM, Dolezal C, Carballo-Dieguez A. Sexual Abuse of Boys: Short- and long term association and implications for HIV. In: Koenig L, Doll LS, O'Leary A, Pequegnat W, eds. *From Child Sexual Abuse to Adult Sexual Risk.* Washington, DC: American Psychological Association; 2004:93–114.
6. Rind B. An empirical examination of sexual relations between adolescents and adults: they differ from those between children and adults and should be treated separately. *J Psychol Hum Sex.* 2004;16(2/3):55–62.
7. Doll LS, Koenig L, Purcell DW. Child Sexual Abuse and Adult Sexual Risk: Where are we now? In: Koenig L, Doll LS, O'Leary A, Pequegnat W, eds. *From Child Sexual Abuse to Adult Sexual Risk.* Washington, DC: American Psychological Association; 2004:3–10.
8. Molnar BE, Buka SL, Kessler RC. Child sexual abuse and subsequent psychopathology: results from the National Comorbidity Survey. *Am J Public Health.* 2001; 91(5):753–760.
9. Rind B, Tromovitch P, Bauserman R. A meta-analytic examination of assumed properties of child sexual abuse using college samples. *Psychol Bull.* 1998;124(1): 22–53.
10. Spiegel J. *Sexual Abuse of Males: The SAM Model of Theory and Practice.* New York, NY: Brunner Routledge; 2003;545.
11. Dube SR, Anda RF, Whitfield CL, et al. Long-term consequences of childhood sexual abuse by gender of victim. *Am J Prev Med.* 2005;28:430–438.
12. Mendel MP. *The Male Survivor: The Impact of Sexual Abuse.* Thousand Oaks, CA: Sage; 1995.
13. Bartholow BN, Doll LS, Joy D, et al. Emotional, behavioral, and HIV risks associated with sexual abuse among adult homosexual and bisexual men. *Child Abuse Negl.* 1994;18:747–761.
14. Doll LS, Joy D, Bartholow BN, et al. Self-reported childhood and adolescent sexual abuse among adult homosexual/ bisexual men. *Child Abuse Negl.* 1992;16: 855–864.
15. Rind B. Gay and Bisexual Adolescent Boys' Sexual Experiences with Men: an empirical examination of psychological correlates in a non-clinical sample. *Arch Sex Behav.* 2001;30(4):345–368.
16. Carballo-Dieguez A, Dolezal C. Association between history of childhood sexual abuse and adult HIV-risk sexual behavior in Puerto Rican men who have sex with men. *Child Abuse Negl.* 1995;19(5):595–605.
17. Paul JP, Catania J, Pollack L, Stall R. Understanding childhood sexual abuse as a predictor of sexual risk-taking among men who have sex with men: The Urban Men's Health Study. *Child Abuse Negl.* 2001;25(4):557–584.

18. CDC. National Survey of Family Growth (cycle 6). *Centers for Disease Control and Prevention* [Web site]. www.cdc.gov/nchs/nsfg.htm. Accessed August 11, 2006.
19. Parsons JT, Bimbi DS, Koken JA, Halkitis PN. Factors related to childhood sexual abuse among gay/bisexual male Internet escorts. *J Child Sexual Abus.* 2005;14(2): 1–23.
20. Kalichman SC, Gore-Felton C, Benotsch E, Cage M, Rompa D. Trauma symptoms, sexual behaviors, and substance abuse: correlates of childhood sexual abuse and HIV risks among men who have sex with men. *J Child Sex Abus.* 2004;13(1):1–15.
21. Kalichman SC, Benotsch E, Rompa D, et al. Unwanted sexual experiences and sexual risks in gay and bisexual men: associations among revictimization, substance use and psychiatric symptoms. *J Sex Res.* 2001;38(1):1–9.
22. Dolezal C, Carballo-Dieguez A. Childhood sexual experiences and the perception of abuse among Latino men who have sex with men. *J Sex Res.* 2002;39(3):165–173.
23. Arreola SG, Neilands TB, Pollack LM, Paul JP, Catania JA. Higher prevalence of childhood sexual abuse among Latino men who have sex with men than non-Latino men who have sex with men: data from the Urban Men's Health Study. *Child Abuse Negl.* 2005;29(3)7:285–90.
24. Relf MV. Childhood sexual abuse in men who have sex with men: the current state of the science. *J Assoc Nurses AIDS Care.* 2001;12(5):20–29.
25. Finkelhor D. Current information on the scope and nature of child sexual abuse. *Future Child.* 1994;4(2):31–53.
26. Freyd JJ, Putnam FW, Lyon TD, et al. The science of child sexual abuse. *Science.* 2005;308(5721):501.
27. Gorey KM, Leslie DR. The prevalence of child sexual abuse: integrative review adjustment for potential response and measurement biases. *Child Abuse Negl.* 1997;21(4):391–398.
28. Bensley LS, Van Eenwyk J, Simmons KW. Self-reported childhood sexual and physical abuse and adult HIV-risk behaviors and heavy drinking. *Am J Prev Med.* 2000;18(2):151–158.
29. Risin LI, Koss MP. The sexual abuse of boys: prevalence and descriptive characteristics of childhood victimizations. *J Interpers Violence.* 1987;2(3):309–323.
30. Briere J, Elliot D. Prevalence and psychological sequelae of self-reported childhood physical and sexual abuse in a general population sample of men and women. *Child Abuse Negl.* 2003;27:1205–1222.
31. Sell R, Wells J, Wypij D. The prevalence of homosexual behavior and attraction in the United States, United Kingdom, and France: results of national population-based samples. *Arch Sex Behav.* 1995;24:235–248.
32. Finlinson HA, Robles RR, Colon HM, et al. Puerto Rican drug users experiences of physical and sexual abuse: comparisons based on sexual identities. *J of Sex Res.* 2003;40(3):277–285.
33. Tjaden P, Thoennes N, Allison CJ. Comparing violence over the life span in samples of same-sex and opposite-sex cohabitants. *Violence Vict.* 1999;14(4):413–425.
34. Duncan DF. Prevalence of sexual assault victimization among heterosexual and gay/lesbian university students. *Psychol Rep.* 1990;66(1):65–66.
35. Goldman JDG, Padayachi UK. Some methodological problems in estimating incidence and prevalence in child sexual abuse research. *J Sex Res.* 2000;37:305–314.

36. Romano E, De Luca RV. Male sexual abuse: a review of effects, abuse characteristics, and links with later psychological functioning. *Aggres Violent Behav.* 2001; 6(1):55–78.

37. Dallam SJ, Gleaves DH, Cepeda-Benito A, Silberg JL, Kraemer HC, Spiegel D. The effects of child sexual abuse: comment on Rind, Tromovitch, and Bauserman. *Psychol Bull.* 2001;127(6):715–733.

38. Ondersma SJ, Chaffin M, Berliner L, Cordon I, Goodman GS, Barnett D. Sex with children is abuse: comment on Rind, Tromovitch, and Bauserman (1998). *Psychol Bull.* 2001;127(6):707–714.

39. Rind B, Tromovitch P, Bauserman R. The validity and appropriateness of methods, analyses, and conclusions in Rind et al. (1998): a rebuttal of victimological critique from Ondersma et al. (2001) and Dallam et al. (2001). *Psychol Bull.* 2001; 127(6):734–758.

40. Finkelhor D. What's wrong with sex between adults and children? Ethics and the problem of sexual abuse. *Am J Orthopsychiatry.* 1979;49(4):692–697.

41. Heiman J, Heard-Davidson A. Child sexual abuse and adult sexual relationships: review and perspectives. In: Koenig L, Doll LS, O'Leary A, Pequegnat W, eds. *From Child Sexual Abuse to Adult Sexual Risk: Trauma, Revictimization, and Intervention.* Washington, DC: American Psychological Association; 2004:13–47.

42. West DJ. Boys and sexual abuse: an English opinion. *Arch Sex Behav.* 1998;27(6): 539–559.

43. Collings SJ. The long-term effects of contact and noncontact forms of child sexual abuse in a sample of university men. *Child Abuse Negl.* 1995;19(1):1–6.

44. Rind B. Adolescent sexual experiences with adults: pathological or functional? *J Psychol Hum Sex.* 2003;15(1):5–22.

45. Supreme Court of Kansas. *State of Kansas vs. Limon* [Web site]. http://www.kscourts .org/kscases/supct/2005/20051021/85898.htm. Accessed March 10, 2006.

46. Stanley JL, Bartholomew K, Oram D. Gay and bisexual men's age-discrepant childhood sexual experiences. *J Sex Res.* 2004;41(4):381–389.

47. Lenderking WR, Wold C, Mayer KH, Goldstein R, Losina E, Seage GR, 3rd. Childhood sexual abuse among homosexual men: prevalence and association with unsafe sex. *J Gen Intern Med.* 1997;12(4):250–253.

48. O'Leary A, Purcell D, Remien RH, Gomez C. Childhood sexual abuse and sexual transmission risk behaviour among HIV-positive men who have sex with men. *AIDS Care.* 2003;15(1):17–26.

49. Ratner PA, Johnson JL, Shoveller JA, et al. Non-consensual sex experienced by men who have sex with men: prevalence and association with mental health. *Patient Educ Couns.* 2003;49:67–74.

50. Feiring C, Taska L, Lewis M. Age and gender differences in children's and adolescents' adaptation to sexual abuse. *Child Abuse Negl.* 1999;23(2):115–128.

51. Saywitz KJ, Mannarino AP, Berliner L, Cohen JA. Treatment for sexually abused children and adolescents. *Am Psychol.* 2000;55(9):1040–1049.

52. Nelson EC, Heath AC, Madden PA, et al. Association between self-reported childhood sexual abuse and adverse psychosocial outcomes: results from a twin study. *Arch Gen Psychiatry.* 2002;59(2):139–145.

53. Desai S, Arias I, Thompson M, Basile K. Childhood victimization and subsequent adult revictimization assessed in a nationally representative sample of women and men. *Violence Vict.* 2002;17:639–653.

54. Stall R, Mills T, Williamson J, et al. Association of co-occurring psychosocial health problems and increased vulnerability to HIV/AIDS among urban men who have sex with men. *Am J of Public Health.* 2003;93:939–942.

55. Dorais M. Hazardous journey in intimacy: HIV transmission risk behaviors of young men who are victims of past sexual abuses and who have sexual relations with men. *J Homosex.* 2004;48(2):103–124.

56. King N. Childhood sexual trauma in gay men: social context and the imprinted arousal pattern. In: Cassese J, ed. *Gay Men and Childhood Sexual Trauma: Integrating the Shattered Self.* Binghamton, NY: The Harrington Park Press/The Haworth Press; 2000:19–35.

57. Lisak D. The psychological impact of sexual abuse: content analysis of interviews with male survivors. *J Trauma Stress.* 1994;7(4):525–548.

58. Dhaliwal GK, Gauzas L, Antonowicz DH, Ross RR. Adult male survivors of childhood sexual abuse: Prevalence, sexual abuse characteristics, and long-term effects. *Clin Psychol Rev.* 1996;16(7):619–639.

59. Millett G, Malebranch D, Mason B, Spikes P. Focusing "down low": Bisexual black men, HIV risk and heterosexual transmission. *J Natl Med Assoc.* 2005;97:52S-59S.

60. Ohene SA. Sexual abuse history, risk behavior, and sexually transmitted diseases: The impact of age at abuse. *Sex Trans Dis.* 2005;32(6):358–363.

61. Bailey JM, Zucker KJ. Childhood sex-typed behavior and sexual orientation: a conceptual analysis and quantitative review. *Dev Psychol.* 1995; 31(1):43–55.

62. Kendall-Tackett KA, Williams LM, Finkelhor D. Impact of sexual abuse on children: a review and synthesis of recent empirical studies. *Psychol Bull.* 1993;113(1):164–180.

63. Bryant SL, Range LM. Type and severity of child abuse and college students' lifetime suicidality. *Child Abuse Negl.* 1997;21(12):1169–1176.

64. Rind B, Tromovitch P. A meta-analytic review of findings from national samples on psychological correlates of child sexual abuse. *J Sex Res.* 1997;34(3):237–255.

65. Harrison A, Cleland E, Gouws E, Frohich J. Early sexual debut among young men in rural South Africa: heightened vulnerability to sexual risk? *Sex Trans Infect.* 2005;81:259–261.

66. Palmer SE, Brown RA, Rae-Grant NI, Loughlin MJ. Survivors of childhood abuse: their reported experiences with professional help. *Soc Work.* 2001;46(2):136–145.

67. Lentsch KA, Johnson CF, Lentsch KA, Johnson CF. Do physicians have adequate knowledge of child sexual abuse? The results of two surveys of practicing physicians, 1986 and 1996. *Child Maltreat.* 2000;5(1):72–78.

68. Broussard SD, Wagner WG. Child sexual abuse: who is to blame? *Child Abuse Negl.* 1988;12(4):563–569.

69. Lab DD, Feigenbaum JD, De Silva P. Mental health professionals' attitudes and practices towards male childhood sexual abuse. *Child Abuse Negl.* 2000;24(3):391–409.

70. Belcher L, Kalichman SC, Topping M, et al. A randomized trial of a brief HIV risk reduction counseling intervention for women. *J Consul Clin Psychol.* 1998;66:856–861.

71. Briere J. Intergrating HIV/AIDS prevention activities into psychotherapy for child sexual abuse survivors. In: Koenig L, Doll LS, O'Leary A, Pequegnat W, eds. *From Child Sexual Abuse to Adult Sexual Risk: Trauma, Revictimization, and Intervention.* Washington, DC: American Psychological Association; 2004:219–232.

4

Prevalence of Primary Mental Health Morbidity and Suicide Symptoms among Gay and Bisexual Men

Susan D. Cochran and Vickie M. Mays

There can be little doubt that social context shapes risk for psychiatric morbidity. This is so whether it be at the level of social advantages conferred by individual characteristics such as gender or race/ethnicity,[1–45] actual or anticipated social interactions such as experiences with discrimination,[6] or even characteristics of the physical environment in which one lives.[7] For gay and bisexual men, the social topography of their lives differs in many important ways from those of their heterosexual counterparts.[8] Thus it should come as no surprise that gay and bisexual men, as compared to heterosexual men, appear to experience differential risk for some psychiatric disorders[9–24] and especially suicide-related morbidity.[10,14,15,17,20,21,25,26]

In this chapter, we seek to accomplish four aims. First, as a way of framing the findings that we will present, we highlight some of the methodological issues that currently influence our understanding of mental health morbidity concerns among gay and bisexual men. Second, we review evidence for disparities in mental health morbidity and suicide phenomenology affecting gay and bisexual men, emphasizing primarily those studies with either heterosexual comparison groups or sophisticated research designs that minimize uncontrolled selection bias. While problematic alcohol and drug use reflect important mental health issues in their own right, Chapter 5 in this book (Ostrow and Stall) devotes itself to covering these particular topics in greater detail. Consequently, our coverage will be limited to the confluence of drugs and alcohol with other primary mental health disorders that might adversely affect the lives of gay and bisexual men. Third, we touch on some of the possible reasons for the differential risk that has been observed in a flurry of relatively recent studies. Finally, we share our thoughts of important future directions for research on the mental health of gay and bisexual men.

While the majority of chapters in this book contain only studies conducted in the United States, we have included, where available, research from both

Europe and Australia, particularly population-based studies of gay men's mental health. This reflects the long history of population-based psychiatric epidemiological studies in these countries and their willingness to measure sexual orientation–related markers. Due to the dearth of population-based studies on the topic of sexual orientation and mental health, we chose to include these findings in our chapter.* They provide both comparative and supportive evidence of the role of sexual minority status in mental disorders.

Conceptualizations of the associations between mental health and homosexuality have changed radically over time.[12] Early "illness models" viewed homosexuality as pathological or indicative of mental illness.[27] When later research pioneered by Evelyn Hooker[28] found few differences in psychiatric morbidity associated with homosexuality, the prevailing view for nearly 30 years was that there were no differences of import.[12] But the onset of the human immunodeficiency virus (HIV) epidemic and increasing interest in the possible harmful effects of anti-gay bias spawned a body of research beginning in the mid-1980s that examined anew mental health concerns of gay and bisexual men. This more recent work treats sexual orientation as similar to other individual indicators (e.g., gender, race, ethnicity) that might be associated with differential risk for the onset, course, or treatment of mental health morbidity and substance use disorders.[12,29] The new-sprung literature finds, in general, that gay and bisexual men represent a vulnerable population for prevalent mental health morbidity, especially major depression, substance use disorders, anxiety disorders, and suicide attempts.[12] As well, studies document higher perceived need for mental health services among gay and bisexual men than their heterosexual counterparts.[30]

Methodological Underpinnings to Research on Gay and Bisexual Men's Mental Health

Four major methodological issues permeate the recent research on mental health morbidity among gay and bisexual men. We have chosen to begin this chapter by making these issues explicit, as they are the methodological context that frames many of the current research findings. The first two issues (how sexual orientation is defined and measured and how respondents are sampled in any particular study) are critical to the appropriateness of generalizing study findings.[8,31] The key question here is the definition of the population of gay and bisexual men. In reality, this is an open population with ill-defined boundaries, but labels can make this population seem more defined than it really is. The latter two issues (identifying the possible effects of

---

*When we cite studies conducted with samples from outside the United States, we have used an asterisk to indicate that the citations include at least one study with a non-US sample. Otherwise, all studies cited are US-based.

response bias among study respondents and specifying key variables that belong in study instrumentation) are equally crucial to interpreting evidence of sexual orientation–related differences in mental health morbidity.

Defining Sexual Orientation

Sexual orientation is a multidimensional concept involving intercorrelated dimensions of sexual attraction, desires, behavior, and fantasies, as well as self-identity and emotional, social, and lifestyle preferences.[32] While all of these dimensions appear to index a single underlying construct,[33] single markers of sexual orientation vary in their sensitivity and specificity in identifying individuals who might be classified as gay or bisexual. For example, in a national household survey of sexual behavior, Laumann[32] found that only 42% of those who reported same-sex sexual partners in adulthood also self-identified as gay, homosexual, or bisexual. The contradictions between sexual behavior and identity have been noted by behavioral scientists for some time.[32–37]* At this point, the question of whether some dimensions of sexual orientation (e.g., sexual behavior) are more closely linked to mental health morbidity than others remains unanswered.

One implication of the heterogeneous nature of sexual orientation is that classification methods may draw from different source populations. Some of the work reported below measures sexual orientation identity; some uses sexual behavior as a proxy for homosexual or bisexual identity. Thus, each method samples a somewhat different subpopulation. Bailey,[38] for example, has suggested that individuals who report same-sex behavior histories include not only gay/lesbian or bisexual individuals but also heterosexuals who have a higher degree of sexual impulsivity. Classification by sexual history alone would then tend to inflate the prevalence of disorders association with sexual impulsivity among those labeled as gay or bisexual. A second difficulty in classification by sexual behavior alone is that respondents who are not sexually active in the time frame measured are not classifiable and must be discarded from further study. This may be upward of 20% of any particular sample.[11] Discarding celibate respondents from analyses may also introduce bias if recent sexual activity is correlated with mental health outcomes of interest.[11] The caution, here, for the reader is that methods of classification may influence study findings.

Drawing Study Samples

Research in this area has typically used one of two major sampling strategies that shape our understanding of the burden of disorders within this population.[31] The first approach, nearly exclusively employed in the published literature until 1998, relies on convenience-based sampling of readily identifiable individuals who label themselves as lesbian, gay, or bisexual.[12] In this tradition, samples are drawn with unknown selection probability usually from those who are reachable through participation in lesbian and gay community venues or through social networks accessible to researchers, such as through advertisements or commercial mailing lists. Sometimes, selection strategies are heavily confounded with study outcomes (e.g., recruitment from bars or bath houses when a study goal is to estimate sexual risk–taking behaviors in the population as a whole). Often there are no comparable heterosexual comparison groups because the methods of sample selection (e.g., recruitment at gay pride events or gay bars) have no obvious counterpart outside the gay community. The limitations of these methods have been noted elsewhere.[12,39,40]

A second sampling strategy emerged as a consequence of the HIV epidemic, which created an urgent need to estimate the prevalence of homosexual risk behaviors among men[32,41–49] and changes in American family structures.[8] Both the nature of the epidemic and the changing American family structure, by chance, resulted in greater opportunities and resources for researchers interested in studying lesbian, gay, and bisexual life in general and willingness by some survey researchers to insert sexual orientation–related questions into several large health and social surveys that sampled respondents irrespective of their sexual orientation. Some of these latter data sets in which these questions have been asked are state of the art in terms of sampling design (e.g., population-based surveys, population-based twin registries, longitudinal cohort studies, US census data). What these data sets all have in common is that each includes at least one potential marker of homosexuality in the survey instrument (e.g., reports of same-gender sexual partners over various time frames; cohabiting in a same-sex marital-equivalent relationship; same-sex attractions; self-identification as lesbian, gay, bisexual, or homosexual) and that samples are selected in ways that minimize possible sexual orientation–related sampling bias.

Population-based surveys in which the primary interest is documenting patterns of sexual behavior[35,36*,50] or sexual development[51,52] often include multiple markers of sexual orientation. However, the great majority of population-based surveys are not designed to examine sexual behavior in detail but to provide the federal government and others estimates on a range of important topics. These surveys typically include a single set of questions about the genders of sexual partners if any measure of sexual activity is taken. Currently, several of these population-based surveys of both types also assess psychiatric variables or substance use. Although their usefulness is somewhat limited due to the very small numbers of lesbian, gay, and bisexual individuals identified in each study, researchers, including our research group, have quickly capitalized on this new information to compare individuals reporting markers of homosexuality to those who do not.[9,10,13–24,30,51,53–68*]

The newer sampling methods associated with this second generation of data sets greatly reduce selection bias and are constructed with relevant heterosexual comparison groups. But they raise other methodological issues. For example, the relatively low prevalence of homosexuality in the population results in extremely small sample sizes for homosexually classified subgroups in many of the studies (generally 2% to 4% of the total sample), generating some uncertainty about the stability of findings.

To overcome these limitations, researchers have crafted new methods of oversampling minority sexual orientation respondents in systematically or probabilistically drawn samples, coupled with better assessment of sexual orientation status. For example, one strategy is to create an initial sampling frame that includes neighborhoods of high gay density (HGD). This can be done by using information from the US Census to map households with two same-gender adults in which one is reported as an unmarried partner. A prominent example is the Urban Men's Health Survey (UMHS),[69] which successfully generated a systematically drawn sample of men who have sex with men (MSM) from four HGD urban environs to examine HIV risk among MSMs (the survey has no heterosexual comparison group). A second method of systematic sampling is venue-based time-space sampling in gay male neighborhoods or socializing locations.[70] A third is a yoked-sampling approach. For example, Solomon and colleagues[71] systematically sampled from the Vermont registry of civil unions to create an initial lesbian and gay sample and then asked couples to recruit friends and siblings for a comparison group. This approach melds systematic sampling with convenience methods, but might be vulnerable to anticipated biases (e.g., trusted siblings will be more likely to be recruited).

Like classification of sexual orientation, sampling determines the population under study. This, then, can have an important effect on observed prevalences.[70] For example, if rates of dysfunctional alcohol use among gay and bisexual men are higher among those living in high gay density urban environments as compared to gay and bisexual men living in suburban environments, then findings from studies using an HGD sampling strategy will likely overestimate levels of dysfunctional alcohol use among gay and bisexual men as a whole.

Accounting for Response Bias

The possible effects of response bias either in acknowledging minority sexual orientation markers or reporting mental health symptoms are not yet well understood[12] and are the source of important continuing debates in the field. As an example, Savin-Williams[72] has argued that current concerns about suicide risk among gay youth are being driven, to some extent, by sexual orientation–related differences in propensity to label events as suicide attempts or not. At this point in the research literature, there are few definitive answers to concerns that sexual orientation–related differences in thresholds for reporting psychological symptoms might be at the heart of recent findings documenting mental health disparities. It may be that the common thread linking sexual orientation and higher rates of morbidity is generated, to some extent, by a lower threshold for disclosing socially stigmatizing information.

Asking the Causal Questions

Homosexuality and its relationship with mental health is an inherently controversial topic.[73] Despite the removal of homosexuality from the *Diagnostic and Statistical Manual of Mental Disorders* more than 30 years ago,[74] many Americans still believe that homosexuality itself is an indication of mental illness.[75] Many in the research community, however, postulate that whatever association is observed between homosexuality and mental illness is generated by a third causal factor, such as minority stress,[29,76] discrimination,[64] or differences in social demography.[57] Some of the work discussed below made concentrated efforts to assess the role of these possible "third factors" in generating mental health disparities affecting gay and bisexual men. But many of the existing general population surveys that have recently been used to examine sexual orientation–related differences in the prevalence of disorders were simply not designed to do so. These data sets might have included a single marker of sexual orientation and extensive measures of psychiatric disorders, but they did not assess sexual orientation–related topics that might be of causal relevance, such as experiences with disclosing homosexuality to others[77] or gay-related discrimination.[64] Like all active research fields, the answers to many of the compelling causal questions await further study. Thus, one last caution to the reader is that the "why" of many of the disparities in morbidity we reviewed are simply unknown at this point, although social and contextual factors, including those mentioned in the latter part of this chapter, are likely to underlie the differences that have been identified in psychiatric morbidity risk for gay and bisexual men.

Disparities in Mental Health Morbidity

Direct evidence for the existence of mental health disparities among gay, bisexual, and heterosexual men comes from several recent surveys in which respondents were sampled irrespective of their sexual orientation. These surveys measured both markers of sexual orientation and indicators of mental health morbidity, often using well-validated, standardized psychiatric instruments. Across studies, the majority of gay and bisexually classified men interviewed did not meet criteria for any of the measured psychiatric disorders. Nevertheless, prevalences of psychiatric morbidity among gay and bisexually classified men were somewhat higher than that seen among similarly sampled heterosexual men.

Prevalence of Psychiatric Disorders

Affective Disorders

Several studies have used information contained in existing population-based[9,10,13,22,30]* or longitudinal cohort[21,78]* data sets to examine links between major depression, as indexed by structured interview protocols, and self-reports of sexual orientation or same-gender sexual behavior. Most have documented higher prevalence of major depression among homosexually experienced men or those who identify as gay or bisexual when compared to heterosexual controls. In one report,[10] evidence was found of perhaps greater lifetime susceptibility to recurrent major depressions among homosexually active men in the NHANES III. Sandfort[22*] found higher one-year and lifetime prevalence of bipolar disorder among Dutch men who reported any male sexual partners in the year prior to interview, as compared to men who reported only female sexual partners.

Given the expectation that adolescence and early adulthood may be a particularly difficult time for those of minority sexual orientation,[79–81] we (and colleagues)[13] also explored the possibility that age at onset of depressive disorders would be earlier in this population. Here, we did find a hint that homosexually experienced men have an earlier onset of major depression than probable heterosexual men, but sample size limitations prevented a convincing test of this hypothesis. Recently, using longitudinal information from the Christchurch Health and Development Study assessing prevalence of major depression in ages 21 to 25 years, Fergusson and colleagues[78*] reported exceptionally high rates (approximately 50%) among young men who indicated at least some homosexuality. In contrast, 14.5% of similar heterosexual men met criteria for major depression. These rates exceed that observed among middle-aged gay and bisexual men in a separate study (31%).[30]

Anxiety Disorders

Over the years, there has been little research examining differential risk for anxiety disorders between gay and bisexual men as compared to heterosexual men, despite the fact that some studies have shown that anxiety is a normative consequence of gay-related victimization.[82] As well, the chronic threat of HIV infection or illness might generate greater vulnerability to anxiety-related disorders. With the new methodologies, researchers had a critical opportunity to examine the burden of anxiety disorders among gay and bisexual men. Initial findings[21*] from a longitudinal cohort study in New Zealand suggested that sexual minority youth suffer higher rates of generalized anxiety disorder in adolescence than their heterosexual peers. These findings were later replicated with more specific measurement of sexual orientation.[78*] In addition, using information from the 1996 National Household Survey on Drug Abuse, we[9] observed higher rates of panic attacks among men reporting past year same-gender sexual partners, as compared to similar men reporting only opposite-gender partners. This finding was replicated in a third study using information available in the Midlife Survey of Adult Development, in which sexual orientation identity was specifically measured.[30] Sandfort,[22*] too, found higher rates of anxiety disorders (panic, obsessive-compulsive disorder, simple phobia, social phobia, and agoraphobia) in homosexually active Dutch men when compared to heterosexually active men. Also, in a fourth study using the National Comorbidity Survey, we (and colleagues) reported that homosexually experienced men were more likely than exclusively heterosexually experienced men to meet criteria for lifetime generalized anxiety disorder.[13] Additional evidence from longitudinal cohort studies also indicates that there may be greater risk for anxiety disorders among gay and bisexual men. Jorm and colleagues[83]* found higher prevalences of anxiety symptoms among 149 homosexual and bisexual individuals of the nearly 5000 persons surveyed at initial cohort formation. Fergusson and colleagues[78]* recently reported that approximately 43% of young men reporting any markers of homosexuality met criteria for an anxiety disorder between the ages of 21 and 25 years, in contrast to 10% of heterosexual men in the same cohort. Estimates of rates of anxiety disorders among middle-aged homosexual and bisexual men from another study[30] are about half that.

Population-based findings examining possible differential risk for post-traumatic stress disorders (PTSD) have not been reported yet, despite an extensive literature emphasizing a higher risk for victimization in this population.[15,16,23,82,84,85] One large survey of homeless and runaway street youth[86] used systematic sampling and sophisticated measurement of PTSD but did not observe higher rates among gay and bisexual males as compared to heterosexual males, despite higher levels of sexual victimization and abuse in the former group. At this point, reasonable suspicions of greater morbidity risk for PTSD await confirmatory evidence.

Prevalence of Suicide Symptoms

The evidence for greater risk for suicide attempts and completions among gay and bisexual adolescent and adult males comes from numerous quarters. Findings from these studies, both convenience-based and the more recent systematic sampling methodologies, have generally documented a higher risk for suicide attempts among both sexual minority youth and adults[10,13–15,17,18,20,21,25,26,59,78,83,84,87–99]* as well as completed adult suicide.[100]* Two longitudinal birth cohort studies from New Zealand in which sampling proceeded before sexual orientation was known[78,98]* assessed both markers of sexual orientation and reports of lifetime suicide attempts among young men in their early twenties. Both found higher rates of attempts among homosexually classified men as compared to heterosexually classified men.

While there has been well-spirited debate as to whether findings on suicide attempts accurately reflect a greater risk for completed suicides,[101] we recently found, using vital statistics data from Denmark, a sixfold increase in age-adjusted risk for completed suicide among men, but not women, who were in registered same-sex domestic partnerships when compared to married persons.[102]* Indeed, the 2001 Surgeons General Report on Suicide has labeled youth with minority sexual orientation as a vulnerable population.[103]

Comorbidity with Substance Use

Dysfunctional substance use, including alcohol and illicit drugs, and substance use disorders are often comorbid with affective and anxiety disorders.[3] Within the gay community, there has been long-standing concern that illicit drug and alcohol use, abuse, and dependency are more prevalent than in heterosexual populations. Further, substance use has important implications for HIV-related sexual risk taking[104–108] whether or not there are disparities in problematic use.

Population-based studies, however, have found little evidence for important disparities in alcohol use patterns or morbidity indicators among gay and bisexual men as compared to similar heterosexual men.[9,11,13,22,30,109,110]* Men, whatever their sexual orientation, tend to be heavier users and misusers of alcohol when compared to women,[3] and although gay and heterosexual men might drink in different contexts, rates of problematic alcohol use are similar.[111]

In contrast, there is fairly good evidence[56, 98]* for higher prevalence of illicit drug use among gay and bisexual men as compared to heterosexual men, including both recent and lifetime use of marijuana and cocaine.[56] But findings concerning drug dependency disorder are contradictory. For example, we observed higher rates of drug dependency disorder among recently homosexually experienced men as compared to exclusively heterosexually experienced men in the National Comorbidity Survey.[13] But these results were not replicated in similar comparisons of homosexually and heterosexually experienced men interviewed in the 1996 National Household Survey on Drug Abuse[9] or in comparisons of homosexual and bisexual identified men to heterosexually identified men assessed in the Midlife Survey on Adult Development.[112] Recently, Fergusson and colleagues,[78]* using cohort data, observed higher rates of illicit drug dependence among young gay and bisexual young men, as compared to heterosexual men, in their early twenties.

As information on psychiatric morbidity among gay and bisexual men has emerged, so too has concern about possible comorbidity of substance use with other disorders.[30] Recently, Sandfort and colleagues[61]* reported higher rates of substance use comorbidity with affective and anxiety disorders among homosexually experienced Dutch men as compared to those who reported only female sexual partners. But overall there has been little work examining this issue. Disparities in the occurrence of comorbidity would have important implications for the need to screen gay and bisexual men for substance abuse and to consider treatment and intervention protocols that address both substance abuse and mental health morbidity.[30]

Disparities in Levels of Psychological Distress

There is additional evidence that gay and bisexual men may experience higher levels of psychological distress than heterosexual men.[113–115]* Findings from a population-based survey[30] that made direct comparisons between middle-aged men who identified as gay or bisexual and middle-aged heterosexual men indicate that sexual minority men report higher current levels of psychological distress, and a greater percentage characterize their mental health at both age 16 and the time of the interview as "poor" or "fair." Similarly, Sandfort and colleagues,[61]* in comparisons of sexually active Dutch men who either reported or did not report any male sexual partners, found several indications of higher distress levels among homosexually classified men, including reports of lower self-esteem and more emotional difficulties with role functioning. In a longitudinal birth cohort study from New Zealand,[98]* young men who reported same-sex attractions were more likely than those who reported only opposite-sex attractions to indicate a period of two weeks of depressed mood in the past year. In one of the few studies measuring psychological distress in African American MSM,[113] we compared scores on the CES-D, a scale assessing depressive distress, with those in published studies of heterosexual African American men. Distress levels were greater among African American gay and bisexual men. Thus, evidence from a number of quarters, with various measurements of both distressed mood and minority sexual orientation, find greater risk among gay and bisexual men when compared to heterosexual men.

Effects of the HIV Epidemic

Few segments of the American population have been as affected by the HIV epidemic as gay men. Repeatedly, studies examining associations between HIV risk and gay men in the United States have documented negative psychological effects of the epidemic among both infected and uninfected men,[113,116–131] including some evidence for higher rates of diagnosable disorders among HIV-infected men.[120,129,131,132] Nevertheless, the majority of the recent studies have not been able to examine the role of HIV infection in driving the greater psychiatric morbidity burden observed. This is so because many of the existing data sets used to examine links between sexual orientation and mental health do not measure HIV infection status. Similarly, those data sets in which the interest was in estimating HIV infection prevalence did not include diagnostic measures of primary mental health disorders.

Social Context as an Explanation of Mental Health Disparities

This brief review of an emerging literature indicates that gay and bisexual men are at somewhat elevated risk for affective, anxiety, and drug use disorders as compared to their heterosexual counterparts. Further, the risk attached to minority sexual orientation seems to cut across ethnic/racial backgrounds[19,90,92,133] and international boundaries.[22,100,134,135]* Whether minority ethnicity/race interacts additively with minority sexual orientation in generating even greater risk for substance abuse/mental health morbidity[92,136,137] is an open question. And methodological concerns, many of which were highlighted at the beginning of this chapter, still temper confidence in any individual study finding. But the accumulating results across different sampling strategies, assessments of sexual orientation, and constructions of comparison groups (despite the still small sample sizes) lends a measure of robustness to the evidence. Why this disparity exists, however, is not as clear.

Underlying much of the recent work is the recognition that sexual orientation has multiple influences on the life course. Some of this is generated by society's profound ambivalence about both homosexuality in general[73] and the rights[138] of persons who themselves identify as lesbian or gay. Thus, one model seeking to explain the greater risk for psychiatric morbidity[29] invokes the notion of minority stress. According to this model, anti-gay stigma generates a social context in which those of minority sexual orientation more commonly experience prejudiced events, develop self-perceptions of possessing a stigmatized identity, and have higher expectations of social rejection. This, then, results in minority stress, which generates higher levels of mental health morbidity. In fact, several high-quality surveys have demonstrated that individuals with minority sexual orientation do report more frequent experiences with everyday discrimination than heterosexual persons.[61,64,65,139]* In one population-based study,[64] for example, we reported that in a middle-aged sample, gay and bisexual men were more likely than heterosexual men to report that discrimination had made life harder and had interfered with having a full and productive life. Further, when differential levels of discrimination were controlled for, the association between sexual orientation and mental health morbidity greatly attenuated.[64] Thus, the need to cope with social adversity may generate greater vulnerability to mental health morbidity.

The effects of this social stressor can be felt throughout the lifespan. In childhood and adolescence, the development of minority sexual orientation may be initially marked by a distressing sense of being different.[140] For example, in a recent study of 182 children in fourth through eighth grades,[141] those children who described themselves as not likely to achieve heterosexual milestones (falling in love with an opposite-sex person, getting married, having a family, being a spouse, having a child) reported greater gender nonconformity, lower levels of self-worth, and poorer social relationships, although independent ratings by other children did not support this latter perception. Minority sexual orientation and gender nonconformity in childhood and adolescence can also be an early magnet for maltreatment from families and peers.[16,24,61,78,80–82,84,85,141–153]* Some of this maltreatment may be in the form of childhood sexual abuse (CSA). Estimates from the Urban Men's Health Survey suggest that perhaps 21% of gay men have positive histories of CSA,[154] a rate that appears to exceed estimates for men in general.[155–157] Among homeless and runaway youth, estimated prevalence of sexual abuse are greater among gay and bisexual males (28%) than heterosexual males

(10%).[152] Maltreatment in the context of a stigmatized sexual orientation status may also have deleterious effects. In surveys of youth with high levels of victimization, sexual minority youth were more likely than others to evidence both substance use and suicidal symptoms.[152,158] Greater exposure to childhood maltreatment can have long-reaching harmful effects. In both the general literature and some research focusing explicitly on individuals with minority sexual orientation, childhood maltreatment is a correlate of early initiation of drug use[159, 160] and adult psychopathology.[61,78,161,162]*

In adulthood, gay and bisexual men continue to face higher risk for discrimination and exposure to hate crimes or violence.[64,95,139] But there are other factors besides social adversity that may shape risk for mental health morbidity. Sexual orientation has many subtle and overt effects on social roles and the course of life events. For example, the family structures of gay men are different from those of heterosexual men,[163] including a lower rate of marriage, cohabitation with a relationship partner, and parenting,[8] all of which are known protective factors for substance use and mental health morbidity.[164] Levels of education appear to be somewhat higher among gay men when compared to heterosexual men.[8] Choices about careers and career paths may lead to different trajectories.[165,166] Sources of social support vary,[167] with many gay and bisexual men seeking out "gay friendly" environments for socializing and the receipt of everyday services and goods. Some move into highly urban, high gay density neighborhoods.[35] Sexual networks, too, vary by sexual orientation in their risk for sexually transmitted diseases, and social networks differ in the extent to which they are impacted by the effects of the HIV epidemic. All of these differences might, in their own right, influence risk for mental health morbidity among gay and bisexual men, apart from the pernicious effects of minority stress. Therefore, it is likely that the underlying causes for the observed disparities arise from multiple sources.

Future Directions

Research in the recent past has documented, fairly convincingly, an apparent disparity in mental health disorders associated with sexual orientation. Unfortunately, it is easier at this point to identify differences in risk among gay, bisexual, and heterosexual men than it is to answer the question of why these differences exist in the first place. Indeed, the number and complexity of questions percolating up through the published literature represent an astounding vitality to the field. Some areas of inquiry, however, are as yet understudied. For example, research examining the possible additive or synergistic effects of multiple stigmatized statuses such as minority sexual orientation and ethnic or racial minority background is sparse.[92,121,133,168–171] Further, we currently have only hints as to what aspects of gay and bisexual men's experiences generate greater vulnerability for mental health morbidity and what factors function to promote resiliency. The majority of gay and bisexual men master the social adversities of anti-gay stigma and successfully navigate the social topography of their lives. Indeed, despite the higher prevalence of mental health disorders observed in recent studies, it is still generally true that the majority of gay and bisexual men studied show no evidence of mental health morbidity on study measures. In fact, an unpublished population-based study[172] found that levels of life satisfaction among homosexually and exclusively heterosexually experienced men interviewed in the General Social Survey did not differ significantly.

More and better research is needed to answer the critical questions associated with mental health morbidity among the subpopulation of gay and bisexual men who do experience increased risk for psychiatric disorders. This can best be achieved by a mixture of study designs and measurement approaches. In this mix, it is key that general population-based surveys be represented, given their attributes of minimizing selection bias and maximizing the availability of heterosexual comparison groups. Yet, of the four major general population-based psychiatric epidemiological studies currently funded by the National Institutes of Health that will document the burden of primary mental health disorders in the United States, two (the National Comorbidity Survey Replication[3] and the National Survey of American Life[173]) did not include the measurement of sexual orientation or sexual behavior. The remaining two (the National Latino and Asian American Study[174] and the California Quality of Life Survey[114]) will be able to provide some insight, but each will be limited in the extent to which they can fully explore the complex causal questions underlying the findings presented in this chapter. Therefore, in this regard, it is encouraging that some periodic national health surveys, such as the National Survey of Family Growth, the National Health and Nutrition Examination Survey, and the National Epidemiologic Survey on Alcohol and Related Conditions, in recognition of the emerging evidence of sexual orientation–linked health disparities, have included sexual orientation assessment in study instruments. This ensures that a growing database will offer researchers numerous opportunities in coming years to tackle the causal questions.

Much has been accomplished in beginning to quantify the mental health morbidity burden in gay and bisexual men in recent times. But, we are a long way from having sufficient empirical information that can serve as the foundation for developing evidence-based interventions or successful methods of primary prevention of mental health disorders. We also cannot assume that the mental health concerns of men of various minority sexual orientations are similar. For example, in a recent population-based study, the California Quality of Life Survey, we observed that homosexually experienced heterosexual men experienced the highest rates of psychological distress when compared to gay, bisexual, or exclusively heterosexual men.[114] In a similar vein, findings from the Urban Men's Health Survey suggest that homosexually active men who do not identify as gay, queer, or homosexual are more likely to evidence higher levels of depressive distress.[95] This suggests that future work may profit from exploring the differences in risk for psychiatric morbidity that are linked to classification differences within sexual orientation identity and behavior. Further clarification of disparities, identifying causal pathways, and developing methods to reduce vulnerability and promote resiliency will all serve to enhance the lives and well-being of gay and bisexual men.

Authors' Note

The development of this chapter was supported in part by grants from the National Institute of Mental Health (R01-MH 61774), the National Institute of Drug Abuse (R01-DA 15539 and R01-DA-20826), and the National Center for Minority Health and Health Disparities (P60-MD 00508).

References

1. Kessler RC, Berglund P, Borges G, Nock M, Wang PS. Trends in suicide ideation, plans, gestures, and attempts in the United States, 1990–1992 to 2001–2003. *JAMA*. 2005;293(20):2487–2495.
2. Kessler RC, Berglund P, Demler O, Jin R, Merikangas KR, Walters EE. Lifetime prevalence and age-of-onset distributions of DSM-IV disorders in the National Comorbidity Survey Replication. *Arch Gen Psychiatry*. 2005;62(6):593–602.
3. Kessler RC, Chiu WT, Demler O, Merikangas KR, Walters EE. Prevalence, severity, and comorbidity of 12-month DSM-IV disorders in the National Comorbidity Survey Replication. *Arch Gen Psychiatry*. 2005;62(6):617–627.
4. Kessler RC, Demler O, Frank RG, Olfson M, Pincus HA, Walters EE, et al. Prevalence and treatment of mental disorders, 1990 to 2003. *N Engl J Med*. 2005; 352(24):2515–2523.
5. Mays VM, Cochran SD, Barnes N. Race, race-based discrimination and negative health outcomes of African Americans. *Annu Rev Psychology*. 2007;58.
6. Kessler RC, Mickelson KD, Williams DR. The prevalence, distribution, and mental health correlates of perceived discrimination in the United States. *J Health and Soc Behav*. 1999;40(3):208–230.
7. Galea S, Ahern J, Rudenstine S, Wallace Z, Vlahov D. Urban built environment and depression: a multilevel analysis. *J Epidemiol Community Health*. 2005;59(10):822–827.
8. Cochran SD, Mays VM, Brown ER, Ponce N. Demography of sexual orientation in California: health and public policy implications. Under review.
9. Cochran SD, Mays VM. Relation between psychiatric syndromes and behaviorally defined sexual orientation in a sample of the US population. *Am J Epidemiol*. 2000;151(5):516–523.
10. Cochran SD, Mays VM. Lifetime prevalence of suicide symptoms and affective disorders among men reporting same-sex sexual partners: results from NHANES III. *Am J Public Health*. 2000;90(4):573–578.
11. Cochran SD, Keenan C, Schober C, Mays VM. Estimates of alcohol use and clinical treatment needs among homosexually active men and women in the U.S. population. *J Consult Clin Psychol*. 2000;68(6):1062–1071.

12. Cochran SD. Emerging issues in research on lesbians' and gay men's mental health: does sexual orientation really matter? *American Psychologist.* 2001;56(11): 931–947.

13. Gilman SE, Cochran SD, Mays VM, Hughes M, Ostrow D, Kessler RC. Risk of psychiatric disorders among individuals reporting same-sex sexual partners in the National Comorbidity Survey. *Am J Public Health.* 2001;91(6):933–939.

14. Remafedi G, French S, Story M, Resnick MD, Blum R. The relationship between suicide risk and sexual orientation: results of a population-based study. *Am J Public Health.* 1998;88(1):57–60.

15. Faulkner AH, Cranston K. Correlates of same-sex sexual behavior in a random sample of Massachusetts high school students. *Am J Public Health.* 1998;88(2): 262–266.

16. Garofalo R, Wolf RC, Kessel S, Palfrey SJ, DuRant RH. The association between health risk behaviors and sexual orientation among a school-based sample of adolescents. *Pediatrics.* 1998;101(5):895–902.

17. Garofalo R, Wolf RC, Wissow LS, Woods ER, Goodman E. Sexual orientation and risk of suicide attempts among a representative sample of youth. *Arch Ped Adol Med.* 1999;153(5):487–493.

18. Lock J, Steiner H. Gay, lesbian, and bisexual youth risks for emotional, physical, and social problems: results from a community-based survey. *J Am Acad Child and Adolesc Psychiatry.* 1999;38(3):297–304.

19. Saewyc EM, Skay CL, Bearinger LH, Blum RW, Resnick MD. Sexual orientation, sexual behaviors, and pregnancy among American Indian adolescents. *J Adolesc Health.* 1998;23(4):238–247.

20. Herrell R, Goldberg J, True WR, Ramakrishnan V, Lyons M, Eisen S, et al. Sexual orientation and suicidality: a co-twin control study in adult men. *Arch Gen Psychiatry.* 1999;56(10):867–874.

21. Fergusson DM, Horwood LJ, Beautrais AL. Is sexual orientation related to mental health problems and suicidality in young people? *Arch Gen Psychiatry.* 1999;56(10): 876–880.

22. Sandfort TG, de Graaf R, Bijl RV, Schnabel P. Same-sex sexual behavior and psychiatric disorders: findings from the Netherlands Mental Health Survey and Incidence Study (NEMESIS). *Arch Gen Psychiatry.* 2001;58(1):85–91.

23. Russell ST, Franz BT, Driscoll AK. Same-sex romantic attraction and experiences of violence in adolescence. *Am J Public Health.* 2001;91(6):903–906.

24. Tjaden P, Thoennes N, Allison CJ. Comparing violence over the life span in samples of same-sex and opposite-sex cohabitants. *Violence and Victimization.* 1999; 14(4):413–425.

25. Lehmann JB, Lehmann CU, Kelly PJ. Development and health care needs of lesbians. *J Women's Health.* 1998;7(3):379–387.

26. Schneider SG, Farberow NL, Kruks GN. Suicidal behavior in adolescent and young adult gay men. *Suicide and Life-Threatening Behavior.* 1989;19(4):381–394.

27. Gonsiorek JC. Mental health and sexual orientation. In: Savin-Williams RC, Cohen KM, eds. *The Lives of Lesbians, Gays, and Bisexuals: Children to Adults.* Ft Worth, TX: Harcourt Brace College Publishers; 1996;462–478.

28. Hooker E. The adjustment of the male overt homosexual. *J Projective Techniques.* 1957;21:17–31.

29. Meyer IH. Prejudice, social stress, and mental health in lesbian, gay, and bisexual populations: conceptual issues and research evidence. *Psychological Bulletin.* 2003; 129(5):674–697.

30. Cochran SD, Mays VM, Sullivan JG. Prevalence of mental disorders, psychological distress, and mental health services use among lesbian, gay, and bisexual adults in the United States. *J Consult Clin Psychol.* 2003;71(1):53–61.

31. Corliss HL, Cochran SD, Mays VM. Sampling approaches to studying mental health concerns in the lesbian, gay, and bisexual community. In: Martin J, Meezan B, eds. *Handbook of Research Methods with Gay, Lesbian, Bisexual, and Transgender Populations*: Haworth Press; in press.

32. Laumann EO, Gagnon JH, Michael RT, Michaels S. *The Social Organization of Sexuality: Sexual Practices in the United States.* Chicago, IL: University of Chicago Press; 1994.

33. Weinrich JD, Snyder PJ, Pillard RC, Grant I, Jacobson DL, Robinson SR, et al. A factor analysis of the Klein sexual orientation grid in two disparate samples. *Arch Sexual Behav.* 1993;22(2):157–168.

34. Diamond LM. What does sexual orientation orient? A biobehavioral model distinguishing romantic love and sexual desire. *Psychol Rev.* 2003;110(1): 173–192.

35. Laumann EO, Ellingson S, Mahay J, Paik A, Youm Y, eds. *The Sexual Organization of the City.* Chicago, IL: University of Chicago Press; 2004.

36. Smith AM, Rissel CE, Richters J, Grulich AE, de Visser RO. Sex in Australia: sexual identity, sexual attraction and sexual experience among a representative sample of adults. *Aust N Z J Public Health.* 2003;27(2):138–145.

37. Doll LS, Beeker C. Male bisexual behavior and HIV risk in the United States: synthesis of research with implications for behavioral interventions. *AIDS Education and Prevention.* 1996;8(3):205–225.

38. Bailey JM. Homosexuality and mental illness. *Arch Gen Psychiatry.* 1999;56:883–884.

39. Solarz A, ed. *Lesbian Health: Current Assessment and Directions for the Future.* Washington, DC: Institute of Medicine, National Academy Press; 1999.

40. Herek GM. Bad science in the service of stigma: a critique of the Cameron group's survey studies. In: Herek GM, ed. *Stigma and Sexual Orientation: Understanding Prejudice Against Lesbians, Gay Men, and Bisexuals.* Thousand Oaks, CA: Sage; 1998. p. 223–255.

41. Anderson JE, Dahlberg LL. High-risk sexual behavior in the general population: results from a national survey, 1988–1990. *Sex Trans Dis.* 1992;19(6):320–325.

42. Smith TW. A methodological analysis of the sexual behavior questions on the General Social Surveys. *J Off Statistics.* 1992;8:309–326.

43. Cottler LB, Helzer JE, Tipp JE. Lifetime patterns of substance use among general population subjects engaging in high risk sexual behaviors: implications for HIV risk. *Am J Drug and Alcohol Abuse.* 1990;16(3–4):207–222.

44. Billy JOG, Tanfer K, Grady WR, Kleponger DH. The sexual behavior of men in the United States. *Fam Plann Perspect.* 1993;25:52–60.

45. Turner CF, Danella RD, Rogers SM. Sexual behavior in the United States 1930–1990: trends and methodological problems. *Sex Trans Dis.* 1995;22(3):173–190.

46. Ross MW. Prevalence of risk factors for human immunodeficiency virus infection in the Australian population. *Med J Austr.* 1988;149(7):362–365.

47. Wadsworth J, Field J, Johnson AM, Bradshaw S, Wellings K. Methodology of the National Survey of Sexual Attitudes and Life-Styles. *J Royal Stat Soc: Statistics in Society.* 1993;156:407–421.

48. Izazola-Licea JA, Gortmaker SL, De Gruttola V, Tolbert K, Mann J. Assessment of non-response bias in a probability household survey of male same-gender sexual behavior. *Salud Publica Mexico.* 2000;42(2):90–98.

49. Johnson AM, Wadsworth J, Wellings K, Bradshaw S, Field J. Sexual lifestyles and HIV risk. *Nature.* 1992;360(6403):410–412.

50. Laumann EO, Gagnon JH, Michael RT, Michaels S. National Health and Social Life Survey [United States]. 1992. http://www.icpsr.umich.edu/archive1.html. Accessed March 2, 2000.

51. Russell ST, Driscoll AK, Truong N. Adolescent same-sex romantic attractions and relationships: implications for substance use and abuse. *Am J Public Health.* 2002; 92(2):198–202.

52. Dickson N, Paul C, Herbison P. Same-sex attraction in a birth cohort: prevalence and persistence in early adulthood. *Soc Sci Med.* 2003;56(8):1607–1615.

53. Saewyc EM, Bearinger LH, Blum RW, Resnick MD. Sexual intercourse, abuse and pregnancy among adolescent women: does sexual orientation make a difference? *Fam Plann Perspect.* 1999;31(3):127–131.

54. Saewyc EM, Pettingell S, Magee LL. The prevalence of sexual abuse among adolescents in school. *J Sch Nurs.* 2003;19(5):266–272.

55. Saewyc EM, Bearinger LH, Heinz PA, Blum RW, Resnick MD. Gender differences in health and risk behaviors among bisexual and homosexual adolescents. *J Adolesc Health.* 1998;23(3):181–188.

56. Cochran SD, Ackerman D, Mays VM, Ross M. Patterns of drug use among homosexually active men and women in the 1996 NHSDA. *Addiction.* 2004;99(8): 989–998.

57. Burgard SA, Cochran SD, Mays VM. Alcohol and tobacco use patterns among heterosexually and homosexually experienced California women. *Drug Alcohol Depend.* 2005;7(77):61–70.

58. Russell ST, Consolacion TB. Adolescent romance and emotional health in the United States: beyond binaries. *J Clin Child Adolesc Psychol.* 2003;32(4):499–508.

59. Russell ST, Joyner K. Adolescent sexual orientation and suicide risk: evidence from a national study. *Am J Public Health.* 2001;91(8):1276–1281.

60. Russell ST, Seif H, Truong NL. School outcomes of sexual minority youth in the United States: evidence from a national study. *J Adolesc.* 2001;24(1):111–127.

61. Sandfort TG, de Graaf R, Bijl RV. Same-sex sexuality and quality of life: findings from the Netherlands Mental Health Survey and Incidence Study. *Arch Sex Behavior.* 2003;32(1):15–22.

62. Tang H, Greenwood GL, Cowling DW, Lloyd JC, Roeseler AG, Bal DG. Cigarette smoking among lesbians, gays, and bisexuals: how serious a problem? *Cancer Causes Control.* 2004;15(8):797–803.

63. Gruskin EP, Hart S, Gordon N, Ackerson L. Patterns of cigarette smoking and alcohol use among lesbians and bisexual women enrolled in a large health maintenance organization. *Am J Public Health.* 2001;91(6):976–979.

64. Mays VM, Cochran SD. Mental health correlates of perceived discrimination among lesbian, gay, and bisexual adults in the United States. *Am J Public Health.* 2001;91(11):1869–1876.

65. Krieger N, Sidney S. Prevalence and health implications of anti-gay discrimination: a study of black and white women and men in the CARDIA cohort. *Int J Health Services.* 1997;27(1):157–176.

66. Diamant AL, Wold C, Spritzer K, Gelberg L. Health behaviors, health status, and access to and use of health care: a population-based study of lesbian, bisexual, and heterosexual women. *Arch Fam Med.* 2000;9(10):1043–1051.

67. Valanis BG, Bowen DJ, Bassford T, Whitlock E, Charney P, Carter RA. Sexual orientation and health: comparisons in the Women's Health Initiative sample. *Arch Fam Med.* 2000;9(9):843–853.

68. Corliss H, Cochran SD, Mays VM, Seeman T, Greenland S. Patterns of health insurance coverage among cohabiting and married individuals in the National Health Interview Survey. under review.

69. Catania JA, Osmond D, Stall RD, Pollack L, Paul JP, Blower S, et al. The continuing HIV epidemic among men who have sex with men. *Am J Public Health.* 2001;91(6):907–914.

70. Pollack LM, Osmond DH, Paul JP, Catania JA. Evaluation of the Centers for Disease Control and Prevention's HIV behavioral surveillance of men who have sex with men: sampling issues. *Sex Transm Dis.* 2005;32(9):581–589.

71. Solomon SE, Rothblum ED, Balsam KF. Pioneers in partnership: lesbian and gay male couples in civil unions compared with those not in civil unions and married heterosexual siblings. *J Fam Psychol.* 2004;18(2):275–286.

72. Savin-Williams RC. Suicide attempts among sexual-minority youths: population and measurement issues. *J Consult Clin Psychol.* 2001;69(6):983–991.

73. Terry J. *An American Obsession: Science, Medicine, and Homosexuality in Modern Society.* Chicago, IL: University of Chicago Press; 1999.

74. Bayer R, Spitzer RL. Edited correspondence on the status of homosexuality in DSM-III. *J Hist Behav Sci.* 1982;18(1):32–52.

75. Washington Post. Americans on Values Followup Survey, 1998. Washington, DC: Kaiser Family Foundation/Washington Post; 1999 8/10/98 to 8/27/98.

76. Meyer IH, Dean L. Patterns of sexual behavior and risk taking among young New York City gay men. *AIDS Educ Prev.* 1995;7(5 Suppl):13–23.

77. Morris JF, Waldo CR, Rothblum ED. A model of predictors and outcomes of outness among lesbian and bisexual women. *Am J Orthopsychiatry.* 2001;71(1): 61–71.

78. Fergusson DM, Horwood LJ, Ridder EM, Beautrais AL. Sexual orientation and mental health in a birth cohort of young adults. *Psychol Med.* 2005;35(7):971–981.

79. D'Augelli AR, Hershberger SL, Pilkington NW. Lesbian, gay, and bisexual youth and their families: disclosure of sexual orientation and its consequences. *Am J Orthopsychiatry.* 1998;68(3):361–371.

80. D'Augelli AR. Developmental implications of victimization of lesbian, gay, and bisexual youths. In: Herek GM, ed. *Stigma and Sexual Orientation: Understanding Prejudice Against Lesbians, Gay Men, and Bisexuals.* Thousand Oaks, CA: Sage; 1998; 187–210.

81. Savin-Williams RC. Verbal and physical abuse as stressors in the lives of lesbian, gay male, and bisexual youths: associations with school problems, running away, substance abuse, prostitution, and suicide. *J Consult Clin Psychol.* 1994;62(2):261–269.

82. Herek GM, Gillis JR, Cogan JC, Glunt EK. Hate crime victimization among lesbian, gay, and bisexual adults. *J Interpersonal Violence.* 1997;12(2):195–212.

83. Jorm AF, Korten AE, Rodgers B, Jacomb PA, Christensen H. Sexual orientation and mental health: results from a community survey of young and middle-aged adults. *Br J Psychiatry.* 2002;180:423–427.

84. Hershberger SL, Pilkington NW, D'Augelli AR. Predictors of suicide attempts among gay, lesbian, and bisexual youth. *J Adolesc Research.* 1997;12(4):477–497.

85. Otis MD, Skinner WF. The prevalence of victimization and its effect on mental well-being among lesbian and gay people. *J Homosex.* 1996;30(3):93–121.

86. Whitbeck L, Chen B, Hoyt X, Adams GW. Discrimination, historical loss and enculturation: culturally specific risk and resiliency factors for alcohol abuse among American Indians. *J Stud Alcohol.* 2004;65(4):409–418.

87. Hammelman TL. Gay and lesbian youth: contributing factors to serious attempts or considerations of suicide. *J Gay and Lesbian Psychother.* 1993;2(1):77–89.

88. Remafedi G, Farrow JA, Deisher RW. Risk factors for attempted suicide in gay and bisexual youth. In: Garnets LD, Kimmel DC, eds. *Psychological Perspectives on Lesbian and Gay Male Experiences.* New York, NY: Columbia University Press; 1993; 486–499.

89. Rotheram-Borus MJ, Hunter J, Rosario M. Suicidal behavior and gay-related stress among gay and bisexual male adolescents. *J Adolesc Res.* 1994;9(4):498–508.

90. Barney DD. Health risk-factors for gay American Indian and Alaska Native adolescent males. *J Homosex.* 2003;46(1–2):137–157.

91. Botnick MR, Heath KV, Cornelisse PG, Strathdee SA, Martindale SL, Hogg RS. Correlates of suicide attempts in an open cohort of young men who have sex with men. *Can J Public Health.* 2002;93(1):59–62.

92. Consolacion TB, Russell ST, Sue S. Sex, race/ethnicity, and romantic attractions: multiple minority status adolescents and mental health. *Cultur Divers Ethnic Minor Psychol* 2004;10(3):200–214.

93. Garcia J, Adams J, Friedman L, East P. Links between past abuse, suicide ideation, and sexual orientation among San Diego college students. *J Am Coll Health.* 2002;51(1):9–14.

94. Huebner DM, Rebchook GM, Kegeles SM. Experiences of harassment, discrimination, and physical violence among young gay and bisexual men. *Am J Public Health* 2004;94(7):1200–1203.

95. Mills TC, Paul J, Stall R, Pollack L, Canchola J, Chang YJ, et al. Distress and depression in men who have sex with men: the Urban Men's Health Study. *Am J Psychiatry* 2004;161(2):278–285.

96. Paul JP, Catania J, Pollack L, Moskowitz J, Canchola J, Mills T, et al. Suicide attempts among gay and bisexual men: Lifetime prevalence and antecedents. *Am J Public Health* 2002;92(8):1338–1345.

97. Safren SA, Heimberg RG. Depression, hopelessness, suicidality, and related factors in sexual minority and heterosexual adolescents. *J Consult Clin Psychol.* 1999; 67(6):859–866.

98. Skegg K, Nada-Raja S, Dickson N, Paul C, Williams S. Sexual orientation and self-harm in men and women. *Am J Psychiatry.* 2003;160(3):541–546.

99. Balsam KF, Beauchaine TP, Mickey RM, Rothblum ED. Mental health of lesbian, gay, bisexual, and heterosexual siblings: effects of gender, sexual orientation, and family. *J Abnorm Psychol.* 2005;114(3):471–476.

100. Qin P, Agerbo E, Mortensen PB. Suicide risk in relation to socioeconomic, demographic, psychiatric, and familial factors: a national register-based study of all suicides in Denmark, 1981–1997. *Am J Psychiatry.* 2003;160(4):765–772.

101. Savin-Williams RC, Ream GL. Suicide attempts among sexual-minority male youth. *J Clin Child Adolesc Psychol.* 2003;32(4):509–522.
102. Mathy RM, Cochran SD, Olsen J, Mays VM. Incidence of suicide among same-sex partners in Denmark: a hidden epidemic among gay men. under review.
103. Surgeon General. *National Strategy for Suicide Prevention: Goals and Objectives for Action.* Washington DC: DHHS; 2001.
104. Seage GR, 3rd, Mayer KH, Wold C, Lenderking WR, Goldstein R, Cai B, et al. The social context of drinking, drug use, and unsafe sex in the Boston Young Men Study. *J Acquired Immune Deficiency Syndromes and Human Retrovirology.* 1998;17(4): 368–375.
105. Knowlton R, McCusker J, Stoddard A, Zapka J, Mayer K. The use of the CAGE questionnaire in a cohort of homosexually active men. *J Stud Alcohol.* 1994;55(6): 692–694.
106. Stall R, McKusick L, Wiley J, Coates TJ, Ostrow DG. Alcohol and drug use during sexual activity and compliance with safe sex guidelines for AIDS: the AIDS Behavioral Research Project. *Health Education Quarterly* 1986;13(4):359–371.
107. Stall R, Paul JP, Greenwood G, Pollack LM, Bein E, Crosby GM, et al. Alcohol use, drug use and alcohol-related problems among men who have sex with men: the Urban Men's Health Study. *Addiction.* 2001;96(11):1589–1601.
108. Shoptaw S, Peck J, Reback CJ, Rotheram-Fuller E. Psychiatric and substance dependence comorbidities, sexually transmitted diseases, and risk behaviors among methamphetamine-dependent gay and bisexual men seeking outpatient drug abuse treatment. *J Psychoactive Drugs.* 2003;35 Suppl 1:161–168.
109. Stall R, Wiley J. A comparison of alcohol and drug use patterns of homosexual and heterosexual men: the San Francisco Men's Health Study. *Drug and Alcohol Dependence.* 1988;22(1–2):63–73.
110. Drabble L, Midanik LT, Trocki K. Reports of alcohol consumption and alcohol-related problems among homosexual, bisexual and heterosexual respondents: results from the 2000 National Alcohol Survey. *J Stud Alcohol.* 2005;66(1):111–120.
111. Trocki KF, Drabble L, Midanik L. Use of heavier drinking contexts among heterosexuals, homosexuals and bisexuals: results from a National Household Probability Survey. *J Stud Alcohol.* 2005;66(1):105–110.
112. Cochran S, Mays V, Sullivan J. Prevalence of mental disorders, psychological distress, and mental health services use among lesbian, gay, and bisexual adults in the United States. *J Consult Clin Psychol.* 2003;71(1):53–61.
113. Cochran SD, Mays VM. Depressive distress among homosexually active African American men and women. *Am J Psychiatry.* 1994;151(4):524–529.
114. Cochran SD, Mays VM. Physical health complaints among lesbians, gay men, bisexuals, and homosexually experienced heterosexuals: results from the California Quality of Life Survey. *Am J Public Health.* Published online April 26, 2007. DOI: 10.2105/AJPH.2006.087254.
115. Sandfort TG, Bakker F, Schellevis FG, Vanwesenbeeck I. Sexual orientation and mental and physical health status: findings from a Dutch population survey. *Am J Public Health.* 2006; 96(6):1119–1125.
116. Dickey WC, Dew MA, Becker JT, Kingsley L. Combined effects of HIV-infection status and psychosocial vulnerability on mental health in homosexual men. *Soc Psychiatry & Psychiatric Epidemiology.* 1999;34(1):4–11.
117. Domino G, Shen D. Attitudes toward suicide in patients with HIV/AIDS. *Omega: J Death and Dying.* 1997;34(1):15–27.

118. Evans S, Ferrando S, Sewell M, Goggin K, Fishman B, Rabkin J. Pain and depression in HIV illness. *Psychosomatics.* 1998;39(6):528–535.

119. Ferrando S, Evans S, Goggin K, Sewell M, Fishman B, Rabkin J. Fatigue in HIV illness: relationship to depression, physical limitations, and disability. *Psychosomatic Medicine.* 1998;60(6):759–764.

120. Atkinson JH, Jr., Grant I, Kennedy CJ, Richman DD, Spector SA, McCutchan JA. Prevalence of psychiatric disorders among men infected with human immunodeficiency virus: a controlled study. *Arch Gen Psychiatry.* 1988;45(9):859–864.

121. Myers HF, Satz P, Miller BE, Bing EG, Evans G, Richardson MA, et al. The African-American Health Project (AAHP): study overview and select findings on high risk behaviors and psychiatric disorders in African American men. *Ethnicity and Health.* 1997;2(3):183–196.

122. Lyketsos CG, Hoover DR, Guccione M, Dew MA, Wesch J, Bing EG, et al. Depressive symptoms over the course of HIV infection before AIDS. *Soc Psychiatry and Psychiatric Epidemiol.* 1996;31(3–4):212–219.

123. Maj M. Depressive syndromes and symptoms in subjects with human immunodeficiency virus (HIV) infection. *Br J Psychiatry.* 1996(30):117–122.

124. Galvan FH, Burnam MA, Bing EG. Co-occurring psychiatric symptoms and drug dependence or heavy drinking among HIV-positive people. *J Psychoactive Drugs.* 2003;35 Suppl 1:153–160.

125. Hays RB, Turner H, Coates TJ. Social support, AIDS-related symptoms, and depression among gay men. *J Consult Clin Psychol.* 1992;60(3):463–469.

126. Kemeny ME, Dean L. Effects of AIDS-related bereavement on HIV progression among New York City gay men. *Aids Educ and Prev.* 1995;7(5 Suppl):36–47.

127. Ostrow DG. Mental health issues across the HIV-1 spectrum for gay and bisexual men. In: Cabaj RP, Stein TS, eds. *Textbook of Homosexuality and Mental Health.* Washington, DC: American Psychiatric Press, Inc; 1996;859–880.

128. Page-Shafer K, Delorenze GN, Satariano WA, Winkelstein W, Jr. Comorbidity and survival in HIV-infected men in the San Francisco Men's Health Survey. *Ann Epidemiol.* 1996;6(5):420–430.

129. Rabkin JG, Ferrando SJ, Jacobsberg LB, Fishman B. Prevalence of Axis I disorders in an AIDS cohort: a cross-sectional, controlled study. *Compr Psychiatry.* 1997;38(3):146–154.

130. Siegel K, Karus D, Epstein J, Raveis VH. Psychological and psychosocial adjustment of HIV-infected gay/bisexual men: disease stage comparisons. *J Comm Psychol.* 1996;24(3):229–243.

131. Kelly B, Raphael B, Judd F, Perdices M, Kernutt G, Burrows GD, et al. Psychiatric disorder in HIV infection. *Austr N Z J Psychiatry.* 1998;32(3):441–453.

132. Berg MB, Mimiaga MJ, Safren SA. Mental health concerns of HIV-infected gay and bisexual men seeking mental health services: an observational study. *AIDS Patient Care STDS.* 2004;18(11):635–643.

133. Balsam KF, Huang B, Fieland KC, Simoni JM, Walters KL. Culture, trauma, and wellness: a comparison of heterosexual and lesbian, gay, bisexual, and two-spirit native Americans. *Cultur Divers Ethnic Minor Psychol.* 2004;10(3):287–301.

134. Pinhey TK, Millman SR. Asian/Pacific Islander adolescent sexual orientation and suicide risk in Guam. *Am J Public Health.* 2004;94(7):1204–1206.

135. Wichstrom L, Hegna K. Sexual orientation and suicide attempt: a longitudinal study of the general Norwegian adolescent population. *J Abnorm Psychol.* 2003;112(1):144–151.

136. Yoshikawa H, Wilson PA, Chae DH, Cheng JF. Do family and friendship networks protect against the influence of discrimination on mental health and HIV risk among Asian and Pacific Islander gay men? *AIDS Educ Prev.* 2004;16(1):84–100.

137. Mays VM, Yancey AK, Cochran SD, Weber M, Fielding JE. Heterogeneity of health disparities among African American, Hispanic, and Asian American women: unrecognized influences of sexual orientation. *Am J Public Health.* 2002;92(4):632–639.

138. Wood PB, Bartkowski JP. Attribution style and public policy attitudes toward gay rights. *Social Science Quarterly* 2004;85(1):58–74.

139. Herek GM, Gillis JR, Cogan JC. Psychological sequelae of hate-crime victimization among lesbian, gay, and bisexual adults. *J Consult Clin Psychol.* 1999;67(6):945–951.

140. Egan SK, Perry DG. Gender identity: a multidimensional analysis with implications for psychosocial adjustment. *Dev Psychol.* 2001;37(4):451–463.

141. Carver PR, Egan SK, Perry DG. Children who question their heterosexuality. *Dev Psychol.* 2004;40(1):43–53.

142. Harry J. Parental physical abuse and sexual orientation in males. *Arch Sex Behav.* 1989;18(3):251–261.

143. Pilkington NW, D'Augelli AR. Victimization of lesbian, gay, and bisexual youth in community settings. *J Community Psychol.* 1995;23(1):34–56.

144. McConaghy N, Silove D. Do sex-linked behaviors in children influence relationships with their parents? *Arch Sex Behav.* 1992;21(5):469–479.

145. Waldo CR, Hesson-McInnis MS, D'Augelli AR. Antecedents and consequences of victimization of lesbian, gay, and bisexual young people: a structural model comparing rural university and urban samples. *Am J Comm Psychol.* 1998;26(2):307–334.

146. Landolt MA, Bartholomew K, Saffrey C, Oram D, Perlman D. Gender nonconformity, childhood rejection, and adult attachment: a study of gay men. *Arch Sex Behav.* 2004;33(2):117–128.

147. Corliss HL, Cochran SD, Mays VM. Reports of parental maltreatment during childhood in a United States population-based survey of homosexual, bisexual, and heterosexual adults. *Child Abuse and Neglect.* 2002;26(11):1165–1178.

148. Bailey JM, Kim PY, Hills A, Linsenmeier JA. Butch, femme, or straight acting? Partner preferences of gay men and lesbians. *J Pers Soc Psychol.* 1997;73(5):960–973.

149. Alley TR, Dillon NE. Sex-linked carrying styles and the attribution of homosexuality. *J Soc Psychol.* 2001;141(5):660–666.

150. Fitzpatrick KK, Euton SJ, Jones JN, Schmidt NB. Gender role, sexual orientation and suicide risk. *J Affect Disord.* 2005;87(1):35–42.

151. Rivers L. Recollections of bullying at school and their long-term implications for lesbians, gay men, and bisexuals. *Crisis* 2004;25(4):169–175.

152. Whitbeck LB, Chen X, Hoyt DR, Tyler KA, Johnson KD. Mental disorder, subsistence strategies, and victimization among gay, lesbian, and bisexual homeless and runaway adolescents. *J Sex Res.* 2004;41(4):329–342.

153. Dolezal C, Carballo-Dieguez A. Childhood sexual experiences and the perception of abuse among Latino men who have sex with men. *J Sex Res.* 2002;39(3):165–173.

154. Paul JP, Catania J, Pollack L, Stall R. Understanding childhood sexual abuse as a predictor of sexual risk-taking among men who have sex with men: the Urban Men's Health Study. *Child Abuse and Neglect* 2001;25(4):557–584.

155. Nelson EC, Heath AC, Madden PA, Cooper ML, Dinwiddie SH, Bucholz KK, et al. Association between self-reported childhood sexual abuse and adverse psychosocial outcomes: Results from a twin study. *Arch Gen Psych.* 2002;59(2):139–145.

156. Pimlott-Kubiak S, Cortina LM. Gender, victimization, and outcomes: reconceptualizing risk. *J Consult Clin Psychol.* 2003;71(3):528–539.

157. Finkelhor D. The international epidemiology of child sexual abuse. *Child Abuse Negl* 1994;18(5):409–417.

158. Bontempo DE, D'Augelli AR. Effects of at-school victimization and sexual orientation on lesbian, gay, or bisexual youths' health risk behavior. *J Adolesc Health.* 2002;30(5):364–374.

159. Relf MV, Huang B, Campbell J, Catania J. Gay identity, interpersonal violence, and HIV risk behaviors: an empirical test of theoretical relationships among a probability-based sample of urban men who have sex with men. *J Assoc Nurses AIDS Care.* 2004;15(2):14–26.

160. Kilpatrick DG, Acierno R, Saunders B, Resnick HS, Best CL, Schnurr PP. Risk factors for adolescent substance abuse and dependence: data from a national sample. *J Consult Clin Psychol.* 2000;68(1):19–30.

161. Arnow BA. Relationships between childhood maltreatment, adult health and psychiatric outcomes, and medical utilization. *J Clin Psychiatry.* 2004;65 Suppl 12:10–15.

162. de Graaf R, Bijl RV, Ten Have M, Beekman AT, Vollebergh WA. Pathways to comorbidity: the transition of pure mood, anxiety and substance use disorders into comorbid conditions in a longitudinal population-based study. *J Affect Disord.* 2004;82(3):461–467.

163. Matthews CR, Lease SH. Focus on lesbian, gay, and bisexual families. In: Perez RM, DeBord KA, Bieschke KJ, eds. *Handbook of Counseling and Psychotherapy with Lesbian, Gay, and Bisexual Clients.* Washington, DC: American Psychological Association; 2000;249–274.

164. Office of Applied Studies-SAMHSA. National Household Survey on Drug Abuse: population estimates, 1999. In: *Office of Applied Studies, SAMHSA.* Rockville, MD: US Department of Health and Human Services; 2000.

165. Badgett MVL. Employment and sexual orientation: disclosure and discrimination in the workplace. In: Ellis AL, Riggle EDB, eds. *Sexual Identity on the Job: Issues and Services.* New York, NY: Harrington Park Press/Haworth Press; 1996;29–52.

166. Badgett MVL. Vulnerability in the workplace: evidence of anti-gay discrimination. In: *Angles: The Policy Journal of the Institute for Gay and Lesbian Studies.* 1997;2(1):1–4.

167. Green RJ. Risk and resilience in lesbian and gay couples: comment on Solomon, Rothblum, and Balsam (2004). *J Fam Psychol.* 2004;18(2):290–292.

168. Crawford I, Allison KW, Zamboni BD, Soto T. The influence of dual-identity development on the psychosocial functioning of African-American gay and bisexual men. *J Sex Res.* 2002;39(3):179–189.

169. Peterson JL, Folkman S, Bakeman R. Stress, coping, HIV status, psychosocial resources, and depressive mood in African American gay, bisexual, and heterosexual men. *Am J Community Psychol.* 1996;24(4):461–487.

170. Siegel K, Epstein JA. Ethnic-racial differences in psychological stress related to gay lifestyle among HIV-positive men. *Psychol Rep.* 1996;79(1):303–312.

171. Matthews AK, Hughes TL. Mental health service use by African American women: exploration of subpopulation differences. *Cultur Divers Ethnic Minor Psychol.* 2001;7(1):75–87.

172. Nellos CE, Cochran SD, Mays VM. Trends in life satisfaction among individuals reporting same-gender sexual behavior in the 1988–2000 General Social Survey.

Paper presented at the 130th Annual Meetings of the American Public Health Association; 2002 November 9–13; Philadelphia, PA; 2002. Available at: http://apha.confex.com/apha/130am/techprogram/paper_43212.htm. Accessed August 28, 2007.

173. Jackson JS, Torres M, Caldwell CH, Neighbors HW, Nesse RM, Taylor RJ, et al. The National Survey of American Life: a study of racial, ethnic and cultural influences on mental disorders and mental health. Int J Methods Psychiatr Res 2004;13(4):196–207.

174. Alegria M, Takeuchi D, Canino G, Duan N, Shrout P, Meng XL, et al. Considering context, place and culture: the National Latino and Asian American Study. *Int J Methods Psychiatr Res.* 2004;13(4):208–220.

5

Alcohol, Tobacco, and Drug Use among Gay and Bisexual Men

David G. Ostrow and Ron Stall

Substance abuse consumes a significant portion of US health care resources and is involved in up to half of the chronic disease morbidity and mortality in the United States. While exact figures are not available for the collective health consequences of substance abuse, it is instructive to consider the health effects of just one substance of abuse alone: alcohol. Recent studies indicate that nearly 19 million Americans (8% of the US population) require treatment for an "alcohol problem," and 16 million drink heavily.[1] One in four children lives with a parent who is dependent on, or abuses, alcohol.[2] Alcohol dependence is responsible for approximately 100,000 deaths each year.[3] Chronic heavy drinking is a leading cause of cardiovascular illnesses, such as cardiomyopathy, coronary artery disease, high blood pressure, dangerous heart rhythms, and stroke. It is the leading cause of illness and death from liver disease in the United States.[4] Consuming four or more alcoholic beverages a day significantly increases the risk of developing any type of cancer.[5] Psychiatric disorders, such as depression, anxiety disorders, sociopathy, and antisocial personality disorder occur more often among alcoholics than in the general population,[6] while similar preexisting psychiatric disorders may predispose an individual to alcohol and drug abuse. Harmful and hazardous drinking is involved in about one-third of suicides, one-half of homicides, and one-third of child abuse cases.[7] In the 2003 National Survey on Drugs and Health by the US Department of Health and Human Services, among heavy alcohol users, 61.7% smoked cigarettes in the past month, whereas only 17.4% of nondrinkers were current smokers.[1] Alcohol abuse and dependence costs the United States $185 billion in direct and indirect social costs per year, with more than 70% of the cost attributed to lost productivity.[4] The addition of the health effects of drugs and/or tobacco would multiply these estimates of the impact of drug abuse on the health of Americans even further, illustrating the enormous health effects of the multiple substance abuse epidemics that exist among Americans.

Long before the HIV/AIDS crisis began in the United States, there was recognition of a variety of medical and psychological sequelae of substance abuse and dependence among men who have sex with men (MSM), and a suspicion that rates of substance use/abuse among gay men might be significantly higher than among heterosexual men. Since the beginning of the AIDS crisis, an increasing number of medical conditions have been recognized as associated with substance abuse, including the myriad HIV-associated conditions, chronic hepatitis C, multiple pulmonary conditions, and other metabolic and cardiovascular conditions.

This chapter will review numerous studies to support the conclusion that the prevalence rates of substance use/abuse and their complications among gay, bisexual, and MSM are generally elevated when compared to those found among men in general population samples. The study of drug, alcohol, and tobacco use by MSM has evolved from a poorly defined subfield of study to become a key component of HIV prevention research and an important "stand alone" topic in behavioral epidemiology. There are several reasons why this evolution has occurred, including the recognition of the continuing importance of bar and bathhouse culture in gay male life, the recent growth of interest in gay men's health in general, and the creation of more rigorous data sets to measure use and abuse of substances by gay men. In addition, some drug use/abuse among MSM may be different in that it is associated with sexual expression, including "risky sex" (currently most appropriately defined as unprotected anal intercourse with partners of unknown or opposite HIV serostatus). Given this context, there is good reason to hypothesize that gay men may suffer a disproportionate burden of substance use when compared to the frequency of substance use in the general population.

Instead of using the limiting term of *recreational drug use* or the awkward term of *non-prescribed psychoactive drugs,* we will use the term *drugs* to refer to all drugs (including alcohol and tobacco) that are used for purposes other than medically supervised treatment of diagnosed conditions. This distinction can be difficult to make at times (e.g., the use of medically prescribed erectile dysfunction drugs [EDDs] by MSM to counteract the side effects of stimulant use). Among MSM, many of the drugs that will be discussed have specific associations with either increasing the motivation to have sex (alcohol and marijuana), increasing the sensation of sexual pleasure in terms of intensity (poppers [volatile nitrites], amphetamines, and ecstasy), duration (crystal methamphetamine, or "Tina;" Viagra® or other erectile dysfunction drugs [EDD]), or the lessening of negative thoughts and associations that might otherwise inhibit sex (downers, alcohol; crystal methamphetamine and other stimulants, heroin and other tranquilizers, and opiate analgesics). Because of these associations, some of these drugs are often thought of as "gay sex drugs." However, their use for other purposes and the frequent lack of information on why they are being used or if they are even used during sex means that we cannot automatically assume that all or even most of the drug use rates cited here are for sexual purposes.

The Epidemiology and Health Disparity Implications of Drug Use among MSM

Prevalence of Drug Use among Men Who Have Sex with Men

Before reviewing the individual studies that have looked at specific rates of drug use among particular samples of MSM, it is important to note that few population-based samples allow for direct comparisons between homosexual and heterosexual adult males in the United States. Among the many studies reviewed for this chapter, only three fit the criteria of being population-based and fairly current.[8–10] A fourth study[11] used a mix of sampling strategies and only included HIV-negative MSM who were not in a mutually monogamous relationship with another HIV-negative man, but did attempt to recruit an otherwise broad and diverse sample of MSM from six US cities (Boston, Chicago, Denver, New York, San Francisco, and Seattle) for an HIV prevention intervention trial (the Explore Study). Prevalence rates of drug class use from these four studies will be used here to estimate average levels of drug and alcohol use among contemporary American MSM.

Specific drug use rates by MSM from all four studies are given in Tables 5-1, 5-2, and 5-3. The focus here is on drugs or drug classes that were assessed across this group of studies, namely alcohol, marijuana, poppers, cocaine, hallucinogens/psychedelics, ecstasy, and amphetamines. Three of the studies also assessed opiate use, while the Explore study combined ecstasy in the hallucinogens category. These more recent studies provide reasonable estimates of drug use among MSM for comparison to point prevalence rates for men in general.

A. Marijuana use rates among MSM: Stall & Wiley[8]: 77.5% (past 6 months); Stall et al.[9]: 42.4% (past 6 months); Cochran et al.[10]: 13.9% (last month); Koblin et al.[11]: 46.3% (past 6 months).

B. Popper use rates among MSM: Stall & Wiley[8]: 57.7% (past 6 months); Stall et al.[9]: 19.8% (past 6 months); Cochran et al.[10]: 30.8% lifetime use of inhalants but no reported recent (past month) use of inhalants; Koblin et al.[11]: 36.6% (past 6 months).

C. Cocaine use rates among MSM: Stall & Wiley[8]: 52% (past 6 months); Stall et al.[9]: 15.2% (past 6 months); Cochran et al.[10]: 37.2% (lifetime) vs. 3.9% (last month); Koblin et al.[11]: 19.3% (past 6 months).

D. Hallucinogens/psychedelics use rates among MSM: Stall & Wiley[8]: 17.6% (past 6 months); Stall et al.[9]: 4.2% (past 6 months); Cochran et al.[10]: 34.7% (lifetime) vs. 1.6% (past month); Koblin et al.[11]: 24% (past 6 months, includes ecstasy).

E. Ecstasy use rates among MSM: Stall et al.[9]: 11.7% (past 6 months).
F. Amphetamines use rates among MSM: Stall & Wiley[8]: 28.1% (past 6 months); Stall et al.[9]: 11.7% (past 6 months, combining "speed" and "other uppers" categories); Cochran et al.[10]: 14.4% (lifetime) vs. 0.7% (past month); Koblin et al.[11]: 12.9% (past 6 months).
G. Opiates/injection use rates among MSM: Stall & Wiley[8]: 3.9% (past 6 months); Stall et al.[9]: 3.2% (past 6 months); Cochran et al.[10]:4.1% (lifetime) vs. 0.8% (past month) for heroin specifically; Koblin et al.[11]: 10% of men reported injection drug use in past 6 months, presumably includes both opiate and amphetamine needle use.

Health Disparities Related to Drug Use by MSM

It should be noted that there are difficulties in comparing the population-based drug use prevalences of MSM cited above with published point-prevalence estimates for heterosexual men or even males in general. Ideally, the studies would contain their own "control" samples of heterosexual men derived from the same population base and utilizing valid and nonbiased methods to identify a representative sample of diverse MSM to compare to the heterosexual male sample. Of the four studies summarized above, the one that comes closest to these criteria is the Stall and Wiley 1988 study,[8] but that study utilized data collected in the latter half of 1984, at the peak of the AIDS epidemic in San Francisco, and was limited to single men residing in the 19 San Francisco census tracts with the highest rates of AIDS cases. Given the catchment area and the early date for the study, it is not surprising that the Stall and Wiley study drug use prevalence rates are uniformly the highest among the four studies examined here. On the opposite end of this spectrum, the Cochran et al. 2004 study[10] utilized the 1996 National Household Survey on Drug Abuse,[12] which relied on a single question about the gender of sexual partners in the last 12 months, rather than asking about sexual orientation or conducting an in-depth sexual behavior assessment. This methodology resulted in a very large sample of adult, sexually active respondents ($n = 9908$), but only 98 of these men (2.5%) and 96 of these women (2%) reported any same sex partners. Again, given the national scope of the study and the post-AIDS date of the study, it is not surprising that this study produced the lowest prevalence rates for recent drug use and failed to detect any recent use of one of the most commonly used gay sex drugs, poppers.

Given these limitations in available population-based data, any conclusions concerning primary drug use health disparities of MSM based on the existing scientific database must be considered preliminary and are best viewed in the context of the accumulated clinical experience of health care providers working with MSM populations, as discussed below. Nonetheless, here are presented the crude relative odds ratios of drug use for each of the categories listed above as contained in the Cochran et al[10] and Stall et al.[9] papers (alcohol and ecstasy use are not included here because alcohol-related health disparities are discussed separately in this chapter, and there is no hetero-sexual comparison data for ecstasy use in any of the published studies):

A. Marijuana: Cochran et al.[10] reported an OR of 3.5 for daily use of marijuana by MSM compared to non-MSM; Stall et al.[9] reported a 3.9-fold higher rate of marijuana use in the past six months among their four-city sample of MSM compared to men 13 years and older from the predominantly heterosexual 1999 NHSDA survey.[13]

B. Poppers: Cochran et al.[10] reported an OR of 3.8 for lifetime use of inhalants by MSM compared to non-MSM; there are no comparable non-MSM popper use data in the Stall et al.[9] report, but the Stall and Wiley San Francisco study[8] reported an overall rate of only 1% for popper use among heterosexual men, compared to rates of 54% to 59% of MSM across age groupings.

C. Cocaine: Cochran et al.[10] reported an OR of 2.5 for lifetime use and 2.2 for daily use of cocaine in the past month; Stall et al.[9] reported a 6.6-fold higher rate of cocaine use in the past 6 months compared to the 1999 NHSDA.

D. Hallucinogens: Cochran et al.[10] reported an OR of 2.3 for lifetime use.

E. Amphetamines- Cochran et al.[10] reported an OR of 2.2 for lifetime use; Stall et al.[9] reported a 12.2-fold higher rate of stimulant use by MSM in the past 6 months compared to the 1999 NHSDA.

F. Opiates: Cochran et al.[10] reported an OR of 2.4 for lifetime use of heroin and 9.5 for heroin use in the last month.

In conclusion, for all of the drug classes for which comparable hetero-sexual or general population data exist, MSM exhibit higher use rates than their heterosexual counterparts, especially if lifetime use rates are compared, as in the Cochran et al.[10] study, and specifically for the most commonly used gay "sex drugs," as in the Stall and Wiley[8] and Stall et al.[9] studies. In view of these important disparities in terms of overall drug use, it is important to mention that there is only one published study comparing a matched sample of HIV-seronegative MSM to HIV-seropositive MSM that determined actual diagnoses among MSM for substance abuse using a well-validated structured clinical instrument, the Structured Clinical Interview for DSM-IV.[14] That study, performed in New York City in the immediate pre-HAART (highly active antiretroviral therapy) era (1995–1997), demonstrated highly elevated lifetime rates of drug abuse diagnoses (3–7+ fold) among both HIV-positive and HIV-negative participants, but current (past month) rates of drug abuse that were approximately 2-fold elevated compared to general male population estimates. These data suggest that despite elevated lifetime drug use disorder rates for both HIV+ and HIV- men in the Cornell Medical School cohort, adaptive changes since the recognition of the severity of the AIDS epidemic among MSM and the potential role of drug use in disease progression had significantly reduced the rates of drug use and abuse disorders by 1995.[15]

Trends in Drug Use Patterns among MSM

It is important to realize that the vast majority of the drug use literature for MSM is in the form of cross-sectional, opportunistic samples that may only provide a "snap shot" of the evolving patterns of individual and group drug use. The rise and fall and rise again of the use of poppers among MSM (see Figure 5-1, top panel) offer a rare longitudinal view into factors that influence drug use social norms. The popularity of poppers in the pre-AIDS era, largely limited to gay men, led to suggestions that the drug might be responsible for the high rates among gay and bisexual men of an otherwise rare AIDS-defining disease, Kaposi's sarcoma (KS). This concern, along with legislation essentially outlawing poppers' sale or manufacture, enhanced a rapid downhill decline in the drug's use as an aid to anal intercourse (by relaxing the smooth muscle of the anal sphincter, inhaled nitrites ["poppers"] reduce the pain of anal penetration). When further epidemiological studies failed to confirm poppers' association with KS, propagation of that seemingly redeeming evidence, along with non-enforcement of state and federal bans, led to an upswing in use. The renewed popularity of poppers, especially when used in combination with other "sex drugs" (EDDs, stimulants, ecstasy) has increased the potential for serious drug-drug interactions with life-threatening sequelae.[16] Trends over time in the use of other drugs, as evidenced in the Multicenter AIDS Cohort Study (MACS) data, may also reflect changes in social norms governing drug use among MSM.

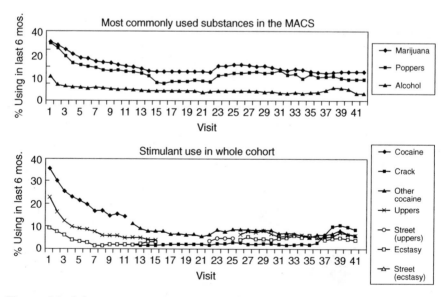

Figure 5-1. Substance use among gay and bisexual men participating in the Multicenter AIDS Cohort Study (MACS).

To assess these cohort effects, one study compared similarly sampled MSM from two distinct cohorts, the SF Men's Health Study (data from 1984) and the SF Young Men's Health Study (data from 1992).[17] They found that alcohol and hallucinogen use were equivalent in both groups, but that rates of marijuana, poppers, cocaine, methamphetamine, "downers," and opiate use were all lower in the latter cohort. Perhaps capturing an important contemporary cohort difference, the prevalence of ecstasy use had doubled from 14.7% use in the 1984 cohort to 31.3% in the 1992 cohort.

Historic Changes in Drug Use by MSM over Time

As is clear from the ordering and data presented from the studies described in Tables 5–1, 5–2, and 5–3, there has been a trend in the literature over time from reporting raw prevalence figures for drug use among "community-based" or opportunistic samples of gay/bisexual men to reporting the sexual risk and other covariates of drug-using MSM. More recently, the literature has focused on studies of "risky" younger MSM attending circuit parties and other extended party venues. Some studies have further focused on users of specific drug classes, such as "club drugs" or crystal methamphetamine.[18] This trend illustrates the increasing emphasis, over the course of the AIDS epidemic, on describing drug use behavioral patterns in the context of HIV transmission risk and potential prevention strategies.[19] Accordingly, the drug use literature reviewed here is organized as follows: Table 5-1, Early AIDS/Pre-HAART Era Studies (1981–1996); 5-2, Middle AIDS/Early HAART Era Studies (1996–2000); and Table 5-3, Post-HAART Era Studies (2000 and beyond), most of which sampled specialized subgroups of MSM or specific venues (i.e., circuit party and other high-risk venue samples). While descriptions of these findings may refer to drug use differences across studies, differences across geographic areas, and differences across cohorts of MSM, it is important to note that such statements are supported by simple, astatistical comparisons of point prevalence rates across studies rather than statistical tests across studies. Despite these methodological limitations and the historical changes in the focus of specific research projects, reviewing the literature permits the identification of important historical trends in drug use patterns over time among MSM.

Early AIDS/Pre-HAART Era Studies

Most of the drug use data presented in Table 5-1 reveal prevalence rates that started out as high or higher than those recorded pre-AIDS[19,20] and rapidly fell to levels that were, in the main, intermediate between those of pre-AIDS-epidemic era levels and rates of heterosexual male samples from equivalent locales, age, and sampling methods. These early downward trends in the use of most drugs during the early AIDS/pre-HAART period (see Figure 5-1) largely paralleled reductions in risky sex, although it is impossible to determine from these studies whether dramatic parallel shifts in drug and sexual behavior are mechanistically linked. For example, Martin and colleagues [20] charted rates of popper use and alcohol abuse or dependence among New York City MSM from highs of 40% and 12% to lows of 7% and 9% between 1980/1981 and 1986/1987. During the same period, the proportion of this random probability sample who reported engaging in anal receptive sex fell from 75% to 6%.

In terms of geographic differences, stimulant use in the early AIDS era was mainly in the form of crystal methamphetamine in the San Francisco samples[17,21] and powder cocaine among Midwest and East Coast samples.[20,22,23] This has changed, over time, to a more equal geographical distribution of the two types of stimulant use among MSM, with, in fact, an enormous increase in the manufacture and distribution of crystal methamphetamine in the Midwest since about 1990.[24] More recently, a more rapid rate of increase in the distribution of crystal methamphetamine has been observed in the Northeast United States, presumably as a result of effective efforts to limit substrate availability and widespread crackdowns on small rural "meth labs," combined with the entry of large Mexican drug cartels into the manufacture and distribution of crystal methamphetamine in the Northeast.[25]

Middle AIDS/Early HAART Era Studies

Examination of both Figure 5-1 and Table 5-2 indicates that drug and alcohol use rates had stabilized by the mid-1990s.[9,10,26,27] Compared to the early AIDS era, there were significant differences in the variety of drugs used by MSM in the late 1990s and early 2000s (Table 5-2). Stimulant use, particularly methamphetamine use, became less regional and appeared in Midwest and East Coast locations as measured in multisite studies such as the Urban Men's Health Study[9] and the National Supplement to HIV/AIDS Surveillance (SHAS) Study.[28] Also striking was the rise in usage of the general category of "club drugs," including, but not limited to, ecstasy, ketamine, gammahydroxybutyrate (GHB), and powder cocaine. Furthermore, one study[26] of a group of HIV-seropositive men recruited in New York City and San Francisco during 2000/2001 identified the erectile dysfunction prescription drug sildenafil (Viagra) as being used by more than 12% of the sample. At the same time, alcohol use, marijuana use, and popper use remained popular among samples of both MSM in general and the HIV+ samples of MSM.[26,27] Some, but not all, samples of MSM in the early 21st century reported higher rates of heroin usage[9] or diagnosed opiate abuse[10] than had been previously observed.

"Post-HAART" Era Studies

Table 5-3 illustrates the continuing evolution of drug use patterns as well as changes in the sampling methods and research objectives. Therefore, direct comparisons of observed prevalence rates cannot be made with the previously discussed studies without careful attention to these specialized sampling issues.

For example, one study[29] took advantage of the increasing popularity of MSM-oriented Internet chat sites by administering an anonymous behavioral questionnaire online to geographically diverse participants in an MSM web chat/dating site. This study found drug use prevalences for the past 6 months that were consistent with the moderate rates found in other diverse "middle AIDS/HAART era" studies. In contrast, a repeat of the Urban Men's Health Study,[30] but limited to San Francisco in 2002–2003, found relatively high rates of crystal methamphetamine use (17%), ecstasy use (16%), and use of other club drugs. These findings suggest either that MSM residing in San Francisco were more likely to be using drugs than the "average" US MSM, and/or that the different sampling strategies used (self-selected Web participants vs. random digit dialing within telephone exchanges with high concentrations of MSMs) selected for groups of men with different drug use levels. The latter explanation is consistent with the concept, discussed in the epidemiological correlates section of this chapter as well as in Chapter 9, that residence in and socializing in an urban "gay ghetto" may be a risk factor for more frequent and polydrug use.

The rest of the studies summarized in Table 5-3 describe data from samples of "high risk" men recruited either on the basis of their consistent "club drug" usage,[18] or young MSM attending all night "circuit parties"[31,32] or other venues[33] where club drug use is expected to be high. Even so, large differences are seen between studies in terms of the rates of use of specific "club drugs." For example ecstasy use was reported by a high of 72% to 75% of men in the Mattison[31] and Mansergh[32] studies; 44% to 55% of men in the New York City "Project Bumps" study,[18] and 10% or less in the four-city study of young MSM[33] and the Internet survey.[29] Of note in these more recent studies, when drug use rates are broken down into general use rates compared to rates of use before/during sex[29,33] we see that the more closely a specific drug is associated with increasing the intensity or duration of sexual intercourse, the closer the general use rates approximate rates of use with sexual partners or during sex (e.g. poppers, crystal methamphetamine). Finally, Mansergh[32] also assessed the drugs most frequently associated with drug "overusage" or overdose episodes; not surprisingly, all "club drugs" but especially GHB (a solution of indeterminate concentration that is notoriously easy to overdose) were found to be associated with recent overusages.[31]

Epidemiological Correlates of Drug Use by MSM

Individual Level Correlates

Sex/drug link and sexual pleasure: In addition to the consistent finding that drug use, in general, is more frequent and used for longer periods of adult life among MSM,[9–10, 34–39] the strong associations between drug use and risky sexual behavior among gay and bisexual men is what differentiates drug use in this group from the general population of heterosexual males. Furthermore, several classes of drugs have become so highly intertwined with sexual expression

Table 5-1. Early AIDS/pre-HAART era studies of drug use among MSM

Study	Sample/Recruitment	Measures/ n	Study period	Alcohol (any)	Alcohol (heavy)	Alcohol (binge)	Marijuana
#20 Martin, Dean, Garcia, & Hall, 1989	Recruited in 1985 using multiple methods to sample NYC MSM	Retrospective substance use prevalences $n = 624$	1981 1987				78% 60%
#54 Ostrow, 1993	Chicago MACS/Coping & Change; recruited through clinics	All use prevalences for last 6 months $n = 384$	1984 1990	95.3% 90%	28% 12–15%		70.2% 43–46%
#17 Crosby, Stall, Paul & Barrett, 1998	SFMHS (25–54 year olds) & SFYMHS (18-29 year olds) recruited San Francisco MSM through multi-stage stratified cluster sampling	SFMHS ($n = 179$) SFYMHS ($n = 268$)	1984 1992	97.2% 92.5%	17.4% 14.7%		85.3% 64.2%
#8 Stall & Wiley, 1988	MSM & single heterosexual men living in same 19 census tracts sampled for SFMHS	MSM ($n = 748$) Hetero men ($n = 286$)	1984	93% 97%	19% 11%		78% 71%
#37 McKirnan & Peterson, 1989	Chicago MSM surveyed in gay venues (9%), health organizations (5%), newspaper insert (55%), & personal or community events (15%)	Substance use in last 6 months $n = 3400$	1985– 1986	86%	19%	23% of MSM have drinking problems vs. 16% of hetero men	Lifetime use rates: 79% for 18–25 yo; 83% for 26–34 yo; 67% for 35+ yo

Poppers	Cocaine	Crack cocaine	Any stimulants	Amphetamines	Hallucinogens	X & MDA	Downers	Opiates	IDU
65%	37%			22%	32%		28%	5%	
23%	28%			4%	10%		8%	2%	
70.6%	33.9%			15–19%	15–19%	15–19%	15–19%	<5%	
43-46%	15%	<2%		4–5%	4–5%	4–5%	4–5%	<5%	
62.2%	71.1%			44.1%	26.6%	14.7%	35%	7.7% (H)	
23.9%	24.3%			25.4%	29.1%	31.3%	11.2%	1.1% (H)	
58%	9%			28%	18%		3%	4%	
1%	2%			17%	12%		0%	5%	
21%	Lifetime use rates: 52% for 18-25 yo; 56% for 26-34 yo; 26% for 35+ yo								

Table 5-1. (*continued*)

Study	Sample/ Recruitment	Measures/ n	Study period	Alcohol (any)	Alcohol (heavy)	Alcohol (binge)	Marijuana
#21 Chesney, Barrett, & Stall, 1998	SFMHS sub-sample of MSM to study HIV seroconversion (SC)	Non -SC ($n = 298$) SC ($n = 39$)	1985–1991	95% 95%	15% 36%		68% 87%
#23 Myers et al., 1992	Talking Sex Project, recruited via multiple community-based venues	$n = 612$, substance use in past month	1988–1989	76.3% at least 1x/week			35.3%
#34 Skinner & Otis, 1996	Gay couples in 2 largest cities in Kentucky recruited via multiple community-based venues; NIDA NHSDA survey	Substance use in past year ($n = 567$) NHSDA substance use prevalence rates ($n = 1250$)	1990 1988	89.7% at least 1x/month 77.5%	31.5% at least 1x/month 16.9%		36.2% 14.7%
#28 Sullivan, Nakashima, Purcell, & Ward, 1998	All HIV+ men SHAS/CDC (supplemental to HIV/STD surveillance) in 12 state and local health deptartments.	Substance use prevalence survey for past 5 years $n = 9735$	1991–1997			29% abuse	51%
#14 Ferrando, et al., 1998	Columbia HIV Center cohort subsample; Psychiatric DSM III diagnosed abuse/de-depend/ ad-diction rates only	HIV$^+$ $n = 183$ HIV$^-$ $n = 84$	1995		34% 23%		23% 18%

Poppers	Cocaine	Crack cocaine	Any stimulants	Amphe-tamines	Halluci-nogens	X & MDA	Downers	Opiates	IDU
44%	40%			17%	13%		6%	2%	
77%	64%			37%	3%		23%	0%	
19.1%	5.5%						10.5%		2.9% in past 5 years
29.7%	9.4%	0.9%	9.3%		5.2%		5.6% sed. 10.2% tranq.	0.2% (H)	
1.9%	6.5%								
14%	31%	16%		15%	8%	8% (Diaz-epam)		5% non-IV	8% (H) 13% (coke) 6% (H +coke) 8% (crystal)
3%	21%		4%		2%				
0%	7%		1%		1%				

Table 5-2. Middle AIDS/early HAART era studies of drug use among MSM, 1996–2000

Study	Sample/ Recruitment	Era/n	Alcohol (any)	Alcohol (heavy)	Alcohol (binge)	Marijuana	Poppers	Cocaine
#9 Stall et al., 2001	Urban Men's Health Survey— Random digit dial telephone interviews in 4 US cities: SF, LA, NYC and Chicago	1996–1998 substance use prevalence for last 6 mnths $n=2172$	87.7%	8.0% 5+ drinks at least 1x/wk		42.4%	19.8%	15.2%
#85 Purcell, et al., 2001	Seropositive Urban Men's Study (SUMS) HIV$^+$ MSM in NYC and SF recruited via outreach and passive recruitment	1997–1998 substance use prevalence for past 3 months $n=456$	63.8%			36%	26.7%	13.2%
#26 Purcell, et al., 2005	Seropositive Urban Men's Intervention Trial (SUMIT) HIV$^+$ MSM in NYC and SF recruited for multi-site RCT	1999–2001 substance use prevalence for past 3 months $n=1168$	75.5%			42.2%	26.1%	17.9%
#10 Cochran et al., 2004	Data from SAMHSA NSHDA comparing sexually active MSM with hetero men	1996 substance prior month MSM ($n=98$)				13.9%	0.0%	3.9%
		Hetero ($n=3922$)				8.4%	0.6%	1.2%

Crack	Any Stimulants	Meth	Downers	Hallucinogens	X	K	GHB	H	Other analgesics	Viagra	IDU
3.0%	2.2% (not inc. Meth)	9.5%	8.8%	4.2%	11.7%			3.2%			1.3%
9.4%		11.6%	8.6%	8.1%	6.6%		2.2%	3.3%			5.3% 16% life-time IDU
NR	6.3%	10.1%	4.9%		7.3%	4.6%	3.7%			12.3%	20% life-time IDU
	0.7%		Sed. 0.0% Tranq. 0.4%	1.6%				0.8%	0%		
	0.9%		Sed. 0.1% Tranq. 0.6%	0.7%				0.1%	1.0%		

Table 5-3. Post-HAART era studies of drug use among MSM, 2001–present

Study	Sample/ Recruitment	Era/n	Alcohol (any)	Alcohol (heavy)	Alcohol (binge)	Marijuana	Poppers
#11 Koblin et al., 2003	EXPLORE randomized HIV risk-reduction trial; HIV⁻ MSM recruited from 6 cities	1999–2001 baseline substance use prevalence in past 6 months $n = 4295$		10.6% at least 4 drinks a day or 6+ drinks per occasion		46.3%	36.6%
#29 Hirschfield et al., 2004	National online anonymous survey of MSM	2001 substance use prevalence in last 6 months $n = 2916$		35% at least 1–3 days/week drink until drunk		30%	19%
#30 Paul et al., 2005	Urban Men's Health Study subsample of San Francisco MSM given RDD interviews and mail surveys	2002–2003 substance use prevalence in last 6 months $n = 879$	83.0%	6.4		43.0	26.0
#33 Celentano, Valleroy, et al., 2005	CDC Young Men's Survey Anonymous multi-site venue-based survey of 15–22 yo MSM in Baltimore, Dallas, LA, NYC, SF, Miami, and Seattle	1994–1998 substance use during sex in last 6 months $n = 3492$	42.8%			28.2%	8.0%
#31 Mattison et al., 2001	Non-random sample of circuit party attendees at 3 events in US and Canada	1998–1999 substance use at circuit parties in last year $n = 1169$	79%			45%	39%
#32 Mansergh et al., 2001	Circuit Party Men's Health Survey of MSM in San Francisco who attended at least one circuit party in last year	1999 substance use at most recent circuit party $n = 295$	56%			26%	9%

Cocaine	Crack	Meth	Downers	Halluci-nogens	X	K	GHB	Heroin	EDD or PDE	IDU
19.3%		12.9%		24.0% (inc. X)				10% recent IDU		IDU recent
7%		6%			10%	4%	3%		9.0%	<1%
10.0%		17.0			16%	12.5% K & GHB combined			29.3%	
		1.0% other amph.								
8.7%	1.5%	9.2%	2.3%	4.1% LSD	7.0%			1.8%		
39%		36%			72%	60%	28%			
19%		36%		4%	75%	58%	25%		12%	8%, last year

that they have assumed the status of "sex-enhancing drugs" within the various subcultures of MSM. While the proportion of drug use that occurs with sex is from 10% to 40% for some of the most commonly used drugs, such as marijuana, these proportions may be even higher for drugs used specifically to enhance intercourse or decrease the pain of anal penetration, such as volatile nitrites (or "poppers") and, increasingly, crystal methamphetamine use.[18,29]

As such, some of the primary variables determining the health effects of drug use among MSM are: the intention to use a particular drug to enhance sexual pleasure, the venue in which drug use and sex are combined, the partner choices that occur when drugs and sex are combined, and the drug(s) effect on male sexual functioning. For example, the use of phosphodiesterase type-5 (PDE5) inhibitors and other erectile dysfunction drugs (EDD) in order to have longer sessions of insertive sex has been rapidly taken up by some groups of MSM to the point that both prescribed and nonprescribed EDDs must now be considered sex-enhancing drugs in this population.[30] Furthermore, in terms of developing measures of dependence or addiction, it should be kept in mind that there may be a stronger potential for addiction to "sex drugs" than to drugs not used in the sexual context, as there are two intense motivations for drug use instead of one.

Age: Age is among the most important determinants of drug use patterns, regardless of the cultural subgroup being examined. For MSM, most studies have shown that the fall-off in drug use that accompanies aging among heterosexual men is attenuated or absent.[4, 8, 21, 34, 35, 40] This difference between homosexual and heterosexual men may be partially related to marital status; because gay men do not have the legal right to marry in our society, they are not exposed to the behavior moderating effects of marriage and child rearing.

Race/class status: Most studies have found that among younger gay and bisexual men, more highly educated and higher socioeconomic status men have higher rates of "club drug" usage (this includes stimulants, powder cocaine, ketamine ["special K"], GHB, and ecstasy). Recent studies have shown a preference for crack cocaine over powder cocaine or crystal methamphetamine among minority MSM.[41,42] Other differences in rates and types of drug usage by race or ethnicity are cited in this chapter. In general, these differences are related to socioeconomic and/or sampling differences. However, some differences (i.e., the preference of black MSM for cocaine or crack cocaine over crystal methamphetamine) persist even after controlling for socioeconomic status.[42,43]

HIV serostatus: Nearly every study reviewed that assessed HIV status shows that HIV seropositive men had higher levels of drug use before becoming infected. For HIV-infected men who stay sexually active with multiple partners, there is also a positive association between drug use and the number of sexual partners post-seroconversion. HIV status may serve as a biological end-point marker for the "fast track" lifestyle of the gay cohort who came of age during the late 1970s and early 1980s, among whom the AIDS and HIV epidemics originally flourished. Similarly, among initially HIV-uninfected men who seroconverted while participating in a prospective seroepidemiological study, the frequency and number of drugs used—especially if the drugs included stimulants, poppers, and EDDs—are associated with higher rates of HIV seroconversion.[16]

Self-perceived threat of HIV/AIDS: Multiple researchers[42,44,45] have shown that reduced concern about HIV/AIDS in the era of HAART is associated with increasing levels of both drug use and risky sex. This is particularly true among MSM who are already HIV-seropositive and those who identify themselves as "barebackers," or men who intentionally engage in unprotected anal sex and self-identify as belonging to an outsider social subgroup.[46,47]

Personality factors, such as sexual sensation seeking and compulsivity: Among the many predisposing factors that link drug use to risky sex, HIV infection, and other risk-taking behaviors, sexual sensation seeking and sexual compulsivity have been the most widely studied.[42,48,49] Proposed early in the AIDS epidemic,[50] enduring personality characteristics such as risk taking, impulsivity, and sensation seeking may be common factors contributing to multiple forms of risky behavior, including drug use. Less well understood among MSM are the roles of negative emotions or affects that have recently been cited by HIV seropositive men as important reasons for using stimulant drugs and engaging in unsafe sex under the influence of drugs.[51]

Contextual/Dyadic or Situational Factors

Type of drug used and mode of consumption: Economics, drug accessibility, and pharmacokinetics appear to account for many of the differences observed in the form and mode of consumption of drugs. For example, drug distribution networks seem to account for the widespread availability of crack cocaine in inner city neighborhoods, while powder cocaine and crystal methamphetamine sales networks predominate among the more affluent and mobile.[52] Differences in the ways in which certain drugs are ingested may have more to do with fear of HIV or hepatitis B or C exposure, causing a shift away from injection of heroin to snorting and smoking. Some gay and bisexual men, long thought to have very low levels (<1% to 2% in studies reviewed) of injection drug use, may be overcoming their fear of needles as the intravenous use of crystal methamphetamine for extended sexual play ("party and play," or PNP, is the Internet buzzword for men seeking sexual partners who will use crystal methamphetamine and other club drugs) increases markedly.[11]

Type of drug use/sexual partner: As mentioned above, certain drugs have assumed nearly mythic reputations as sexual enhancements for MSM, particularly men who desire prolonged sex sessions. While poppers and crystal methamphetamine are frequently cited as favorite "sex drugs" among MSM, other drugs such as marijuana, cocaine, ketamine (or "special K"), and gammahydroxybutyrate (or GHB) have all been reported as being used for sexual enhancement by gay and bisexual men. Currently, several groups of researchers are observing increasing use of prescription EDDs and over-the-counter "herbal" sexual enhancers (such as yohimbine, ephedrine, and guarana preparations) among men who party and play (i.e., combine substance use with sex).[16,53] Furthermore, the impact of drug use on the loosening of sexual inhibitions and promoting unprotected anal sex appears to be dependent on the type of partner involved. Ostrow and colleagues[54] showed that increasing popper use was associated with increasing levels of unprotected receptive anal intercourse (URAI) only with casual and not with primary partners. More recently, the SUMIT intervention study for HIV+ MSM observed that drug use during sex was associated with unprotected anal sex with known seropositive or unknown HIV-status partners, but not with known HIV-negative partners.[26] These observations suggest that the use of drugs during sex *per se* does not confer increased risk of sexually transmitted infections (STI), except under specific circumstances with specific types of partners.

Geographical considerations: Studies summarized in Table 5-1 are sampled across various geographic or urban/rural locations and thus provide insight into specific and general geographic differences among drug-using MSM. Most notable among the geographically based differences are two specific patterns that have been observed since the start of the AIDS epidemic. First, injection drug use and its overlap with homosexual behavior was primarily an East Coast phenomenon, although Chicago and rural Midwestern areas as well as the Pacific Northwest have all had their share of HIV spread through sharing of contaminated injection paraphernalia among MSM.[55] This epidemiological overlap and regional variations would apply to both the regional population of injection drug users (IDUs) who share paraphernalia as well as to the smaller numbers of MSM who share drugs with IDUs. Second, the illicit manufacture and sale of methamphetamine began in the San Francisco to San Diego, California, coastal corridor in the late 1960s and gradually has worked its way across middle America. More recently (since the mid-to-late 1990s), it has become a major drug abuse factor among MSM in the Eastern United States.[24]

Gay bar/Internet orientation: Much of the pre-AIDS data on gay men's drug and alcohol use patterns was obtained using convenience samples from gay bars, bathhouses, and other venues, which functioned as both social clubs and places to meet sexual partners. Obviously, bar samples will include men who use alcohol and other drugs more frequently and/or more problematically. When population-based or multiple sampling frame methods and strict clinical diagnostic criteria are used, the rates of drug use/abuse among younger gay men are not very different from that of similarly sampled heterosexual men,[8] suggesting that a strong orientation to gay bar life is a marker for greater drug abuse. More recently, increasing numbers of MSM are meeting new sexual partners on the Internet; most important for this chapter is the use of Internet chat and dating Web sites to meet partners wanting to use stimulants or other drugs with sex partners ("party and play," or PNP). Hirshfield and colleagues[29] explored the drugs used by 2916 MSM who visited a gay chat and hook-up site in 2001. Unprotected anal intercourse (which was reported by 56% of the respondents during the past 6 months) was associated with the use of poppers, methamphetamine, cocaine, marijuana and Viagra® before or during sex. Unfortunately, the representativeness of any sample of MSM obtained through such Web sites is unclear. For a variety of reasons, men who use crystal methamphetamine and other stimulants, as well as men engaging in extended and group sex play, appear to be overrepresented in such samples.

Social/Cohort Factors

Social norms: One of the greatest shifts ever observed in intimate behaviors was the sexual and drug-use counterrevolution that accompanied the recognition of AIDS and the response catalyzed by the gay and bisexual communities in response to AIDS-associated mortality. More recently, researchers are observing a smaller but significant increase in both risky sex and sex-drug usage by MSM whose fear and concern about the threat of HIV has radically changed in the era of highly active antiretroviral therapy (HAART).[42,56] These changing attitudes are the result of the combination of changed perceptions of personal vulnerability to HIV/AIDS and changing social norms among MSM. Similarly, the rise of the barebacker subculture depends, in part, on the perceived social norm that engaging in unprotected anal sex is an entirely personal matter and does not necessitate obtaining permission from or warning potential sexual partners about one's HIV serostatus.

Concluding Remarks: Drug Use

The data presented in the figure and tables are consistent with continued relatively high rates of drug use among MSM, with differences from general population samples most notable in the area of sex-specific drugs, such as poppers, crystal methamphetamine, and the full range of "club drugs," including ecstasy, cocaine, ketamine and GHB. While generally not as high as the drug use levels reported just prior to or at the start of the AIDS epidemic (late 1970s to mid-1980s), overall current drug use levels among MSM are still elevated when compared to relevant general male population samples. Despite sharp reductions in drug use seen in the first decade of the AIDS epidemic, drug use rates have either stabilized or increased somewhat in recent years. These increases may well be related to reduced concern about HIV since the advent of HAART, as has recently been shown for increases in risky sexual behavior since HAART among the MACS sample of MSM.[56] With the exception of newly popular drugs, such as ecstasy and crystal methamphetamine, these rates have not yet reached rates seen at the start of the AIDS epidemic. Further, a new class of "sex drugs," erectile dysfunction drugs used to enhance sexual pleasure and endurance, has entered the compendium of drugs used relatively frequently by MSM. These factors, as well as the specific epidemiological covariates of drug usage among MSM discussed above, continue to contribute to the drug-related morbidity and mortality of MSM.

While all of these interwoven factors should raise concern among researchers, clinicians, public health workers, and the public about the urgent need for intense primary prevention efforts at preventing the initiation of stimulant and other "hard" drug use among MSM, recent history also shows us that socially imposed restrictions on the consumption of one drug are usually followed by increased use of another drug.[24] In conclusion, the consistent finding across studies that gay men have used many different kinds of drugs at high prevalence rates since at least the late 1970s—and at rates far greater than those reported by comparable samples of the general population of men—is notable, particularly given the enormous cultural, behavioral, and epidemiological changes that have occurred during this same time period.

The Epidemiology of Alcohol Use among MSM

Prevalence of Alcohol Use and Heavy Drinking among MSM

Heavy alcohol use is related to a wide series of physical health problems among men, notably cardiovascular disease,[57] cirrhosis,[58] trauma,[59] and a wide array of social problems. A presumption of heavy drinking among gay men has existed in the scientific literature since at least the 1970s[60] and has been a stereotypical portrayal of gay men in fiction and other art forms during far earlier periods. This presumption is due in part to the fact that gay bars have functioned historically as de facto community centers and have served as one of the primary places where gay men could congregate prior to the birth of the US gay civil rights movement. The fact that the dominant location of the public gay male world was situated in alcohol-selling venues, in combination with the need of individual men to cope with the daily effects of homophobia and discrimination, was also widely presumed to encourage pervasive heavy drinking among gay men. For all of these reasons it seems reasonable to hypothesize that a subculture that annually celebrates Gay Freedom Day on the anniversary of a riot against police harassment at the Stonewall Tavern in New York City would have a high prevalence of alcohol-related health problems. However, the questions remain: (1) do gay men indeed report a higher prevalence of alcohol consumption and/or heavy drinking compared to heterosexual men?, (2) do gay men suffer from a disproportionate burden of alcohol-related medical and psychological problems compared to heterosexual men?, and (3) do gay men with alcohol-related problems have particular issues in terms of access to culturally tailored alcohol and drug interventions?

Given the historical importance of gay bars in gay culture, it is not surprising that the first pioneering research on gay men's health tended to oversample or even sample exclusively from among gay bar patrons. This early body of work tended to confirm suspicions that there was a high prevalence of heavy drinking and/or alcohol abuse among gay men. The estimates of alcohol abuse and/or alcoholism from this early work tended to cluster in the 30% range,[36,60,61] an alcohol dependency rate that would rank among the highest reported for any other American population. However, the methodological flaw of using samples of bar patrons to generate estimates of heavy drinking for an entire population now seems glaring. That said, this pioneering work did make the important contribution of drawing attention to the importance of substance abuse as a health issue among gay men and lesbians and did so with very few resources. In retrospect, it is difficult to imagine how this research focus could have been started in any other way.

The advent of the AIDS crisis forced the first serious funding of research on gay men's health concerns. Alcohol use and other forms of substance use were typically measured in these early research studies as a hypothesized cause of immune function collapse. The inclusion of these measures in large samples of gay men that were not restricted to gay bar samples allowed a more careful look at alcohol use and heavy drinking among gay men.[8,34,37,62] Although the research conducted in the context of the AIDS epidemic was not without flaws of its own,[63] it tended to generate data to show that gay men reported rates of heavy drinking that were rather similar to those reported among men in the general population. For example, Stall and Wiley[8] reported data from the household-based sample of gay and heterosexual men drawn from the neighborhoods adjoining the Castro district in San Francisco. They found that patterns of overall alcohol consumption were not significantly different between gay men and their heterosexual neighbors, although there was a higher reported prevalence of heavy drinking (19%) by gay men than that reported by heterosexual male residents (11%) of the same residential district in San Francisco. A contemporaneous study reported data from New York City to show that there were no differences in the rates of alcohol abuse and dependence disorders between gay men and heterosexual men.[62]

Consistent with these general findings, Stall and colleagues[9] reported the alcohol use consumption patterns and heavy drinking rates within a large household-based sample ($n = 2172$) of MSM residents of San Francisco, Los Angeles, Chicago and New York. Alcohol consumption in the past 6 months was very common within the sample (88%); however, prevalence rates for 3 or more alcohol-related problems (12%) or drinking 5 or more drinks at one sitting at least once a week (frequent/heavy alcohol use, 8%) was far less common. The frequent/heavy drinking rate among MSM in this sample for the past 6 months was roughly comparable to that reported among men from a large national household survey aged 12 or greater in the past 30 days (9%) drawn from the general population.

Two additional studies have advanced this field even further by taking large-scale samples of the general population and making direct comparisons between rates of heavy drinking, problem drinking, and alcohol dependency between gay/bisexual men and heterosexual men sampled under the same protocol. Cochran and Mays[64] analyzed data from the large-scale, population-based 1996 National Household Survey of Drug Abuse in which a supplemental questionnaire asked for the gender of respondents' sexual partners. Their analysis of these data yielded roughly equivalent rates of alcohol dependency between the men reporting any same-gender (10.6%) and exclusive opposite-gender partners (7.6%), which in turn generated a nonsignificant unadjusted odds ratio estimate of 1.45 (95% CI=0.62–3.41) of differences in rates of alcohol dependency between the two groups of men. Similarly, Drabble, Midanik, and Trocki[65] reported data from the population-based 2000 National Alcohol Survey, which also included measures of sexual behavior, orientation, and identity. Again, the measures of heavy drinking, alcohol-related problems, and dependency were roughly equivalent between heterosexual men, bisexual men, and homosexual men, although in the case of one measure (drunk > 2 times in the past year), homosexual men were marginally more likely to report drinking at this level than were heterosexual men (p < .05, 67.2% vs. 42%). However, the mean number of drinks per year, mean number of days drinking 5+ drinks, > 2 social consequences, and rates of ever seeking help for alcohol-related problems were equivalent between exclusively heterosexual men and bisexual and homosexual men. Of special importance were the similarities in rates of DSM-IV alcohol dependency, which were not significantly different between exclusively heterosexual (5.6%), bisexual (5.6%), and homosexual (10.4%) men in this sample. Interestingly, in a separate analysis of this same data set, Trocki, Drabble, and Midanik[66] reported that while gay men spent more time in heavy-drinking bar environments than did heterosexual men, their alcohol consumption when in these environments did not seem to increase from usual consumption patterns.

Finally, it should also be pointed out that the bulk of the literature examining rates of use and misuse among gay men adopted a cross-sectional research design. It may be that with measurement over longer periods of the life course, rates of problematic use of alcohol by gay men would increase and possibly become significantly different from those found among heterosexual men. Relevant to this point are data from a small-scale five-year prospective study of HIV seropositive and seronegative gay men conducted during the pre-HAART era.[15] The analysis of these data showed a significant decline in problematic alcohol and drug use during the 1980s, and that men used a series of strategies outside of formal treatment to reduce alcohol and drug use.

These data suggest that long-term measures of substance use may uncover important increases and decreases in alcohol and other forms of drug use over the life course, as well as documentation of non-treatment-based techniques that work to help men reduce use over long periods of time. Replication of this design with a larger sample of men drawn from a community-based sample would advance our understandings of how alcohol and drug use patterns change across the life course in important ways. In addition, temporal gay community events cannot be excluded as the causes of changes in drinking patterns over time, as the start of the AIDS epidemic and the development of HAART have already shown in terms of drug use and risky sexual patterns.

Correlates of Problematic Alcohol Use and/or Alcohol Dependence

Although the literature on alcohol use among gay men has tended to emphasize the question of point prevalence rates of use and abuse, a cluster of papers have emerged to report associations with heavy or problematic alcohol consumption among gay men. As a general rule, however, these studies have not been theory-based studies specifically designed to explain alcohol abuse among gay men; rather this body of literature consists of a set of secondary data analyses of existing data sets that were designed to address other scientific questions. Nevertheless, the cluster of significant associations reported in this literature could be incorporated into a theory of alcohol abuse among gay men that would in turn serve as a useful guide to treatment and prevention efforts.

Greenwood and colleagues[67] analyzed data from the San Francisco Young Men's Health Study to test for demographic associations with frequent/heavy alcohol use. They found that men who were frequent/heavy drinkers were more likely to be employed in nonprofessional occupations, to attend gay bars more frequently, and to report greater numbers of male sexual partners. Ghindia and Kola[68] included a broader mix of variables in their analysis of an opportunistic sample of gay men in the Cleveland area. They found that a familial history of substance use and a measure of self-esteem were associated with alcohol abuse among gay men. Stall and colleagues[9] reported a correlational analysis of frequent/heavy drinking and three or more alcohol problems within a large household-based sample of gay men. They found that a set of variables was associated with both alcohol abuse measures: a history of parental substance abuse, greater bar attendance, and less frequent reading of the gay print media. Other variables associated only with frequent/heavy drinking included lower educational attainment, less harassment for being gay, a bimodal relationship to affiliation with the gay community (with the lowest and highest levels of affiliation being positively related to frequent/ heavy drinking), and having a middle range of friends/family or lovers currently living with HIV. Variables associated only with three or more alcohol-related problems included having a low sense of well-being, fewer visits to sex clubs, lower perceived exclusivity on the part of gay culture, and expiring anti-gay verbal harassment. Finally, Crosby and colleagues[17] described reductions in heavy alcohol use across cohorts of gay men, reductions that they attributed, in part, to the effects of the AIDS epidemic, an analysis also offered by Remien and colleagues.[15] Together, the associations reported in this set of papers can be taken to mean that variables having to do with socialization to alcohol use (e.g., history of parental substance abuse), class-based demographics (e.g., occupation and educational attainment), connection to specific ways of accessing gay culture (e.g., greater bar attendance, readership of gay media), sexual practice (e.g., greater number of sex partners), experience of homophobic attacks (e.g., greater experience of anti-gay harassment), and the experience of historical events especially important to gay men (e.g., the AIDS epidemic) shape alcohol consumption among MSM. The identification of independent associations with substance abuse that are specific to gay male culture in the list given above may mean that standard alcohol abuse prevention and treatment programs may need to be modified so that they address unique factors driving substance abuse among gay men.

Alcohol Use among Gay Men: Concluding Remarks

Alcohol use is pervasive among gay men, and participation in bar culture remains an important aspect of many gay men's lives over the life course. Nevertheless, the proportion of the gay male population that experiences alcohol-related problems at any one point in time does not appear to be appreciably higher for gay men than for heterosexual men (see also [63,69,70] for separate reviews of this same literature). This finding may point to the possibility that gay men may have important resources and/or coping mechanisms to avoid or resolve alcohol-related problems and that a better understanding of such strategies, if they exist, could inform community-based prevention and treatment programs.

In conclusion, the fact that the bulk of the evidence points to a rough comparability in the prevalence of alcohol-related problems or heavy drinking between gay men and men drawn from the general population does not mean that the misuse of alcohol is not a health threat within the gay male population. Access to effective alcohol treatment and prevention services are an important priority for gay and bisexual men, much as they are for heterosexual men.

The Epidemiology of Tobacco Smoking among MSM

The Prevalence of Tobacco Smoking among MSM

Tobacco smoking is prominent among the greatest preventable causes of morbidity and mortality,[71] with adverse outcomes to health not only in increased risk for lung cancer and emphysema, but also for cardiovascular health and other neoplasms.[72] The fact that gay men have specifically been targeted by tobacco companies as a target audience,[73] along with evidence that tobacco use can further impact the health of HIV positive individuals in negative ways,[74] may amplify the harm to health caused by tobacco use among gay male populations. Answering the question of whether gay men smoke at higher rates than those found among American men in general is a first step in support of efforts to reduce the burden of tobacco-related disease among gay men in the United States.

A series of community-based studies published over the past decade have consistently reported findings to suggest that gay men smoke at higher rates than men in the general US population. For example, Skinner[35] used a set of mailing lists of gay male and lesbian organizations that served residents of a southern US state to generate a prevalence rate of 39.7% for current smoking among gay men. The data reported by Skinner were consistent with a set of earlier reports derived from opportunistic sampling methods that presented data showing rates of smoking among gay men were in the 40% range.[38] Amplifying this work, Stall and colleagues[75] used a time-series sample of gay bar patrons ($n = 1897$) and a household-based telephone list serve sample ($n = 696$) of gay men in Portland, Oregon, and Tuscon, Arizona, to generate an overall rate for current smoking of 48%. Modal consumption was about one pack of cigarettes per day in both the bar and community sample, with approximately two-thirds of the men in both samples smoking one pack per day or more. About half (50.1%) of the men in the bar sample smoked, while the rate of smoking in the community sample (41.5%) was significantly lower, a finding that suggests that an over-reliance on bar sampling methods may artificially inflate estimates of smoking among gay men. The overall rate of smoking in both the Tucson and Portland samples for gay men was significantly higher than concurrent surveillance estimates of smoking among male residents of Oregon (22.9%) or Arizona (26.8%).

Taking into account that household-based samples of gay men may avoid biases in smoking rates introduced by the use of gay bar samples, Greenwood and colleagues[76] conducted a follow-up of the Urban Men's Health Study, a household-based telephone sample of gay male residents of New York, Chicago, San Francisco and Los Angeles ($n = 2402$), to measure current and past smoking practices. Using this sampling frame, Greenwood and colleagues generated a rate of current smoking among MSM of 31.4%, significantly higher than that concurrently reported among a comparable sample of men in the general US population (24.7%). The modal smoking pattern was one pack of cigarettes per day. In addition, they found that a substantial proportion of the gay men had a significant prior history of tobacco use (27% of the sample), but were no longer smoking. The finding that approximately one-quarter of all urban gay men are former smokers suggests that well-designed and fielded tobacco control efforts within this population could well be effective.

Both the Stall[75] and Greenwood[76] approach of comparing household-based samples of specific communities to smoking rates reported in the general population can be faulted on methodological and analytical grounds, primarily having to do with the weaknesses of comparing rates of smoking across sampling frames. Tang and colleagues[77] took advantage of the very rare opportunity of analyzing data on tobacco use from a very large household-based behavioral surveillance survey of the general population that included questions about same-sex behavior and attraction. Tang and colleagues analyzed data from the California Health Interview Survey ($n = 44,606$) that included subsamples of self-identified gay male ($n = 593$) and bisexual male ($n = 282$) respondents to generate a rate of current smoking among MSM of 33.2% compared to a rate of 22.3% among heterosexual male California residents. Controlling for demographic variables in a multivariate analysis, gay men in the California Health Interview Survey were more likely to be current smokers than were the heterosexual male respondents drawn from the same sample (OR = 1.95; 95% CI = 1.66–2.73). In addition to the findings regarding tobacco use, the success of the California Health Interview Survey in creating data to support comparisons between heterosexual male and homosexual male respondents suggests that other large household-based sampling strategies could and should include measures of same-sex behavior and attraction so that this and other analyses of health disparities concerning gay men can be extended and/or replicated. Finally, taken together, the household-based sampling data strongly suggests that gay men are significantly more likely to smoke than are heterosexual men and that the extent of this enhanced rate of smoking is substantial.

Correlates of Tobacco Smoking among Gay Men

In addition to increased rates of smoking, the literature has also identified a set of associations with smoking within gay male samples. For example, Stall and colleagues[75] found that heavy drinking, frequent bar attendance, greater AIDS-related losses, HIV seropositivity, lower self-reported health rating, lower educational attainment, and lower income were all associated with smoking among gay men. Tang and colleagues[77] reported that being in the 35–44 age cohort, being non-Hispanic, having lower educational attainment, and having a household income less than $30,000 a year was associated with current smoking among California gay men. Thus, across these two studies, lower education attainment and lower income were associated with current smoking, with other variables associated with gay bar culture, HIV seropositivity, and greater experience of the AIDS epidemic, and with specific age cohorts and ethnic status also possibly associated with current smoking among gay men. These findings suggest that tobacco cessation programs may need to address or tailor activities to incorporate "gay-specific" variables (including some of the variables listed above) to improve programmatic effectiveness.

Tobacco Smoking among Gay Men: Concluding Remarks

In sum, the household-based sampling data strongly suggests that gay men are significantly more likely to smoke than are heterosexual men and that the extent of this enhanced rate of smoking is substantial (see also Ryan et al.[78] for an additional review of this literature). In addition, some relatively unique associations with smoking may be found among gay men. Specific tailoring of prevention and treatment programs that take such variables into account may increase the penetration and effectiveness of such programs within gay male populations.

Promising Responses to Resolving Health Disparities Associated with Substance Use among MSM

Given the direct morbidities and mortalities associated with excess drug, alcohol, and tobacco use among MSM, improved primary and secondary drug prevention efforts would seem to be of the highest priority. However, the literature contains several negative reports of focused drug use prevention programs for MSM that were no more effective than "control" conditions (for example, see [19,27]). We focus here on promising interventions for the most difficult to treat types of drug and/or alcohol abuse and dependence among MSM, noting those interventions that are specifically designed to reduce the sexual and STD risk that often accompanies drug abuse problems.

As summarized in Miller, Gold and Smith[79] and further elaborated for MSM in the 2001 CSAT Monograph "A Provider's Introduction to Substance Abuse Treatment for Lesbian, Gay, Bisexual and Transgender Individuals,"[39] these intervention modalities include:

1. 12-Step Programs (AA, NA, etc.). Emphasizing complete abstinence through psychosocial and spiritual involvement in 12-step self-help groups, these programs have relatively high rates of one-year abstinence (45% to 80%),[79] especially if combined with other modalities of treatment.
2. Individual Supportive Psychotherapy (ISP). Nonspecific in nature, such therapy is often employed in conjunction with 12-step and other forms of treatment to support the individual's attempts to recover. Most efficacy studies have been with alcoholics, where moderate efficacy is noted.[79]
3. Standard Cognitive-Behavioral Treatment (CBT). Widely varying techniques to help individuals identify high-risk situations that may lead to substance use and to develop alternative cognitions and behaviors for such situations. Shown effective in preventing single lapses in substance use from developing into full-blown relapse.[39,79]
4. Gay Culturally Sensitive Cognitive Behavioral Therapy (G-CBT). As described in Shoptaw et al.,[80] this is essentially modifying standard CBT to include specific training for MSM to avoid sexual and other situations in which substance use may play a role in substance use lapses and relapse. This therapy emphasizes the links between drug use and high-risk sexual behavior as described in this chapter.

5. Contingency Management Interventions (CMI). Based on contracting with participants for specific positive and/or negative consequences to abstinence or relapse, such as escalating payments for "clean" urines indicating drug-free periods between treatment sessions. The effectiveness of CMI in the treatment of methamphetamine abusing MSM is discussed below.

6. Pharmacological Interventions (Rx). A mixed bag of drug treatments that either use aversive agents (e.g., antabuse for alcohol use), substitution for the abused agent (i.e., methadone or bupernorphine for opiate addiction), blocking agents that modify or eliminate the "high" from abused drugs (i.e., lithium for cocaine, acomprasate for alcohol), and antidepressants to treat any depression that might underlie drug use. In addition, transdermal patches that deliver a steady dose of nicotine or narcotic analgesic can be used to eliminate the harm associated with the smoking of tobacco and the injection of opiates, respectively. Used either alone or in combination with 12-step, ISP, CBT or CMI, pharmacological interventions have not been tested specifically in MSM populations. However, their growing popularity and data indicating that they are at least equivalent to CBT or ISP in varied populations[39,79] would suggest their usefulness as part of a multidimensional approach to drug abuse among MSM.

7. Harm Reduction (HR). Popular since the advent of AIDS among intravenous drug users, these modalities are used at the individual and social level to decrease the physical harms related to drug use, such as the distribution of clean syringes and needles to avoid HIV and HCV infection among intravenous drug users (IVDUs), and the use of transdermal patches as mentioned above. The effectiveness of harm reduction approaches is very controversial and difficult to ascertain, as they are mostly fielded in anonymity to protect the addicted individuals, who continue to be dependent on illegal drug(s).

8. Combined modalities from the above list. Since substance use/abuse is a multifactorial condition, multiple treatment modalities that are tailored to an individual's level of need and state of motivation to change can be more effective than any single treatment modality. However, the cost efficacy of such approaches has been difficult to prove in controlled clinical trials.

9. In addition to these specific and targeted forms of drug abuse treatment, the concept of syndemics described in detail in Chapter 9 would suggest that structural changes in the larger society that limit or eliminate the stigma, abuse, and discrimination that are commonly described by gay and bisexual men might have a significant impact on the rates of initiation of drug use that is related to self-medication and relief from the negative psychological impacts of anti-gay stigma, abuse, and discrimination. Natural experiments of structural interventions and their impact on drug abuse among MSM are in process as

some states legalize gay marriage and others include sexual orientation in their anti-discrimination statutes.

While trials of standardized drug interventions that directly compare the various modalities listed above are beginning to emerge, there are few data to suggest that specific types of drug abuse intervention are more or less effective among MSM. For example, Shoptaw and colleagues directly compared four of the above treatment modalities for crystal methamphetamine dependent MSM in the Los Angeles area.[80] One hundred sixty-two men were randomly assigned to 16 weeks of treatment with either CBT ($n = 40$), CM ($n = 42$), G-CBT ($n = 40$), or combined CBT and CM ($n = 40$), with follow-up assessments at 6 and 12 months post treatment. During treatment, CM and CBT plus CM showed greater effectiveness in reducing methamphetamine usage, while the G-CBT treated men had significantly reduced rates of unprotected anal sex during the first four weeks of treatment. These between-group differences disappeared at longer follow-up times, but all groups continued to show overall reductions in methamphetamine use over the full one-year period of follow-up assessment. This is one of the first published studies to demonstrate the efficacy of CM interventions for crystal methamphetamine–dependent MSM, as well as showing the importance of standard treatment modalities for this most difficult to treat group of drug-abusing MSM.

Gay and bisexual drug and alcohol abusers tend to react to most available interventions in the same manner as their heterosexual counterparts; few tend to take advantage of interventions with an abstinence goal, and for other interventions, there are generally poor adherence and follow-up rates.[19] There is a pressing need for more community-based interventions that appeal to persons who are not yet using but are thinking about it and also to persons who have not yet acknowledged that they have a "problem" with their drug use. Such interventions must combine the best of drug-specific interventions with culturally sensitive interventions that take into account the special nature of drug use among MSM populations. A related innovation would be to include assessment of commercial and other venues where MSM obtain and learn about the use of substances (e.g., "circuit parties", gay bars and bathhouses, etc.), with the overall goal of developing interventions that can be fielded and evaluated in such settings. Finally, it bears repeating that structural interventions that reduce the stigma, abuse, and discrimination experienced by MSM have an enormous but untested potential for synergizing the effectiveness of targeted substance-abuse interventions.[81]

Moving the Field of Alcohol, Tobacco, and Drug Studies among MSM Forward

On the research front, there are several directions that will likely yield important new insights toward understanding how MSM use drugs, tobacco, or alcohol and how these use patterns translate into health problems. To make a very broad generalization, we have now probably reached the point of diminishing return in terms of the progress to be made by fielding additional stand-alone cross-sectional descriptive studies of substance use patterns. However, there are several exceptions to this broad statement that are likely to yield important insights: studies to describe drug, tobacco, or alcohol use patterns among ethnic minority MSM and/or specific age cohorts of MSM; and the inclusion of sexual orientation and sex behavior questions in large samples of the general American population to permit direct comparisons of substance use patterns between MSM and their fellow citizens. That said, the use of stand-alone cross-section samples of the gay male communities to study drug, tobacco, and alcohol use patterns has been the dominant research design for the past third of a century, and the findings that have accrued from recent applications of this design have been remarkably consistent.

Where the field can move forward in productive ways is in the study of how use patterns change over time among gay men, not only through the use of serial cross-sectional studies (to capture changing trends in drug, tobacco, or alcohol use over historical time) but also through the use of longitudinal natural history studies (to capture changes in drug, tobacco, or alcohol use patterns as men age). Neither of these designs has enjoyed sufficient use in the field, which means that we now have only a very poor sense of how use patterns change as men age or of the correlates of new use patterns as these waves pass through gay communities. One such focus that might be particularly promising would be the study of the evolution of problematic use patterns, such as may exist in the progression of crystal methamphetamine use from occasional to frequent snorting of the drug, to smoking and drug injection. In addition, identifying the social and psychological characteristics of men most likely to be caught up in new waves of problematic drug use as they crest in gay communities would also be a valuable contribution.

None of this work should move forward without careful attention to theory development to explain patterns of drug, tobacco, or alcohol use and abuse by gay men. In particular, this theory development should take into account variables that are very likely to be unique to or especially important among MSM in explaining problematic use. While problematic substance use among MSM is shaped by many of the same variables that influence drug, tobacco, or alcohol use among heterosexual men, such variables as homophobia and internalized homophobia, the connection between substance abuse and sexual sensation seeking, the remaining importance of gay bars as de facto community centers, alcohol and drug use norms specific to gay male culture, and syndemic interplays between mental health, violence, and substance abuse epidemics are also important to explaining problematic substance abuse among gay men. Although each of these variables has been shown in individual analyses to be important to understanding problematic substance use among gay men, a theoretical synthesis that includes all of these variables in one explanatory paradigm has yet to be achieved. An integrative theoretical model would contribute toward improving not only the description and prediction of substance abuse problems among MSM but would also provide an important blueprint for the design of community-based prevention and treatment services.

On the treatment program front, we have very little in the way of rigorously controlled data to demonstrate that standard approaches to substance abuse treatment are effective among MSM, much less programs that have been specifically translated to meet their needs. In view of the general lack of rigorous data to show the efficacy of tobacco treatment, or alcohol or substance abuse treatment regimens among MSM, this agenda should probably start first with a collaborative statement of "best practices" by front-line treatment providers (see prior section on treatment innovations). Work could then begin to test innovative treatment regimens designed for MSM to measure the efficacy of such programs, an agenda that would work to improve the quality of programs available to men who wish to control problematic use. A similar trajectory of work could begin to inform the primary prevention agenda and would likely yield important insights toward the design of community-based responses to control problematic use before it requires clinical attention.

Even after effective substance abuse treatment programs have been fielded, issues of treatment access will remain important. As has been known for many years on both the research and programmatic front, a substantial gap exists between the number of gay men who might reasonably be determined to require treatment for addiction to drugs, tobacco, or alcohol and those who actually access it. To date, little work has been done to identify the specific barriers to accessing care for MSM. A replication of the test of "Hart's Law of Inverse Access" (i.e., that those at greatest need for preventive services are the least likely to receive them[82]) in terms of substance abuse treatment and preventive services would be a good first start toward addressing this agenda.[83] These issues may be particularly important for HIV-positive MSM.[85]

While there is little question that MSM communities suffer higher rates of tobacco and drug use and/or abuse than those found among men in general, the characteristic of resilience in handling substance abuse problems by gay men should also be highlighted. Examples of resilience are found throughout the literature on substance use among MSM: the high rates of successful cessation of tobacco use by gay men, the consistent finding of no difference in heavy drinking rates between gay and heterosexual male samples, and high rates of successful cessation of substance use careers over the life course. These findings, and others, would not be possible were there not strong mechanisms in place among gay men to manage drug abuse careers and problems associated with drug use. As yet, these mechanisms of resilience and strength in handling substance abuse careers are not well understood and may be the greatest single gap in our knowledge concerning gay men and substance use. Work that also emphasizes the resilience of gay men in dealing with the various substance abuse epidemics would improve not only our understandings of these epidemics but also the provision of effective substance abuse and prevention services to gay men.

References

1. Substance Abuse and Mental Health Services Administration. *2003 National Survey on Drug Use and Health: Results.* Rockville, MD: Office of Applied Studies; 2004.

2. Grant BF, Dawson DA, Stinson FS, Chou SP, Dufour MC, Pickering RP. The 12-month prevalence and trends in DSM-IV alcohol abuse and dependence: United States, 1991–1992 and 2001–2002. *Drug Alcohol Depend.* 2004;74:223–234.

3. Garbutt JC, West SL, Carey TS, Lohr KN, Crews FT. Pharmacological treatment of alcohol dependence: a review of the evidence. *JAMA.* 1999;281:1318–1325.

4. National Institute on Alcohol Abuse and Alcoholism. *Tenth Special Report to the U.S. Congress on Alcohol and Health.* NIH Publication No. 00–1583. Bethesda, MD: National Institutes of Health; 2000.

5. Bagnardi V, Blangiardo M, Vecchia C, Corrao G. Alcohol consumption and the risk of cancer: a meta-analysis. *Alcohol Res Health.* 2001;25:263–270.

6. Modesto-Lowe V, Kranzler HR. Diagnosis and treatment of alcohol-dependent patients with comorbid psychiatric disorders. *Alcohol Res Health.* 1999;23:144–149.

7. National Council on Alcoholism and Drug Dependence (NCADD), Inc. Recovery: it's a family affair. Let's talk about it. Fact sheet. Community Anti-Drug Coalition of America. 2002. http://www.ncadd.org/programs/awareness/aam02factsheet.html. Accessed September 4, 2007.

8. Stall R, Wiley J. A comparison of alcohol and drug use patterns of homosexual and heterosexual men: the San Francisco Men's Health Study. *Drug Alcohol Depend.* 1988;22:63–73.

9. Stall R, Paul JP, Greenwood G, et al. Alcohol use, drug use and alcohol-related problems among men who have sex with men: the Urban Men's Health Study. *Addiction.* 2001;96:1589–1601.

10. Cochran SD, Ackerman D, Mays VM, Ross MW. Prevalence of non-medical drug use and dependence among homosexually active men and women in the US population. *Addiction.* 2004;99:989–998.

11. Koblin BA, Chesney MA, Husnik MJ, et al. High-risk behaviors among men who have sex with men in 6 US cities: baseline data from the EXPLORE Study. *Am J Public Health.* 2003;93:926–932.

12. Office of Applied Studies, Substance Abuse and Mental Health Services Administration (SAMHSA). National Household Survey on Drug Abuse (1966) Public Use Data File [CD-ROM]. Rockville, MD: SAMSHA; 1996.

13. Office of Applied Studies, SAMHSA. *1999 National Household Survey on Drug Abuse. Public Use Data File* [CD-ROM]. Rockville, MD: SAMSHA; 2000.

14. Ferrando S, Goggin K, Sewell M, et al. Substance use disorders in gay/bisexual men with HIV and AIDS. *Am J Addict.* 1998;7:51–60.

15. Remien RH, Goetz R, Rabkin JG, et al. Remission of substance use disorders: gay men in the first decade of AIDS. *J Stud Alcohol.* 1995;56: 226–232.

16. Ostrow DG. Sex, drugs and attitudes: searching for the common underlying causes of risk-taking among gay/bisexual men in the Multicenter AIDS Cohort Study (MACS). *PDE5 Inhibition and HIV Risk: Current Concepts and Controversies;* 2005 September 25–27; Potomac, MD (conference abstract).

17. Crosby GM, Stall RD, Paul JP, Barrett DC. Alcohol and drug use patterns have declined between generations of younger gay-bisexual men in San Francisco. *Drug Alcohol Depend.* 1998;52:177–182.

18. Halkitis PN, Green KA, Mourgues P. Longitudinal investigation of methamphetamine use among gay and bisexual men in New York City: findings from Project BUMPS. *J Urban Health.* 2005;82(suppl. 1):i18–i25.
19. Ostrow DG. The role of drugs in the sexual lives of men who have sex with men: continuing barriers to researching this question. *AIDS Behav.* 2000;4:205–219.
20. Martin JL, Dean L, Garcia M, Hall W. Barbara Snell Dohrenwend Memorial Lecture. The impact of AIDS on a gay community: changes in sexual behavior, substance use, and mental health. *Am J Community Psychol.* 1989;17:269–293.
21. Chesney MA, Barrett DC, Stall R. Histories of substance use and risk behavior: precursors to HIV seroconversion in homosexual men. *Am J Public Health.* 1998; 88:113–116.
22. Ostrow DG. Substance use and HIV-transmitting behaviors among gay and bisexual men. In: Battjes RJ, Sloboda Z, Grace WC, eds. *The Context of HIV Risk Among Drug Users and Their Sexual Partners.* Rockville, MD: Department of Health and Human Services; 1994:88–103. NIDA Research Monograph, No. 143.
23. Myers T, Rowe CJ, Tudiver FG, et al. HIV, substance use and related behaviour of gay and bisexual men: an examination of the talking sex project cohort. *Br J Addict.* 1992;87:207–214.
24. Case P. The history of methamphetamine: an epidemic in context. Presentation at 1st National Conference on Methamphetamine, HIV and HCV, August 2005, Salt Lake City, UT. http://www.harmredux.org/conferencemedia.html. Accessed September 4, 2007.
25. Anonymous. New drug replaces old. *New York Times,* January 23, 2006, p. A1.
26. Purcell DW, Moss S, Remien RH, Woods WJ, Parsons JT. Illicit substance use, sexual risk, and HIV-positive gay and bisexual men: differences by serostatus of casual partners. *AIDS.* 2005;19(suppl. 1):s37-s47.
27. Ostrow DG, Kalichman S. Methodological issues in HIV behavioral research. In: Peterson J, DiClemente R, eds. *Handbook of HIV Prevention.* New York, NY: Plenum Press; 2000:67–80.
28. Sullivan PS, Nakashima AK, Purcell DW, Ward JW. Geographic differences in noninjection and injection substance use among HIV-seropositive men who have sex with men: Western US versus other regions. Supplement to HIV/AIDS surveillance study group. *J Acquir Immune Defic Syndr Hum Retrovirol.* 1998;19:266–273.
29. Hirshfield S, Remien RH, Humberstone M, Walavalkar I, Chiasson MA. Substance use and high-risk sex among men who have sex with men: a national online study in the USA. *AIDS Care.* 2004;16:1036–1047.
30. Paul JP, Pollack L, Osmond D, Catania JA. Viagra (sildenafil) use in a population-based sample of U.S. men who have sex with men. *Sex Transm Dis.* 2005;32:531–533.
31. Mattison AM, Ross MW, Wolfson T, et al. Circuit party attendance, club drug use, and unsafe sex in gay men. *J Subst Abuse.* 2001;13:119–126.
32. Mansergh G, Colfax GN, Marks G, Rader M, Guzman R, Buchbinder S. The Circuit Party Men's Health Survey: findings and implications for gay and bisexual men. *Am J Public Health.* 2001;91:953–958.
33. Celentano DD, Valleroy LA, Sifakis F, et al. Associations between substance use and sexual risk among very young men who have sex with men. *Sex Transm Dis.* 2005;33:265–271.
34. Skinner WF, Otis MD. Drug and alcohol use among lesbian and gay people in a southern US sample: epidemiological, comparative, and methodological findings from the Trilogy Project. *J Homosex.* 1996;30:59–92.

35. Skinner WF. The prevalence and demographic predictors of illicit and licit drug use among lesbians and gay men. *Am J Public Health.* 1994;84:1307–1310.

36. Morales E, Graves M. Substance abuse: patterns and barriers to treatment for gay men and lesbians in San Francisco. *Report to Community Substance Abuse Services,* San Francisco Department of Public Health; 1983.

37. McKirnan DJ, Peterson PL. Alcohol and drug use among homosexual men and women: epidemiology and population characteristics. *Addict Behav.* 1989;14:545–553.

38. EMT Associates, Inc. *San Francisco Lesbian, Gay and Bisexual Substance Abuse Needs Assessment: Executive Summary.* Sacramento, CA: EMT Associates, Inc; 1991.

39. US Dept. of Health and Human Resources, Center for Substance Abuse Treatments. *A Provider's Introduction to Substance Abuse Treatment for Lesbian, Gay, Bisexual, and Transgender Individuals.* DHHS Publication No. (SMA) 01–3498. Rockville, MD: US Department of Health and Human Services; 2001.

40. McKirnan DJ, Peterson PL. AIDS-risk behavior among homosexual males: the role of attitudes and substance abuse. *Psychol Health.* 1989;3:161–171.

41. Ostrow DG, Plankey MW, 2005. Stimulant use in the MACS and WIHS cohorts and current efforts to understand the effects of methamphetamine use on HIV seroconversion and natural history of infection. Presentation at 1st National Conference on Methamphetamine, HIV and HCV; 2005 August 19–20; Salt Lake City, UT. http://www.harmredux.org/conferencemedia.html. Accessed August 22, 2007.

42. Ostrow DG, Silverberg MJ, Cook RL, Chmiel JS, Johnson L, Jacobson L. Prospective study of attitudinal and relationship predictors of sexual risk in the Multicenter AIDS Cohort Study. *AIDS and Behavior.* In press.

43. Plankey MW, Ostrow DG, Stall R, et al. The relationship between methamphetamine and popper use and risk of HIV seroconversion in the Multicenter AIDS Cohort Study. *J Acquir Immune Defic Syndr.* 2007;45:85–92.

44. Ostrow DE, Fox KJ, Chmiel JS, et al. Attitudes towards highly active antiretroviral therapy are associated with sexual risk taking among HIV-infected and uninfected homosexual men. *AIDS.* 2002;16:775–780.

45. Crepaz N, Hart TA, Marks G. Highly active antiretroviral therapy and sexual risk behavior: a meta-analytic review. *JAMA.* 2004;292:224–236.

46. Shernoff M. Without Condoms: unprotected sex, gay men and barebacking. New York, NY: Routledge; 2006.

47. Halkitis PN, Wilton L, Wolitski RJ, Parsons JT, Hoff CC, Bimbi DS. Barebacking identity among HIV-positive gay and bisexual men: demographic, psychological and behavioral correlates. *AIDS.* 2005;19(suppl. 1):S27–35.

48. Heckman T, Kalichman SC, Kelly JA. Sensation seeking as an explanation for the association between substance use and HIV-related risky sexual behavior. *Arch Sex Behav.* 1996;25:141–154.

49. DiFranceisco W, Ostrow DG, Chmiel JS. Sexual adventurism, high-risk behavior, and human immunodeficiency virus-1 seroconversion among the Chicago MACS-CCS Cohort, 1984 to 1992: a case-control study. *Sex Transm Dis.* 1996;23:453–460.

50. Stall R, McKusick L, Wiley J, Coates TJ, Ostrow DG. Alcohol and drug use during sexual activity and compliance with safe sex guidelines for AIDS: the AIDS Behavioral Research Project. *Health Educ Q.* 1986;13:359–371.

51. Diaz RM. *Latino Gay Men and HIV: Culture, Sexuality, and Risk Behavior.* New York, NY: Routledge; 1998.

52. Friedman SR, Curtis R, Neaigus A, Jose B, Des Jarlais DC. *Social Networks, Drug Injectors' Lives, and HIV/AIDS.* New York, NY: Kluwer Academic; 1999.

53. Rosen RC, Catania JA, Ehrhardt AA, et al. The Bolger Conference on PDE-5 Inhibition and HIV Risk: Summary and Recommendations. *J Sex Med.* 2006;3:960–975.

54. Ostrow DG, Beltran ED, Joseph JG, DiFranceisco W, Wesch J, Chmiel JS. Recreational drugs and sexual behavior in the Chicago MACS/CCS cohort of homosexually active men. Chicago Multicenter AIDS Cohort Study (MACS)/Coping and Change Study. *J Subst Abuse.* 1993;5:311–325.

55. Clatts MC, Welle DL, Goldsamt LA. Reconceptualizing the interaction of drug and sexual risk among MSM speed users: notes toward an ethno-epidemiology. *AIDS Behav.* 2001;5:115–130.

56. Jacobson LP, Ostrow DG, Hylton J, Gore ME, Weisberg M, Silvestre A. Unsafe sexual behavior among homosexual men increases in the era of highly active antiretroviral therapy. 15th International AIDS Conference; 2004 July 11–16; Bangkok, Thailand.

57. Klatsky AL. Alcohol, coronary disease and hypertension. *Annu Rev Med.* 1996;47: 149–160.

58. Klatsky AL, Armstrong MA, Friedman GD. Alcohol and mortality. *Ann Intern Med.* 1992;117:646–654.

59. Hingson RW, Heeren T, Zakocs RC, Kopstein A, Wechsler H. Magnitude of alcohol-related mortality and morbidity among US college students aged 18–24. *J Stud Alcohol.* 2002;63:136–144.

60. Fifield L, Lathan J, Phillips C. *Alcoholism in the Gay Community: The Price of Alienation, Isolation and Oppression.* Los Angeles, CA: Gay Community Services Center; 1977.

61. Lohrenz LJ, Connelly JC, Coyne L, Spare KE. Alcohol problems in several midwestern homosexual communities. *J Stud Alcohol.* 1978;39:1959–1963.

62. Martin J. Drinking patterns and drinking problems in a community sample of gay men. In Seminara D, ed. *Alcohol, Immunodulation and AIDS.* New York, NY: Alan R. Liss; 1990:27–34.

63. Bux D. The epidemiology of problem drinking in gay men and lesbians: a critical review. *Clin Psychol Rev.* 1996;16:277–298.

64. Cochran SD, Mays VM. Relation between psychiatric syndromes and behaviorally defined sexual orientation in a sample of the US population. *Am J Epidemiol.* 2000;151:516–523.

65. Drabble L, Midanik LT, Trocki K. Reports of alcohol consumption and alcohol-related problems among homosexual, bisexual and heterosexual respondents: results from the 2000 National Alcohol Survey. *J Stud Alcohol.* 2005;66:111–120.

66. Trocki KF, Drabble L, Midanik L. Use of heavier drinking contexts among heterosexuals, homosexuals and bisexuals: results from a National Household Probability Survey. *J Stud Alcohol.* 2005;66:105–110.

67. Greenwood GL, White EW, Page-Shafer K, et al. Correlates of heavy substance use among young gay and bisexual men: the San Francisco Young Men's Health Study. *Drug Alcohol Depend.* 2001;61:105–112.

68. Ghindia DJ, Kola LA. Co-factors affecting substance abuse among homosexual men: an investigation within a Midwestern gay community. *Drug Alcohol Depend.* 1996;41:167–177.

69. Paul JP, Stall R, Bloomfield KA. Gay and alcoholic: epidemiological and clinical issues. *Alcohol Health Res World.* 1991;15:151–160.

70. Stall R, Purcell DW. Intertwining epidemics: a review of research on substance use among men who have sex with men and its connection to the AIDS epidemic. *AIDS Behav.* 2000;4:181–192.

71. Murray CJ, Lopez AD. Alternative projects of mortality and disability by cause 1990–2020: Global Burden of Disease Study. *Lancet.* 1997;349:1498–1504.

72. Peto R, Lopez AD, Boreham J, Thun M, Heath C Jr. Mortality from tobacco in developed countries: indirect estimation from national vital statistics. *Lancet.* 1992;339:1268–1278.

73. Smith EA, Malone RE. The outing of Philip Morris: advertising tobacco to gay men. *Am J Public Health.* 2003;93:988–993.

74. Clifford GM, Polesel J, Rickenbach M, et al. Cancer risk in the Swiss HIV Cohort Study: associations with immunodeficiency, smoking, and highly active antiretroviral therapy. *J Natl Cancer Inst.* 2005;97:425–432.

75. Stall RD, Greenwood GL, Acree M, Paul J, Coates TJ. Cigarette smoking among gay and bisexual men. *Am J Public Health.* 1999;89:1875–1878.

76. Greenwood GL, Paul JP, Pollack LM, et al. Tobacco use and cessation among a household-based sample of US urban men who have sex with men. *Am J Public Health* 2005;95:145–151.

77. Tang H, Greenwood GL, Cowling DW, Lloyd JC, Roeseler AG, Bal DG. Cigarette smoking among lesbians, gays, and bisexuals: how serious a problem? (United States). *Cancer Causes Control.* 2004;15:797–803.

78. Ryan H, Wortley PM, Easton A, Pederson L, Greenwood G. Smoking among lesbians, gays and bisexuals: a review of the literature. *Am J Prev Med.* 2001;21:142–149.

79. Miller NS, Gold MS, Smith DE. *Manual of Therapeutics for Addictions.* New York, NY: Wiley-Liss; 1997.

80. Shoptaw S, Reback CJ, Peck JA, et al. Behavioral treatment approaches for methamphetamine dependence and HIV-related sexual risk behaviors among urban gay and bisexual men. *Drug Alcohol Depend.* 2005;78:125–134.

81. Stall R, Mills TC, Williamson J, et al. Association of co-occurring psychosocial health problems and increased vulnerability to HIV/AIDS among urban men who have sex with men. *Am J Public Health* 2003;93:939–942.

82. Hart JT. The inverse care law. *Lancet.* 1971;1:405–412.

83. Ostrow DG, Vanable PA, McKirnan DJ, Brown L. Hepatitis and HIV risk among drug-using men who have sex with men: demonstration of Hart's Law of Inverse Access and application to HIV. *J Gay Lesb Med Assoc.* 1999;3:127–136.

85. Purcell, D., Parsons, J., Halkitis, P., Mizuno, Y., Woods, W. Substance use and sexual transmission risk behavior of HIV-positive men who have sex with men. *J Subst Abuse* 2001 13(1–2):185–200.

6

Sexually Transmitted Infections among Gay and Bisexual Men

Ronald O. Valdiserri

In 1997, when the Institute of Medicine issued its groundbreaking analysis of sexually transmitted diseases (STD) in the United States, *The Hidden Epidemic*, the report estimated that approximately $10 billion were spent annually in the United States on major STDs other than AIDS (acquired immunodeficiency syndrome).[1] More recent estimates suggest annual direct medical costs for STDs, including human immunodeficiency virus (HIV), as high as $15.5 billion dollars.[2] Notably, these estimates do not include indirect costs, such as lost productivity, lost wages, and out-of-pocket expenses—which would drive the economic cost even higher. Undeniably, STDs continue to represent a major threat to the health of many Americans.

As this chapter will document, STDs are an especially important health concern for gay and bisexual men. Compared to heterosexual men, gay and bisexual men in the United States are at disproportionate risk for many STDs, including HIV. Reasons for disparate STD rates are multiple and complex, and cannot be explained solely on the basis of differences in sexual practices or number of sexual partners. A variety of social, behavioral, and physiological factors also contribute to these disparities and will be described in subsequent sections of this chapter. Certainly, one cannot minimize the fact that within the already stigmatized domain of sexually transmitted diseases, the added burden of anti-gay prejudice and stigma[3] engenders further barriers to effective STD prevention and control efforts.

The first part of this chapter will present information about the prevalence of various STDs among gay and bisexual men in the United States—compared to their heterosexual counterparts. With the exception of HIV and hepatitis A, B, and C, which are covered in separate chapters within this volume, descriptive epidemiology will be provided for all major sexually transmitted diseases. Next will follow an analysis of what is known about the genesis of these disparities—with an emphasis on promising approaches to resolving them. To conclude the chapter, research questions that address major gaps in knowledge will be posed. For ease of communication, the term "men who have sex with men," or MSM, will be used to describe men who engage in same sex activities— regardless of their sexual identification.

Prevalence of STDs among Men Who Have Sex with Men (MSM)

As will soon become apparent to the reader, there are many significant gaps in public health's ability to accurately describe the incidence and prevalence of STDs among MSM—particularly among various subgroups. A major reason for this significant information deficit is the fact that nationally notifiable surveil-lance data do not routinely include information on sexual practices—nor the gender of sexual partner. Therefore, much of the MSM-specific information that is available comes from clinic- or community-based samples, enhanced sur-veillance projects, and specific research studies.[4] Some population-based studies are reported in the literature, but these are the exception rather than the rule.

Despite less than complete data, the preponderance of available evidence supports the finding that many STDs occur at disproportionately high rates among MSM. Further, after a period of substantial declines in STDs among MSM in the early 1980s—due to AIDS-related decreases in sexual risk behaviors—an increasing number of MSM now appear to be acquiring STDs.[5–10]

Bacterial STDs

As stated above, information on the incidence and prevalence of STDs in the United States is far from complete, and varies in quality, depending upon the source of the data.[11] Even national health surveys, designed to provide na-tionally representative samples, include relatively small numbers of STDs in their samples—thus leading to wide confidence intervals in various subpop-ulations.[11] Data limitations are especially pronounced when we consider in-cidence and prevalence estimates of STDs for the subset of MSM. Therefore, MSM-specific data are often derived from special studies or from samples of men attending clinics for the treatment of STDs. Of the three bacterial dis-eases reviewed in this section, there is substantial evidence for disparate rates of gonorrhea and syphilis among MSM (Table 6-1). In the case of chlamydia, specific serovars, or strains, appear to be disproportionately higher among MSM—although many cases of rectal chlamydia may remain undiagnosed in MSM (see Table 6-1).

Gonorrhea

Before the onset of widespread sexual behavior changes brought about in response to the AIDS epidemic, MSM in the United States typically had higher

Table 6-1. Prevalence of selected bacterial STDs in men who have sex with men (MSM) vs. men who have sex with women (MSW), selected studies

STD	Setting	Year(s)	Prevalence (MSM vs MSW)	Reference #
Gonorrhea	STD clinic	1977–1978	30.3% vs. 19.8% ($p < .001$)	16
Gonorrhea	STD clinic	1980	25% vs. 12% ($p < .01$)	17
Gonorrhea	STD clinic	1996–2001	12.9% vs. 6.9% ($p < .0001$)	8
Gonorrhea	STD clinic	1997	44.6% vs. 25.6% ($p < .001$)	28
Syphilis	STD clinic	1977–1978	1.08% vs. 0.34% ($p < .001$)	16
Syphilis	STD clinic	1981–1982	7.1% vs. 2.2% ($p <. 001$)	34
Syphilis	Early syphilis cases, San Francisco	2003	94.4% vs. 5.6%*	43
Chlamydia	STD clinic	1980	5% vs. 14% ($p <. 01$)	17
Chlamydia	STD clinic	1996–2001	6.7% vs. 12.7% ($p <. 0001$)	8

*Includes heterosexual female cases

rates of gonorrhea compared to the general population.[12–14] Among some four thousand MSM surveyed in 1977, 39% reported a previous gonorrhea infection.[15] Judson and colleagues compared MSM to heterosexual men visiting an STD clinic in Denver between July 1977 and December 1978 and found the prevalence of gonorrhea to be 30.3% (1601/5282) for MSM compared to 19.8% (2360/11,903) for heterosexual clients ($p < 0.001$).[16] Similarly, among men presenting to a Seattle STD clinic in 1980 with new symptoms or for screening, 25% (40/161) of MSM had positive gonorrhea cultures, compared to 12% (53/435) of heterosexual men ($p < 0.01$).[17]

But in the years immediately following the onset of AIDS in the United States, several metropolitan areas, including New York,[18] Denver,[19] Seattle,[20] Los Angeles,[21] and San Francisco[21] reported declines in gonorrhea rates among MSM. These declines were broadly attributed to increased publicity about the deadly epidemic, behavior changes in response to fear of AIDS, and community-based programs to encourage the adoption of safer behaviors among sexually active MSM.[22–25] This trend began to reverse itself in the 1990s, when several US cities reported increases in gonorrhea rates among MSM[6–8]; furthermore, reported gonorrhea increases among MSM were taking place in the face of continuing overall declines in gonorrhea in the United States.[4]

Results from a national sentinel surveillance system to monitor trends in antimicrobial resistance in *Neisseria gonorrhoeae* reported that, between the years of 1992 and 1999, MSM accounted for an "increasing proportion of gonococcal urethritis cases" collected annually from participating STD clinics in 29 US cities.[26] Whereas in 1992, MSM accounted for 4.5% of annual cases collected through a protocol blinded to sexual orientation, that proportion had increased to 13.2% by 1999 ($p < .001$).[26] Of note, because the Gonococcal Isolate Surveillance Project (GISP) includes only men with urethral gonorrhea, these figures likely underestimate the true scope of the increase in MSM—excluding, as they do, cases of pharyngeal and rectal gonorrhea.[27]

Reminiscent of disparities noted in the pre-AIDS era, most recent reports indicate rates of gonorrhea among STD clinic attendees that are higher for MSM compared to heterosexual men. Among men coming to the Denver Metro Health STD Clinic for services between 1996 and 2001, the gonorrhea positivity rate for MSM (from all anatomic sites) was 12.9%, compared to 6.9% among heterosexual men ($p < .0001$).[8] Reviewing data from 1997 for men presenting to the San Francisco City Clinic with urethritis, the isolation of *Neisseria gonorrhoeae* in MSM was 44.6% (112/251) compared to an isolation rate of 25.6% (212/829) among heterosexual men ($p < .001$).[28] In a separate analysis, reported by Katz and his colleagues, rates of male rectal gonorrhea in San Francisco increased from 72 per 100,000 in 1992 to 160 per 100,000 in 1996.[29] Coincidental with increasing rates of rectal gonorrhea were increasing self-reports of unprotected (i.e., no condom used) anal sex and multiple male partners, collected from cross-sectional surveys of MSM in San Francisco.[29] The increased incidence of male rectal gonorrhea described in San Francisco in the mid- to late 1990s was seen in all racial/ethnic and age groups but was reported to be highest among men aged 25–34 years.[7]

Several recent analyses have documented that among MSM diagnosed with gonorrhea, a disproportionate number are also infected with HIV.[30–32] Data from eight US cities (Chicago, Denver, District of Columbia, Houston, Long Beach, Philadelphia, San Francisco, and Seattle), reporting on gonorrhea among MSM attending STD clinics in those cities in 2002, described the median gonorrhea positivity among MSM as 17.1% (clinic range 11.4% to 23.0%).[30] Whether for urethral, rectal, or pharyngeal gonorrhea, positivity rates were higher for HIV-infected MSM (21%, 10.3%, and 7.7%, respectively) compared to MSM who were HIV negative or who did not know their serostatus (12.5%, 5.5%, and 3.9%, respectively).[30]

Syphilis

In the 1970s, MSM were overrepresented among persons diagnosed with infectious syphilis in the United States. One telling analysis reckoned that the proportion of patients with infectious syphilis who named same-sex contacts, largely male, had risen from 25% in 1970 to nearly 49% in 1980.[33] Two large studies comparing STD rates among clients attending STD clinics carried out in the late 1970s and the early 1980s, respectively, showed significantly higher rates of syphilis among MSM versus heterosexual men: 1.08% versus 0.34% (p < 0.001)[16] and 7.1% versus 2.2% ($p < 0.001$).[34] And in a survey of over four thousand MSM conducted in 1977, men with "four or more years of homo-sexual experience" reported past syphilis infections at rates ranging from 11% to 21.4% depending, respectively, on whether they lived in small cities or large metropolitan areas.[15]

Much like the trends observed for gonorrhea, rates of syphilis among MSM declined in the years following the onset of AIDS in the United States.[35] Although the overall incidence of primary and secondary syphilis increased in the United States between 1981 and 1989, significant declines in the incidence of syphilis among white men—from 10 cases per 100,000 persons in 1982 to 3.2 cases per 100,000 in 1989—were largely attributed to fewer cases among MSM.[36] This same report indicated that similar, albeit smaller, decreases may have occurred among black MSM.[36]

Following syphilis declines among MSM, reported during the 1980s and the early to mid-1990s, several US cities, including New York,[9,37] Seattle,[10] San Francisco,[38] Los Angeles,[38,39] and Chicago[40] reported significant increases in the number and proportion of primary and secondary syphilis cases occurring among MSM. National trends corroborated this reversal. After a decade of overall national declines in primary and secondary syphilis beginning in 1990, the national rates of primary and secondary syphilis in the United States in-creased in 2001, 2002, 2003, and 2004.[4,41] Further, overall increases in rates during 2000–2004 were observed only among men.[4] A model developed to determine the proportion of all nationally reported cases of primary and sec-ondary syphilis occurring among MSM estimated that the proportion had increased from 5% in 1999 to 47% in 2002.[42] The model revealed that the increases were "most dramatic" among white MSM—but also "large" among Hispanic and African American MSM.[42] In San Francisco, of 522 cases of early syphilis reported in 2003, 97% of all reported cases were male, 94% of all reported cases were among MSM, and only 6% were among heterosexual men and women.[43]

Epidemiologic investigations into syphilis outbreaks among MSM have re-vealed several associated factors. Among the most prominent is the emerging use of the Internet as a "virtual venue" for sexually active MSM to meet male sex partners. Of the 434 cases of early syphilis among MSM reported to the San Francisco Department of Public Health in 2002, 33% of the men reported meeting sex partners on the Internet[44]; similar findings have been reported from outbreak investigations in Los Angeles.[45,46] Among MSM diagnosed with syphilis in California between 2001 and 2003, those who reported meeting partners through the Internet had higher numbers of partners and greater numbers of nonlocatable partners, compared to those who had not used the Internet.[47]

Increases in illegal methamphetamine use, reported in the western United States in the 1990s,[48] have been associated with high risk sexual behavior among MSM[49] and, in some analyses, higher rates of STDs—including syphilis.[50] A nested case-control study of some twenty-six hundred MSM, using data collected online in 2001, showed that men with an incident STD were twice as likely to report methamphetamine use.[51]

Another significant observation is that MSM with primary and secondary syphilis are more likely to be infected with HIV. Investigation of a syphilis outbreak among MSM in southern California in 2000 revealed that, of the men who knew their HIV serostatus, 60% were positive.[52] A chart review of MSM receiving syphilis testing at a New York City STD clinic in 2002 found that syphilis seropositivity was nearly five times higher among men infected with HIV compared to men who were not.[53] Another New York City study compared 88 MSM with syphilis to 176 controls, finding that HIV prevalence among those with syphilis was 48% compared to 15% among the controls ($p < .001$).[54] Epidemiologists, estimating the rate of primary and secondary syphilis in persons living with HIV in the United States in 2002, concluded that the rate of primary and secondary syphilis in persons with HIV is considerably higher than the rate among the general population—with extraordinarily high estimated syphilis rates among HIV positive MSM: 336 cases per 100,000, compared to a general population rate of 2.4 cases per 100,000.[55]

Chlamydia

Chlamydia trachomatis is the most commonly reported notifiable disease in the United States.[56] Generally, rates for genital chlamydia infection in women are higher than rates among men,[4] but chlamydia trends among MSM have not been well described. A handful of clinic-based surveys conducted prior to the onset of the AIDS epidemic showed that MSM with urethritis were usually less likely to have urethral chlamydia infection, compared to heterosexual men with urethritis.[17,57]

In the late 1990s, some STD clinics began to report increases in rates of laboratory-confirmed chlamydia infections among MSM.[10,58] For example, Geisler and colleagues reported that anorectal chlamydia infection increased from 4% (1994–1996) to 7.6% (1997–1999) among MSM attending an STD clinic in Seattle ($p < .005$).[58]

A survey of 4860 MSM who presented to San Francisco's Municipal STD Clinic in 2002 found that, overall, 5.3% had urethral chlamydia and 9.2% had rectal chlamydia.[59] And surveillance data collected in 2003 from MSM visiting STD clinics in health departments and in community-based organizations in ten U.S. cities (Boston, Chicago, Denver, Houston, Long Beach, New York City, Philadelphia, San Francisco, Seattle, and Washington, DC) revealed substantial rates of chlamydia infection.[4] A median of 82% of men visiting participating clinics were tested, and the median urethral chlamydial positivity was 6% (range: 5% to 8%).[4]

Although the evidence is not extensive, rates of chlaymdia urethritis generally appear to be higher among heterosexual men attending STD clinics compared to MSM in those same settings[8,17] (see Table 6-1). Non-STD-clinic based samples of men also support the finding that chlamydia urethritis is more common among heterosexual men compared to MSM.[60-62] But this does not mean that chlamydia is an insubstantial problem for MSM. Of some 3,400 San Francisco MSM tested for pharyngeal, urethral, and rectal chlamydia in 2003, most of the infections were detected in the rectum (8%), followed by the urethra (4%) and the pharynx (1%).[63] Furthermore, nearly 85% of rectal chalymdia infections were asymptomatic. This clinical fact, along with the knowledge that, at the time of this writing, culture (which is expensive and cumbersome) is the only approved FDA chlaymdia test for rectal specimens—suggests that many cases of rectal chlamydia infection among MSM remain undiagnosed.[63]

Where one does observe significant chlamydia disparities between heterosexual and homosexual men is with reported cases of lymphogranuloma venereum (LGV). LGV is a systemic, sexually transmitted disease caused by one of three specific serovars, or strains, of *Chlamydia trachomatis*: L1, L2, and L3.[64] LGV occurs rarely in North America and Europe, though it is endemic in some parts of the world, including West Africa, India, and parts of Southeast Asia.[64] It should be noted that non-LGV strains of chlamydia can produce proctitis,[58] but these cases are generally less severe than the intense inflammatory proctitis seen with LGV-specific strains of chlaymdia.[65]

In late 2004 and early 2005, health departments in San Francisco,[66] New York City,[67] Boston,[68] and Atlanta[69] issued health alerts/advisories warning of documented cases of LGV among sexually active MSM—several of whom were infected with HIV. These LGV outbreaks, still under investigation at the time of this writing, follow recent reports of outbreaks of LGV in MSM from the Netherlands, Belgium, France, and Sweden.[70] In 2004, 27 cases of LGV were reported to the US Centers for Disease Control and Prevention.[4]

Viral STDs

This section will address human papillomavirus (HPV), genital herpes simplex virus (HSV), and human herpesvirus 8 (HHV-8); HIV and hepatitis A, B, and C viruses will be addressed separately, in subsequent chapters. While numerous studies have documented the disproportionate impact of HIV on MSM, it would be a mistake to ignore or minimize the health impact of other sexually transmitted viral pathogens (see Table 6-2). Among all men in the United States, both homosexual and heterosexual, viral diseases (including HIV) account for the majority of sexual behavior–attributed health burden.[71]

And two of the pathogens discussed in this section, HPV and HHV-8, are associated with the development of malignancies in MSM—especially men whose immune systems are compromised.

Human Papillomavirus (HPV)

Human papillomavirus (HPV) is the most common sexually transmitted infection in the United States[72]—with an estimated three-quarters of reproductive-aged persons having been infected with genital HPV.[11] A small percentage of infected men and women will develop anogenital warts as a consequence of HPV infection,[73] but the far more serious consequence is the development of anogenital cancers among a subset of persons infected with oncogenic HPV types,[74] especially type 16.[72] Although a vaccine against HPV (effective against the two HPV strains that account for most uterine cervical cancer and the two strains that cause almost all genital warts) was licensed in June 2006, at the time of this writing, it is only recommended for females.[75]

Because of inadequate patient education efforts and incomplete media coverage, many sexually active US women do not fully understand the link between HPV and uterine cervical cancer.[76] Perhaps even more poorly understood, or recognized, is the link between HPV and anal cancer—especially among MSM. Higher rates of anal cancer among "never married" men have long suggested an epidemiological association between HPV and male-to-male sexual behavior[77–79]—especially the strong association of anal cancer with the specific sexual practice of receptive anal intercourse.[80] While, overall, rates of

Table 6-2. Prevalence of selected viral STDs in men who have sex with men (MSM) versus men who have sex with women (MSW), selected studies

STD	Setting	Year(s)	Prevalence (MSM vs. MSW)	Reference
HPV-16	Population-based survey	1991–1994	37.7% vs. 8.1% ($p < .05$)	72
HSV-2	Community-based survey	1988–1989	40% vs. 20%	96
HSV-2	HIV test site	1997–2000	24.1% vs. 13%	97
HSV-2	Population-based survey	1999–2002	23.9% vs. 12.8%	*
HHV-8	Population-based sample	1984–1985	37.6% vs. 0% ($p < .001$)	111
HHV-8	Cross-sectional survey	1997–1998	6% vs. 5%	116

* unpublished data, Dr. Gerry McQuillan, NCHS, CDC

anal cancer are higher among US women than men,[79] when one considers sexual orientation, MSM have annual incidence rates of anal cancer approaching 35/100,000—"which approximates the incidence of cervical cancer in women before the advent of routine cervical pap smear screening."[81]

HPV is not a reportable disease in the United States, and estimates of prevalence and incidence are complicated by the fact that the majority of persons who are infected with the virus have neither clinical signs nor symptoms.[73] Fortunately, important information on the seroprevalence of HPV-16, perhaps the most common oncogenic viral type associated with anal cancer,[82] is available from a population-based survey of American adolescents and adults.[72] Examining sera from a nationally representative sample of the US population, collected between 1991 and 1994, Stone and colleagues demonstrated extremely high rates of HPV-16 seropositivity for MSM.[72] Overall, HPV-16 seroprevalence was higher among women (17.9%) than men (7.9%). Men who reported never having sex with another man had an HPV-16 seroprevalence of 8.1% compared to a 37.7% seroprevalence among men who reported ever having sex with another man; controlling for other factors, including race and age, MSM were over six times as likely to be infected with HPV-16 compared to heterosexual men.[72]

A 2001–2002 study of 1218 HIV-negative MSM from four American cities (Boston, Denver, New York, San Francisco) found that 57% of the participants had anal HPV infection and that 26% were infected with a viral type associated with the development of cancer.[83] HPV infection was independently associated with a history of receptive anal intercourse and more than five sex partners during the preceding six months.[83] Other studies have documented a strong association between HIV and HPV[84–86]—which may be due, in part, to reactivation of previous HPV infection.[87] Reactivation of previous HPV infection secondary to HIV is suggested by a study of over eighteen hundred HIV-positive women, which showed that "a substantial fraction of incident HPV detection . . . is not related to recent sexual activity."[88]

Given that HIV infection can influence the progression of HPV infection, it is not surprising that HIV-infected persons, including HIV-infected MSM, are at increased risk for anogenital HPV-associated cancers.[89,90] Data from 11 state and metropolitan AIDS and cancer registries were linked between 1995 and 1998, showing that for men who contracted HIV through homosexual contact, anal cancer occurred in "extreme excess," with a relative risk of 99.8 for in-situ cancer and 59.5 for invasive anal cancer.[89] An analysis of anal cancer trends in California between 1973 and 1999 showed a near doubling of incidence, between 1988 and 1999, among men who lived in San Francisco County.[90] Although information on sexual orientation was not available, the researchers noted that a high proportion of men from San Francisco with anal cancer were single and never married—suggesting that the men were likely homosexual. The researchers opined that "HIV-related immunosuppression may have accelerated the development of anal cancer and that longer survival of HIV positive men may have allowed cancers with a longer latency to develop."[90]

Herpes Simplex Virus (HSV)

Genital herpes, caused by herpes simplex virus type 2 (HSV-2) and, less frequently, by HSV-1,[91] is one of the three most prevalent STDs in the U.S.[11,92] Population-based surveys estimate that nearly one in five Americans older than age 12 have been infected with HSV-2,[93] with women exhibiting higher rates of infection compared to men.[94] Not surprisingly, higher rates of HSV-2 seroprevalence have been found in persons attending STD clinics. A sample of 4128 heterosexual men and women recruited in the mid-1990s from five inner-city US STD clinics found an overall HSV-2 seroprevalence of 40.8%; seroprevalence was higher in women (52.0%) than men (32.4%) and in blacks (48.1%) compared to non-blacks (29.6%).[95]

Seroprevalence surveys of HSV-2 infection among MSM show rates ranging from 26% in a cohort of 578 HIV negative Seattle men[62] to 40% in a cross-sectional community-based survey conducted in three San Francisco neighborhoods.[96] In the latter study, 20% of heterosexual men were positive for HSV-2, compared to 40% of MSM.[96] Among 987 persons seeking anonymous HIV testing in San Francisco, two or more times between 1997 and 2000, 23.5% were seropositive for HSV-2 antibodies; by sexual orientation: 13% of heterosexual men were positive for HSV-2 compared to 24.1% of MSM and 28.7% of women.[97] An age-adjusted analysis of the National Health and Nutrition Examination Survey (NHANES), a population-based survey conducted during 1999–2002, revealed an HSV-2 prevalence of 23.9% for MSM compared to 12.8% for heterosexual men (unpublished data, Dr. G. McQuillan).

Rates of HSV-2 infection are even higher among MSM who are infected with HIV. Among 109 MSM recruited from a Seattle AIDS project in the mid-1980s, HSV-2 antibodies were found among 73% of 49 men with HIV infection, compared to 32% of 60 men who were HIV seronegative ($p < .0001$).[98] A large case-control study conducted prospectively among MSM in six U.S. cities (Boston, Chicago, Denver, New York, San Francisco, Seattle) during the 1990s demonstrated that previous HSV-2 infection was associated with a nearly twofold increased likelihood of HIV acquisition—independent of other risk factors.[99] Also, it has been shown that acute infection with HSV, as well as a recurrent outbreak, can increase retroviral load among those infected with HIV.[100]

Human Herpesvirus 8 (HHV-8)

Human herpesvirus 8, also known as the Kaposi's sarcoma-associated herpesvirus, was first identified in 1994, when unique viral DNA fragments were isolated from Kaposi's sarcoma (KS) tissues obtained from AIDS patients.[101] But even prior to the identification of HHV-8, a sexually transmitted factor, other than HIV, was long suspected in the etiology of Kaposi's sarcoma—because of the disproportionate occurrence of the malignancy among MSM with AIDS, compared to persons who acquired HIV through nonsexual routes.[102–104] Subsequent research strengthened the supposition of a causative role of HHV-8 in the development of KS. British researchers demonstrated that the detection of HHV-8 in peripheral blood cells of HIV-infected persons, without KS, predicted the subsequent development of KS lesions.[105] A retrospective analysis of stored sera from 40 HIV-infected MSM who eventually developed KS showed that most (80%) developed antibodies to HHV-8 before the clinical development of KS.[106]

While the study of HHV-8 is far from complete, current evidence suggests that infection is uncommon among the general US population. Overall, it is estimated that approximately 3% of US blood donors are seropositive for HHV-8.[107] In addition to the strong association of HHV-8 infection among persons with KS,[105,106,108,109] relatively high rates of HHV-8 infection have been found among women with multiple sex partners,[110] injection drug users,[104,110] and MSM.[111–115] Among US MSM, studies have shown prevalences of HHV-8 infection ranging from 20% to 48%, with the highest rates being observed among men who are also infected with HIV.[111–113,115] However, a 1997–1998 serosurvey of young MSM, aged 15 to 22 years, revealed a much lower rate of HHV-8 seroprevalence—6%—comparable to rates observed among similarly aged young heterosexual men, recruited in the same venues.[116] The authors suggested that past estimates of HHV-8 seroprevalence among MSM may have been higher because of a number of factors, including differences in laboratory methods and declining rates of HHV-8 infection among MSM—after a peak in the 1980s. [116]

Although the precise mode of HHV-8 transmission is unknown, the fact that HHV-8 seroprevalence is higher among MSM with increased numbers of male sex partners[111,112] and evidence of past STDs,[113,117] strongly suggests a sexual mode of transmission. However, other potential modes of transmission, including exposure to infectious saliva, have been suggested.[118] What is known is that MSM who are dually infected with HIV and HHV-8 are at high risk of developing Kaposi's sarcoma[104,113]—although widespread use of highly active antiretroviral therapy in the United States has been associated with significant declines in the incidence of KS among HIV-infected MSM.[119]

Enteric STDs

A wide variety of pathogens can be sexually transmitted among MSM as a result of oral-anal sexual activity or fecal contamination in the context of oral-genital sex (i.e., indirect oral-anal contact). Thus, infections typically associated with fecally contaminated food or water, such as shigellosis,[120–122] typhoid fever,[123] giardiasis,[124–125] and amebiasis,[126–127] can be sexually transmitted among MSM. Hepatitis A, another important enterically transmitted pathogen, will be discussed in Chapter 7.

For most sexually transmitted enteric infections among MSM, detailed prevalence and incidence data are not available. However, a number of studies conducted in the late 1970s and early 1980s documented high rates of infection with various enteric pathogens among MSM. Stool specimens from a convenience sample of 89 sexually active MSM attending an STD treatment facility in New York City in 1977 revealed that 26% harbored pathogenic protozoa.[128] A subsequent study of 180 consecutive male and female patients at an STD clinic in New York City, carried out between 1978 and 1979, showed that exclusively homosexual men had a prevalence of *Giardia lamblia* and/or *Entamoeba histolytica* of 21.5%, compared to 6.2% in bisexual men; none of the heterosexual men or women in this study were infected with these pathogens.[129] In the early 1980s, a survey of MSM with intestinal symptoms[130] and another one studying MSM recruited from a medical practice setting[131] revealed even higher rates of infection with enteric pathogens.

More recent reports suggest that sexually transmitted *Shigella* infection remains a health problem for at least some populations of MSM. An analysis of 228 culture-confirmed cases of shigellosis in San Francisco during 1996, by HIV status and sexual orientation, showed substantially elevated incidence rates for persons who were infected with HIV—especially gay men.[132] Annual incidence rates, per 100,000 population, were determined to be 12.4 for HIV-negative heterosexuals (men and women); 60.1 for HIV-negative gay men; 378 for HIV-positive heterosexuals; and 442 for HIV-positive gay men.[132]

In 2000–2001, public health officials in San Francisco reported an outbreak of *Shigella sonnei* infection, largely among men.[122] Upon further investigation, it was determined that 61% of men with positive cultures were homosexual; 8% were heterosexual; and sexual behavior was unknown for 31%.[122] Consistent with the previous study, about half of the men were also infected with HIV.[122] Outbreaks of *S. sonnei* were also reported among MSM from Massachusetts and New York City, during that same time period (i.e., 2000–2001).[133]

Understanding Disparate Rates of STDs among MSM

Because of the manner in which they are contracted, that is, through intimate sexual relations, STDs continue to carry substantial stigma.[1] This stigma may be further amplified by strong negative attitudes about homosexuality and homosexual practices,[3] thus interfering with an objective assessment of the various factors that result in disparate rates of STDs observed among some populations of MSM. For example, while increased numbers of partners is a major variable influencing STD risk, and some MSM report large numbers of sexual partners,[12,15,16] settling on indiscriminant sexual behavior as the sole reason for increased STDs among MSM is overly simplistic and ignores the influence of other individual and societal determinants of sexual behavior. In order to identify effective strategies to reduce STD disparities among MSM, it is critical that we consider, in detail, the panoply of factors, including increased partner number, that contribute to disparate rates of infection. The following discussion will briefly review these variables; readers should note that several are covered, in depth, in other chapters in this volume.

Physiological Factors

Compared to the female sex organs, the penis is highly "effective" at inoculating pathogens during the process of ejaculation, and this physiological reality has been cited as one reason for increased rates of STD transmission among men who have sex with other men.[134] Also, as noted by Daniel William— an American pioneer in the diagnosis and treatment of STDs among gay and bisexual men—"the functional overlap between the human genital and excretory systems poses a further disease hazard to gay men in regard to an important part of their sexual activity."[135] Unlike the vagina, which is lined by a thick layer of stratified squamous epithelium, the more delicate columnar epithelium of the rectum proves a far less formidable physical barrier to pathogenic microorganisms it might encounter during the act of anal intercourse.

MSM Sexual Behaviors and STD Disparities

Accurate descriptions of sexual behaviors among US MSM are limited, in part, by incomplete estimates of the size of this population. Earlier studies, which did not rely on representative samples, estimated that as many as 8% of US men may be exclusively homosexual.[136] However, more recent estimates suggest that same gender sexual contact among US men ranges from 2% to 5%, depending upon the time frame studied and the behavioral definitions employed.[136–140]

Studies conducted in the 1970s, prior to the onset of the AIDS epidemic and in the first decade of the US "gay liberation" movement, indicated that homosexual men "were more likely than heterosexual men to have had a very large number of sexual partners."[136] Although these early studies were often based on convenience samples,[141] more recent analyses, with better sampling strategies, continue to document some differences in partner number when comparing homosexual to heterosexual men. For example, a 1997 national survey of over 13,000 US college students found that, compared to heterosexual males, men with same sex partners were significantly more likely to report two or more sexual partners in the 30 days prior to survey.[139] For college men with only female partners, 8.6% reported two or more recent partners, compared to 15.9% of bisexual men reporting two or more partners and 20.4% of exclusively homosexual men reporting two or more partners ($p < 0.001$).[139]

While it is plausible to surmise that negative societal reactions to homosexual attraction, as witnessed by the widespread absence of legal recognition of same sex partnerships, contribute to multiple sexual partnerships and thus elevated rates of STDs among MSM,[142,143] a more fundamental reason may lie in the fecund domains of sex and gender. The International Sexuality Description Project, a cross-cultural survey of some 16,000 people across ten major world regions, has demonstrated that "sex differences in the desire for sexual variety are culturally universal."[144] This international collaboration documented that men, regardless of sexual orientation or culture, consistently desired larger numbers of sexual partners than women.[144] Further, compared to women, men required less time to elapse before consenting to sexual intercourse with a new partner and were more likely to seek short-term "mateships" than women.[144] Therefore, even in the circumstance of a neutral societal reaction to same sex attraction, one might predict that two men would be more likely to have larger partner numbers, on average, than a male-female pair bond—and thus be more likely to become exposed to sexual pathogens.

Sexual Networks and STD Disparities

Of course, we do not live in a society that is neutral on the issue of homosexuality.[145] Undoubtedly, stigma plays a role in the expression of sexual behaviors among MSM. Perhaps the most distinctive manifestation of stigma's impact on MSM sexual behavior is seen in the phenomenon of "public sex environments" (PSEs). PSEs are typically public (e.g., public toilets, parks, etc.) and sometimes commercial (e.g., adult bookstores, bathhouses) venues where men can meet other men for furtive, often anonymous, sex.[146,147] According to gay historian Allan Berube, legal sanctions against homosexuality forced MSM to become "sexual outlaws" who developed special expertise in "stealing moments of privacy and at finding the cracks in society where they could meet and not get caught."[148] In Berube's analysis, PSEs fulfill an important social function for some MSM.

Some of the men who meet male partners in PSEs, including bathhouses, do not identify themselves as gay—and a substantial percentage report having female partners.[149] Given the mix of anonymity, risky sexual behavior, and multiple partners, it is not surprising that meeting sexual partners in PSEs is associated with an increased risk for acquiring or transmitting STDs.[150,151] Thus, another contributor to the disparate risk of STDs for some MSM relates to the fact that they meet their partners in venues where high-risk sexual activities take place and/or partners who are at high risk for transmitting STDs are likely to be encountered.[152]

The Internet is an interesting, evolving example of a "sexual risk" venue for some MSM. As mentioned earlier, meeting partners online has been associated with outbreaks of syphilis among MSM.[44–47,153] While it is unclear how much the Internet may actually increase or potentiate unsafe sexual behavior, it is clear that some MSM are using the Internet to seek sexual partners with whom to engage in high risk sexual activities.[154–156] As such, from a sexual network perspective, the Internet can be considered as an effective mechanism through which "core transmitters" of STDs (in this instance, MSM at high risk of transmitting STDs) can rapidly acquire new, susceptible partners.

Sexual network characteristics are considered increasingly germane to understanding the spread of STDs and, by extension, conceptualizing interventions to prevent or interrupt the spread of infection. An early study of HIV transmission among MSM in Iceland suggested that sexual contact in the community was disassortative (i.e., sexual contact occurring between men of disparate sexual activity levels), with the prediction of an extensive spread of HIV throughout the MSM community.[157] Laumann and Youm hypothesized that highly disassortative partner choice with regard to risk (i.e., the pairing of high risk with low risk partners), along with more racially segregated partnering (i.e., African Americans are more likely to choose other African American sexual partners), results in "substantially higher" STD rates for African Americans, compared to other racial/ethnic groups in the United States.[158] Similar dynamics have been invoked to explain the high rates of HIV observed in African American MSM: specifically, the pairing of younger MSM, at lower risk for infection, with older MSM—who are more likely to have been previously exposed to HIV.[159–160]

As observed by Wohlfeiler and Potterat, "MSM have created efficient ways of finding sexual partners,"[161] including the Internet and "traditional" public sex environments like bathhouses and adult bookstores. While further study is needed to better understand them, mounting evidence suggests that sexual networks are a potent variable influencing disparate risk for STD acquisition and transmission among MSM.[152,161]

Developmental and Psychological Factors

In general, US adolescents and young adults are at high risk for acquiring STDs[4]; this observation may be especially true for young MSM. Although data are patchy, studies suggest that young MSM initiate same sex sexual contact earlier than their heterosexual counterparts.[136,162,163] If young MSM seek older, more sexually experienced partners, who have higher levels of risky behavior and are more likely to be infected with STDs, youths' risk of STD exposure will increase. In fact, this may often be the case. A community-based sample of 156 gay, lesbian, and bisexual youth recruited in the early 1990s in New York City revealed that, for male youths, "their first male partners were, on average, approximately six years older than they were." [163]

Sexual relations between younger and older MSM are not just imbalanced in terms of disparate risk of past STD exposure. They may also be imbalanced in terms of younger men's ability to adopt—or insist upon—protective behaviors that could reduce their risk of acquiring an STD, should they be exposed to a pathogen. Compared to older MSM, young MSM have less experience discussing, negotiating, or planning for safer sex. Also, some young MSM, coming to terms with their sexuality, may bear the additional burden of lower self-esteem and internalized homophobia.[136,164,165] Although the published literature does not report a consistent relationship between gay identity and sexual risk (i.e., both increases and decreases in safer sex have been reported),[166] it is not unreasonable to assume that some younger MSM may have difficulty accepting their sexual orientation—which could lead to less willingness to insist upon safer sexual practices.[167]

Finally, as has been extensively covered in Chapter 3 in this volume, a history of childhood sexual abuse among MSM is associated with high risk sexual behaviors—often mediated through the use of alcohol and other drugs.[168, 169]

Contribution of Alcohol and Drug Use to Disparate STD Rates

At the time of this writing, crystal methamphetamine use has garnered widespread attention as a serious public health problem, especially—though not exclusively—among MSM.[170–173] Particularly pronounced has been the association between "crystal meth" use and syphilis outbreaks among MSM—especially on the West Coast of the United States.[50–52,174] Use of the erectile dysfunction drug sildenafil has also been associated with syphilis outbreaks among MSM.[174]

Recent increased attention to crystal methamphetamine use among MSM is understandable, but readers should realize that this is not the only substance of concern. Alcohol and drug use are common among US MSM (see Chapter 5). A venue-based study of nearly 3500 young MSM, conducted between 1994 and 1998 in seven US urban areas (Baltimore, Dallas, Los Angeles, Miami, New York, San Francisco, Seattle), revealed that 88% reported alcohol use in the past six months and two-thirds reported using illegal drugs in the past six months.[175] In 2001, an online survey of 2916 MSM revealed that 45% of the overall sample reported any illicit drug use, and about half reported drinking alcohol before or during sex.[176]

Recreational alcohol and drug use has been clearly shown to be associated with increased sexual risk[176–182] and thus mediates, in part, disparate rates of STDs among MSM. What is less clearly appreciated is the role that substance use may play in the sexual lives of some MSM, especially in terms of decreasing anxiety and blunting awareness of the omnipresent association between highly pleasurable sexual acts and stigma—including the persistent associations between gay sexuality and disease.[183,184]

Promising Approaches to Resolving Disparate Rates of STDs among MSM

Given the multiplicity of factors influencing the disparate rates of STDs among MSM, it is highly unlikely that a single approach will effectively resolve these disparities. However, a comprehensive approach that encompasses improved surveillance, increased diagnostic and treatment capabilities, strengthened prevention efforts, and a vigorous community response could help to substantially narrow STD disparities. This section will highlight interventions and approaches that show promise, and will identify areas where additional study, or investment, is needed to further reduce disparities.

Enhanced Surveillance

Surveillance is the foundation of effective public health action. Because national notifiable STD surveillance data reported to the US Centers for Disease Control and Prevention (CDC) have not historically included information on gender of sexual partners, national trend data on MSM are not available. Recommendations from the recent past have noted this deficiency,[5] and advocacy groups have called for the inclusion of "sexual orientation and gender identity measures" in the STD surveillance data reported to CDC by state and local health departments.[185]

Although, at the time of this writing, our nation still lacks complete STD surveillance data on MSM, important progress has been made in closing this information gap. Most notably, in March 2005, CDC requested that health department STD program directors confidentially provide information on the gender of sex partners for each reported STD case.[186] Although these data are not yet available for analysis, this action represents an important step forward in being able to monitor national STD trends among MSM.

Another effort that will provide much-needed information is the CDC's implementation, in 2002, of a national behavioral surveillance system to monitor high risk sexual behaviors among MSM. Men, aged 18 years and older, are systematically sampled from randomly selected venues where MSM congregate, including bars, clubs, and other community venues, in seventeen U.S. cities.[187] Using ethnographic techniques, venues are first observed to develop sampling time frames that allow for optimal MSM recruitment.[188] Results from this system have been used to direct HIV prevention services to high risk sexually active MSM, and will likely inform future STD prevention efforts, as well.

Significant improvements notwithstanding, it is important to recognize that lack of adequate information about STD trends among MSM is a serious impediment to timely and targeted public health responses at both a community and a national level.[189] Equally important is the need for surveillance information to inform public health actions targeted to racial/ethnic subpopulations of MSM. Nor should we limit ourselves to surveillance information from traditional sources such as STD clinics and doctors' offices. Community and institutional venues, like correctional facilities, are important potential sources of useful information about STD prevalence and incidence among MSM.[190]

Improved and Expanded Testing and Treatment Services

A number of innovative approaches have been described for improving and expanding STD testing and treatment services for MSM. These can be broadly divided into services that are based in health care facilities and those found in community-based settings. Although advances in diagnostic testing, STD therapies, and preventive vaccines will also contribute to improved efforts to prevent and treat STDs in MSM, their enumeration is beyond the scope of this chapter and will not be covered in this section.

Health Care Facility–Based STD Services

In the mid-1990s, only about one-quarter of US adults reported being asked about STDs during routine medical checkups, representing many missed opportunities for STD prevention.[191] A survey of 48 ambulatory clinics (mostly STD clinics) in 29 US states conducted in 2000–2003 showed that, even in clinics devoted primarily to STD care, "fewer than one in five clinics asked questions designed to elicit risk histories from MSM specifically."[192] Failure to take an accurate sexual history may be especially problematic when considering younger MSM who may be loath to spontaneously discuss same-sex behaviors with health care providers.[193]

Improved sexual history taking will result in more complete and accurate clinical assessments—including improved screening for STDs—for both heterosexuals and homosexuals. Given societal attitudes about homosexuality, clinicians should keep in mind that a straightforward, nonjudgmental approach to sexual history taking among MSM clients is especially important.[194] STD treatment guidelines issued by the CDC in 2006 call for routine inquiry about the sex of patients' partners and, for sexually active MSM, at least annual screening for HIV, gonorrhea, chlamydia and syphilis.[195]

One way to encourage the clinical adoption of routine sexual history taking is to employ written or electronic protocols. A survey of 48 HIV primary care clinics in Los Angeles revealed that clinics with written or electronic STD screening protocols were "significantly more likely to report questioning patients at each visit regarding their sexual practices."[196] Although not specific to MSM populations, another encouraging approach to improving STD screening practices employs the Internet to provide continuing medical education modules to practicing physicians who might not otherwise have the time to receive this updated clinical information.[197] Finally, during specific outbreaks of STDs among MSM, health departments have found that direct communication with medical providers, via email, FAX, regular mail, and other communication strategies, can successfully alert providers to the need for increasing screening rates among their gay and bisexual patients.[198]

In response to syphilis outbreaks among MSM, several US metropolitan public health departments have supplemented traditional "partner notification" efforts by placing Disease Intervention Specialists (DIS) in the offices of physicians who diagnose large numbers of MSM with syphilis.[199] As such, patients can be interviewed about their sexual partners, who have been potentially exposed to infectious syphilis, in a convenient and comfortable setting. From the health department's perspective, this approach may result in a more timely identification of infected partners.

Another partner service under evaluation at the time of this writing is "expedited partner therapy."[200] Expedited partner therapy (EPT) "bypasses" the traditional requirement that partners receive a complete medical examination prior to therapy; instead, sexual contacts may receive therapy from public health personnel, designated pharmacy staff, or from patients themselves.[200] Although patient-delivered partner therapy may be an effective approach to reducing STD disparities for some MSM, it may also conflict with existing state laws and, as such, be difficult to implement beyond narrowly defined circumstances.

Community-Based STD Services

Providing STD services in nonmedical venues frequented by MSM is not a new idea. Descriptions of programs to screen for syphilis and gonorrhea in gay bathhouses can be found in the public health literature of the late 1970s.[201,202] Despite the fact that intensive screening for STDs in sex venues, by itself, may not be capable of reducing prevalence of infection,[203] offering STD screening and treatment services in high risk venues is an important component of a comprehensive approach to reducing STD disparities among MSM and may reach some men who might not otherwise be encountered in medical settings.

Unfortunately, STD screening services are often not available in high risk gay venues. A 1996–1997 survey of 63 US gay bathhouses and sex clubs found that while 40% provided HIV testing on site, only 21% provided some type of on-site STD testing.[204] Even in cities with large, well-organized gay populations, community-based STD services may be deficient. For example, a 2003 survey of gay sex clubs in San Francisco reported that none offered ongoing HIV or syphilis counseling and testing on-site.[205]

Somewhat more encouraging are the 2005 findings of Ciesielski and colleagues, who surveyed health departments in Chicago, Houston, Miami, Fort Lauderdale, Los Angeles, New York, and San Francisco to learn more about the scope and yield of MSM-targeted syphilis screening taking place in nonmedical settings.[206] These health departments reported a variety of targeted screening efforts in response to syphilis outbreaks among MSM, including screening in bathhouses and other commercial sex venues, mobile vans, and jails. Although the yield was relatively low (105 new cases of early syphilis among 14,143 syphilis screening tests), the investigators suggested that secondary public health benefits, such as increased community awareness, may be substantial.[206]

New opportunities for improving access to community-based STD services are also emerging from the domain of the Internet. Innovations, including using the Internet to facilitate partner notification[207] and "online" syphilis testing (i.e., printing lab requisitions and receiving results online)[208] hold great promise for increasing the uptake of STD services among MSM who use the Internet to find sexual partners. Other nontraditional approaches include street outreach with client education, followed by self-collection of rectal specimens for chlamydia and gonorrhea screening among MSM attending gay community street fairs.[209]

Improved Health Promotion

In a nationally representative telephone survey of adolescents conducted in 2001–2002, 51% of 15- to 17-year-olds indicated that they would like to know more about how to bring up sexual health issues, such as STDs, with health care providers.[210] When US office–based physicians serving adolescent patients were surveyed in the late 1990s, only 5% reported that they included any risk reduction counseling on HIV/STD transmission during adolescents' visits for general medical/physical examination.[211] A nationally representative survey of office and outpatient medical visits from the late 1990s found that only "35% of visits had documented evidence of HIV/STD counseling at the time when HIV or STD testing was done."[212] One strongly suspects that this number would be lower still were it possible to determine the frequency of MSM-specific counseling.

Yet, rigorously evaluated studies have demonstrated that health care providers can prevent new STDs through short counseling interventions—especially interventions that focus on personalized risk reduction plans.[213,214] However, because time constraints may limit the ability of health care providers to deliver effective health promotion interventions,[215] health care delivery systems may need to be reconfigured to fully achieve the benefits of clinically mediated health promotion.[216]

Enhancing and enabling the health promotion practices of medical care providers is not the only means of improving risk reduction among sexually active MSM. Community-based organizations must play a critical role in educating MSM clients about the ways in which they can prevent or reduce their risk of sexually transmitted infections. Here again, the Internet is proving to be an important component of outreach and education.[217–219] Other important dimensions of health promotion for sexually active MSM include: creating "safe spaces" where gay youth can receive comprehensive and sensitive health promotion services[220]; implementing policies and structural interventions that minimize risk, especially in public sex venues[221]; and ensuring that services for the prevention and treatment of drug and alcohol use are available to MSM clients who need them.[222]

Social marketing campaigns are another important way to address STD disparities, especially campaigns that aim to raise awareness, including symptom recognition, and prompt testing for STDs. In response to syphilis outbreaks among MSM, health departments from several American cities have worked closely with community representatives to develop and implement syphilis awareness campaigns for sexually active MSM.[223] Based on formative market research, the campaigns varied from "Syphilis is Back" to the "Healthy Penis"; preliminary evaluation results suggest an increase in syphilis testing among MSM in Chicago, Houston, Los Angeles, and San Francisco following the campaigns.[223]

Strengthened Community Response

Some policy analysts suggest that community participation in health is the "cornerstone of modern public health."[224] As such, perhaps the most important ingredient of a comprehensive approach to reducing STD disparities among MSM is the recognition, by MSM communities themselves, of the disproportionate health toll of these preventable infections. Undeniably, the history of the US AIDS epidemic is replete with well-documented examples where gay community mobilization resulted in measurable reductions in viral transmission and other positive health impacts.[25]

A recent example of the essential role of community in reducing STD disparities was cited above, that is, syphilis awareness campaigns developed with strong community input and endorsement.[223,225] A further manifestation of community mobilization in support of reducing STD disparities among MSM comes from the Pacific Northwest. A community group, known as the "MSM HIV/STD Prevention Task Force," issued a manifesto in the Fall of 2003, calling for increased community recognition *and responsibility* for prevention of the transmission of HIV and other STDs.[226] The manifesto emphasized the need for all gay and bisexual men to begin a "community dialogue" on the importance of stopping the transmission of STDs, including HIV.

Conclusion

A critical mass of information is currently available to practitioners and policy makers who seek strategies to prevent and control STDs among men who have sex with men. However, as highlighted in this chapter, important research questions about the disproportionately high rates of STDs among MSM remain unanswered or understudied. Table 6-3 summarizes key epidemiological, behavioral, medical and social research priorities that, when addressed, will help to eliminate STD disparities by filling important gaps in our knowledge base.

Table 6-3. Research Priorities to Decrease Disparate Rates of STDs among MSM

- Improve estimates of the incidence and prevalence of STDs among MSM—especially for racial-ethnic subpopulations
- Better characterize the social determinants of STD risk for MSM and develop and test policy and program interventions to mediate risk
- Develop and test community-specific interventions to increase STD awareness, promote STD prevention, and encourage early diagnosis of sexually acquired infections—including Internet-based interventions
- Develop and test practical interventions to improve health care providers' capacity to assess and address the sexual health needs of MSM clients
- Evaluate structural interventions to reduce risk in public sex environments
- Develop and test new approaches to partner notification, diagnosis and treatment—especially approaches based on social network constructs
- Continue to develop improved methods to prevent (e.g., vaccines and rectal microbicides), diagnose and treat STDs among MSM

No single sector or constituency can solve this complex problem on its own. Further, approaches that are monolithic will be doomed to failure. Finally, it would be wise to recognize that when it comes to reducing and eventually eliminating STD disparities among MSM, we must think of "health" in its broadest possible embodiment. Not just as "the absence of disease or infirmity," but as "a state of complete physical, mental, and social well-being."[227] This will require that public health and medical professionals actively engage and support MSM communities in their own vision of what it means to be healthy. Successful efforts to reduce STD disparities among MSM must use societal resources to promote healthy, safe, and fulfilled persons—not just disease-free genital tracts.

Author's Note

The findings and conclusions in this chapter are those of the author and do not necessarily represent the views of the US Department of Veterans Affairs.

References

1. Institute of Medicine. *The Hidden Epidemic: Confronting Sexually Transmitted Diseases.* Washington, DC: National Academy Press; 1997.
2. Chesson JW, Blandford JM, Gift TL, Tao G, Irwin KL. The estimated direct medical cost of sexually transmitted diseases among American youth, 2000. *Persp Sex Repro Health.* 2004;36:11–19.
3. Herek GM. Beyond "homophobia": thinking about sexual prejudice and stigma in the twenty-first century. *Journal of NSRC.* 2004;1:6–24.
4. Centers for Disease Control and Prevention. *Sexually Transmitted Disease Surveillance, 2004.* Atlanta, GA: US Department of Health and Human Services, September 2005.
5. Wolitski RJ, Valdiserri RO, Denning PH, Levine WC. Are we headed for a resurgence of the HIV epidemic among men who have sex with men? *Am J Public Health.* 2001;91:883–888.
6. Centers for Disease Control and Prevention. Gonorrhea among men who have sex with men—selected sexually transmitted diseases clinics, 1993–1996. *MMWR.* 1997;46:889–892.
7. Centers for Disease Control and Prevention. Increases in unsafe sex and rectal gonorrhea among men who have sex with men—San Francisco, California, 1994–1997. *MMWR.* 1999;48:45–48.
8. Rietmeijer CA, Patnaik JL, Judson FN, Douglas JM. Increases in gonorrhea and sexual risk behaviors among men who have sex with men: a 12-year trend analysis at the Denver Metro Health Clinic. *Sex Trans Dis.* 2003;30:562–567.
9. Centers for Disease Control and Prevention. Primary and secondary syphilis among men who have sex with men—New York City, 2001. *MMWR.* 2002;51:853–856.
10. Centers for Disease Control and Prevention. Resurgent bacterial sexually transmitted diseases among men who have sex with men—King County, Washington, 1997—1999. *MMWR.* 1999;48:773–777.

11. Cates W and the American Social Health Association Panel. Estimates of the incidence and prevalence of sexually transmitted diseases in the United States. *Sex Trans Dis.*1999;26:S2-S7.

12. Zenilman J. Sexually transmitted diseases in homosexual adolescents. *J Adol Health Care.* 1988;9:129–138.

13. Ostrow DG. Gonococcal infections. In: Ostrow DG, Sandholzer TA, Felman YM, eds. *Sexually Transmitted Diseases in Homosexual Men: Diagnosis, Treatment, and Research.* New York, NY: Plenum; 1983:57–78.

14. Owen WF. Sexually transmitted diseases and traumatic problems in homosexual men. *Ann Intern Med.* 1980;92:805–808.

15. Darrow WW, Barrett D, Jay K, et al. The Gay Report on Sexually Transmitted Diseases. *Am J Public Health.* 1981;71:1004–1011.

16. Judson FN, Penley KA, Robinson ME, Smith JK. Comparative prevalence rates of sexually transmitted diseases in heterosexual and homosexual Men. *Am J Epidemol.* 1980;112:836–843.

17. Stamm WE, Koutsky LA, Benedetti JK, Jourden L, Brunham RC, Holmes KK. *Chlamydia trachomatis* urethral infections in men. *Ann Intern Med.*1984; 100:47–51.

18. Centers for Disease Control and Prevention. Declining rates of rectal and pharyngeal gonorrhea among males—New York City. *MMWR.* 1984;33:295–297.

19. Judson FN. Fear of AIDS and gonorrhoea rates in homosexual men. *Lancet.* 1983;II:159–160.

20. Handsfield HH. Decreasing incidence of gonorrhea in homosexually active men—minimal effect on risk of AIDS. *West J Med.* 1985;143:469–470.

21. Doll LS, Ostrow DG. Homosexual and bisexual behavior. In: Holmes KK, Sparling PF, Mardh PA, Lemon SM, Stamm WE, Piot P, Wasserheit JN, eds. *Sexually Transmitted Diseases.* New York, NY: McGraw Hill Health Professions Division; 1999:151–162.

22. Centers for Disease Control and Prevention. Self-reported behavioral change among gay and bisexual men—San Francisco. *MMWR.* 1985;34:613–615.

23. Martin JL. The impact of AIDS on gay male sexual behavior patterns in New York City. *Am J Public Health.* 1987;77:578–581.

24. Centers for Disease Control and Prevention. Changes in sexual behavior and condom use associated with a risk-reduction program—Denver, 1988—1991. *MMWR.* 1992;41:412–415.

25. Valdiserri RO. HIV/AIDS in historical profile. In: Valdiserri R, ed. *Dawning Answers: How the HIV/AIDS Epidemic Has Helped to Strengthen Public Health.* Oxford: Oxford University Press; 2003:3–32.

26. Fox KK, del Rio C, Holmes KK et al. Gonorrhea in the HIV era: a reversal in trends among men who have sex with men. *Am J Public Health.* 2001;91:959–964.

27. Mark KE and Gunn RA. Gonorrhea surveillance. *Sex Trans Dis* 2004;31:215–220.

28. Ciemins EL, Flood J, Kent CK et al. Determining the prevalence of *Chlamydia trachomatis* infection among gay men with urethritis. *Sex Trans Dis.* 2000;27:249–251.

29. Katz MH, Schwarcz SK, Kellogg TA, et al. Impact of highly active antiretroviral treatment on HIV seroincidence among men who have sex with men: San Francisco. *Am J Public Health* 2002;92:388–394.

30. McLean CA, Hutchins K, Mosure DJ et al. Gonorrhea positivity among men who have sex with men attending STD clinics in the United States, 2002. Abstract D04A; 2004 National STD Prevention Conference, Philadelphia, PA.

31. Cherneskie T, Shao M, Labes K. Prevalence of Neisseria gonorrhea and HIV among men who have sex with men; report from a New York City sexually transmitted disease clinic. Abstract P015; 2004 National STD Prevention Conference, Philadelphia, PA.

32. Mayer KH, Goldhammer H, Grasso C, et al. STI trends among MSM at the largest health center caring for gay men in New England, 1997–2002. Abstract P144; 2004 National STD Prevention Conference, Philadelphia, PA.

33. Felman YM. Syphilis. In: Ostrow DG, Sandholzer TA, Felman YM, eds. *Sexually Transmitted Diseases in Homosexual Men: Diagnosis, Treatment, and Research.* New York, NY: Plenum; 1983:37–56.

34. Short SL, Stockman DL, Wolinsky SM, Trupei MA, Moore J, Reichman RC. Comparative rates of sexually transmitted diseases among heterosexual men, homosexual men, and heterosexual women. *Sex Trans Dis.* 1984;11:271–274.

35. Ciesielski CA. Sexually transmitted diseases in men who have sex with men: an epidemiologic review. *Curr Infec Dis Reports.* 2003;5:145–152.

36. Rolfs RT and Nakashima AK. Epidemiology of primary and secondary syphilis in the United States, 1981 through 1989. *JAMA.* 1990;264:1432–1437.

37. Blank S, Schillinger JA, Neylans L, et al. Trends in primary and secondary syphilis in NYC, 1998–2002. Abstract P173; 2004 National STD Prevention Conference, Philadelphia, PA.

38. Centers for Disease Control and Prevention. Trends in primary and secondary syphilis and HIV infections in men who have sex with men—San Francisco and Los Angeles, California, 1998–2002. *MMWR.* 2004;53:575–578.

39. Taylor MM, Hawkins K, Gonzalez A, et al. The Serologic Testing Algorithm for Recent HIV Seroconversions (STARHS) to identify recently acquired HIV infections in men with early syphilis in Los Angeles County. *J Acquir Immune Defic Syndr.* 2005;38:505–508.

40. Centers for Disease Control and Prevention. Transmission of primary and secondary syphilis by oral sex—Chicago, Illinois, 1998–2002. *MMWR.* 2004;53:966–968.

41. Centers for Disease Control and Prevention. Primary and secondary syphilis—United States, 2002. *MMWR.* 2003;52:1117–1120.

42. Heffelfinger JD, Swint EB, Weinstock HS. Estimates of the number of cases of primary and secondary syphilis occurring among men who have sex with men in the United States, 1999–2002. Abstract P143; 2004 National STD Prevention Conference, Philadelphia PA.

43. Klausner JD, Kent CK, Wong W, McCright J, Katz MH. The public health response to epidemic syphilis, San Francisco, 1999–2004. *Sex Trans Dis.* 2005;32:S11-S18.

44. Centers for Disease Control and Prevention. Internet use and early syphilis infection among men who have sex with men—San Francisco, California, 1999–2003. *MMWR.* 2003;52:1229–1232.

45. Taylor M, Aynalem G, Smith L, Bemis C, Kenney K, Kerndt P. Correlates of Internet use to meet sex partners among men who have sex with men diagnosed with early syphilis in Los Angeles County. *Sex Trans Dis.* 2002;31:552–556.

46. Aynalem G, Bemis C, Smith LV, et al. The Internet: emerging venue for syphilis epidemics among men who have sex with men in Los Angeles. Abstract C05D; 2004 National STD Prevention Conference, Philadelphia PA.

47. Lo T, Samuel M, Kent C, et al. Characteristics of MSM syphilis cases using the Internet to seek male sex partners, California, 2001–2003. Abstract D04D; 2004 National STD Prevention Conference, Philadelphia, PA.

48. Reback CJ, Grella CE. HIV risk behaviors of gay and bisexual male methamphetamine users contacted through street outreach. *J Drug Issues.* 1999;29:155–166.

49. Shoptaw S, Reback CJ, Freese TE. Patient characteristics, HIV serostatus, and risk behaviors among gay and bisexual males seeking treatment for methamphetamine abuse and dependence in Los Angeles. *J Addic Dis.* 2002;21:91–105.

50. Mitchell SJ, Wong W, Kent CK, Chaw JK, Klausner JD. Methamphetamine use, sexual behavior, and sexually transmitted diseases among men who have sex with men seen in an STD clinic, San Francisco, 2002–2003. Abstract D04C; 2004 National STD Prevention Conference, Philadelphia PA.

51. Hirshfield S, Remien RH, Walavalkar I, Chiasson, MA. Crystal methamphetamine use predicts incident STD infection among men who have sex with men recruited online: a nested case-control study. *J Med Internet Res.* 2004;6:1–7.

52. Centers for Disease Control and Prevention. Outbreak of syphilis among men who have sex with men—Southern California, 2000. *MMWR.*2001; 50:117–120.

53. Whiteley J, Blank S, Shao M, Rubin S, Labes K, Cherneskie T. Seroprevalence of syphilis among men who have sex with men attending a New York City sexually transmitted disease clinic. Abstract P148; 2004 National STD Prevention Conference, Philadelphia, PA.

54. Paz-Bailey G, Meyers A, Blank S, et al. A case-control study of syphilis among men who have sex with men in New York City: association with HIV infection. *Sex Trans Dis.* 2004;31:581–587.

55. Chesson HW, Heffelfinger JD, Voigt RF, Collins D. Estimates of primary and secondary syphilis rates in persons with HIV in the United States, 2002. *Sex Trans Dis.* 2005;32:265–269.

56. Centers for Disease Control and Prevention. Summary of notifiable diseases—United States, 2003. Published April 22, 2005, for *MMWR* 2003;52 (54):1–85.

57. Felman YM, Holmes KK. Nongonoccocal urethritis. In: Ostrow DG, Sandholzer TA, Felman YM, eds. *Sexually Transmitted Diseases in Homosexual Men: Diagnosis, Treatment, and Research.* New York, NY: Plenum; 1983;79–84.

58. Geisler WM, Whittington WL, Suchland RJ, Stamm WR. Epidemiology of anorectal chlamydial and gonococcal infections among men having sex with men in Seattle. *Sex Trans Dis.* 2002;29:189–195.

59. Kent CK, Chaw JK, Klausner JD. Substantial prevalence of urethral and rectal chlamydial infection detected among gay and bisexual men seen in the municipal STD clinic: San Francisco, 2002. Abstract P145; 2004 National STD Prevention Conference, Philadelphia, PA.

60. Ku L, St. Louis M, Farshy C, et al. Risk behaviors, medical care, and chlamydial infection among young men in the United States. *Am J Public Health.* 2002; 92:1140–1143.

61. Cook RL, St. George K, Silvestre AJ, Riddler SA, Lassak M, Rinaldo CR. Prevalence of chlamydia and gonorrhoea among a population of men who have sex with men. *Sex Transm Infect.* 2002;78:190–193.

62. Tabet SR, Krone MR, Paradise MA, Corey L, Stamm WE, Celum CL. Incidence of HIV and sexually transmitted diseases (STD) in a cohort of HIV-negative men who have sex with men (MSM). *AIDS.* 1998;12:2041–2048.

63. Kent CK, Chaw JK, Wong W, et al. Prevalence of rectal, urethral, and pharyngeal chlamydia and gonorrhea detected in 2 clinical settings among men who have sex with men: San Francisco, California, 2003. *Clin Infec Dis.* 2005;41:67–74.

64. Perine PL, Stamm WE. Lymphogranuloma venereum. In: Holmes K, Sparling PF, Lemon S, Stamm WE, Piot P, Wasserheit J, eds. *Sexually Transmitted Diseases.* New York, NY: McGraw Hill Health Professions Division; 1999:423–432.

65. Quinn TC, Goddell SE, Mkrtichian E, et al. Chlamydia trachomatis proctitis. *N Engl J Med.* 1981;305:195–200.

66. San Francisco Department of Public Health. Health Alert: Lymphogranuloma venereum (LGV) infection in San Francisco. December 22, 2004. www.sfcityclinic .org/providers. Accessed June 4, 2005.

67. New York City Department of Health and Mental Hygiene. DOHMH Alert # 4: Confirmed Lymphogranuloma venereum (LGV) infection in two HIV+ New York City residents. February 2, 2005. www.hivguidelines.org/public_html/health-bulletins/health-alert-4.doc. Accessed June 4, 2005.

68. Smith S. A foreign STD sets off worry in Hub: may signal return of risky sex habits. Boston Globe. May 30, 2005. www.boston.com/yourlife/health/diseases/articles/2005/05/30. Accessed June 6, 2005.

69. Georgia Department of Human Resources. Health advisory: appearance of rare Form of Chlamydia (LGV) in Atlanta. February 18, 2005. www.health.state .ga.us/publications/pressrelease/021705.asp. Accessed June 4, 2005.

70. Centers for Disease Control and Prevention. Lymphogranuloma venereum among men who have sex with men—Netherlands, 2003–2004. *MMWR.* 2004;53:985–988.

71. Ebrahim SH, McKenna MT, Marks JS. Sexual behaviour: related adverse health burden in the United States. *Sex Trans Infec.* 2005;81:38–40.

72. Stone KM, Karem KL, Sternberg MR, et al. Seroprevalence of *Human papillomavirus* type 16 infection in the United States. *J Infect Dis.* 2002;186:1396–1402.

73. Koutsky LA, Kiviat NB. Genital Human papillomavirus. In: Holmes K, Sparling PF, Lemon S, Stamm WE, Piot P, Wasserheit J, eds. *Sexually Transmitted Diseases.* New York, NY: McGraw Hill Health Professions Division; 1999:347–359.

74. Kiviat N, Koutsky LA, Paavonen J. Cervical neoplasia and other STD-related genital tract neoplasias. In: Holmes K, Sparling PF, Lemon S, Stamm WE, Piot P, Wasserheit J, eds. *Sexually Transmitted Diseases.* New York, NY: McGraw Hill Health Professions Division; 1999:811–831.

75. Brown D. HPV vaccine advised for girls. *Washington Post.* June 30, 2006, p. A05.

76. Anhang R, Stryker JE, Wright TC, Goldie SJ. News media coverage of Human papillomavirus. *Cancer.* 2004;100:308–314.

77. Daling JR, Weiss NS, Klopfenstein LL, Cochran LE, Chow WH, Daifuku R. Correlates of homosexual behavior and the incidence of anal cancer. *JAMA.* 1982; 247:1988–1990.

78. Peters RK, Mack RM. Patterns of anal carcinoma by gender and marital status in Los Angeles County. *Br J Cancer.* 1983;48:629–636.

79. Melbye M, Rabkin C, Frisch M, Biggar RJ. Changing patterns of anal cancer incidence in the United States, 1940–1989. *Am J Epidemiol.* 1994;139:772–780.

80. Daling JR, Weiss NS, Hislop G, et al. Sexual practices, sexually transmittted diseases, and the incidence of anal cancer. *N Engl J Med.* 1987;317:973–977.

81. Goldstone ST, Winkler B, Ufford LJ, Alt E, Palefsky JM. High prevalence of anal squamous intraepithelial lesions and squamous cell carcinoma in men who have sex with men as seen in a surgical practice. *Dis Colon Rectum.* 2001;44:690–698.

82. Palefsky J. Human papillomavirus infection and anogenital neoplasia in human immunodeficiency virus-positive men and women. *J Natl Cancer Inst Monogr.* 1998; 23:15–20.

83. Chin-Hong PV, Vittinghoff E, Cranston RD, et al. Age-specific prevalence of anal human papillomavirus infection in HIV-negative sexually active men who have sex with men: The Explore Study. *J Infec Dis.* 2004; 190:2070–2076.

84. Critchlow CW, Hawes SE, Kuypers JM, et al. Effect of HIV infection on the natural history of anal human papillomavirus infection. *AIDS.* 1998;12:1177–1184.

85. Palefsky JM, Holly EA, Ralston ML, Jay N. Prevalence and risk factors for human papillomavirus infection of the anal canal in human immunodeficiency virus (HIV)-Positive and HIV-negative homosexual men. *J Infec Dis.* 1998;177:361–367.

86. Friedman HB, Saah AJ, Sherman ME, et al. Human papillomavirus, anal squamous intraepithelial lesions, and human immunodeficiency virus in a cohort of gay men. *J Infec Dis.* 1998;178:45–52.

87. Caussy D, Goedert JJ, Palefsky J, et al. Interaction of human immunodeficiency and papilloma viruses: association with anal epithelial abnormality in homosexual men. *Int J Cancer.* 1990;46:214–219.

88. Strickler HD, Burk RD, Fazzari M, et al. Natural history and possible reactivation of human papillomavirus in human immunodeficiency virus-positive women. *J Natl Cancer Inst.* 2005;97:577–586.

89. Frisch M, Biggar RJ, Goedert JJ. Human papillomavirus-associated cancers in patients with human immunodeficiency virus infection and acquired immunodeficinecy syndrome. *J Natl Cancer Inst.* 2002;92:1500–1510.

90. Cress RD, Holly EA. Incidence of anal cancer in California: increased incidence among men in San Francisco, 1973–1999. *Prev Med.* 2003;36:555–560.

91. Lafferty, WE, Downey L, Celum C, Wald A. Herpes simplex virus type 1 as a cause of genital herpes: impact on surveillance and prevention. *J Infec Dis.* 2000;181:1454–1457.

92. Corey L, Handsfield HH. Genital herpes and public health: addressing a global problem. *JAMA* 2000;283:791–794.

93. Fleming DT, McQuillan GM, Johnson RE, et al. Herpes simplex virus type 2 in the United States, 1976–1994. *N Engl J. Med.* 1997;337:1105–1111.

94. McQuillan GM, Kruszon-Moran D, Kottiri BJ, Curtin LR, Lucas JW, Kington RS. Racial and ethnic differences in the seroprevalence of 6 infectious diseases in the United States: data from NHANES III, 1988–1994. *Am J Public Health.* 2004; 94:1952–1958.

95. Gottlieb SL, Douglas JM, Schmid DS, et al. Seroprevalence and correlates of herpes simplex virus type 2 infection in five sexually transmitted diseases clinics. *J Infec Dis.* 2002;186:1381–1389.

96. Siegel D, Golden E, Washington E, et al. Prevalence and correlates of herpes simplex infections: The Population-Based AIDS in Multiethnic Neighborhoods Study. *JAMA.* 1992; 268:1702–1708.

97. Turner KR, McFarland W, Kellogg TA, et al. Incidence and prevalence of herpes simplex virus type 2 infection in persons seeking repeat HIV counseling and testing. *Sex Trans Dis.* 2003;30:331–334.

98. Stamm WE, Handsfield H, Rompalo AM, Ashley RL, Roberts PL, Corey L. The association between genital ulcer disease and acquisition of HIV infection in homosexual men. *JAMA.* 1988;260:1429–1433.

99. Renzi C, Douglas JM, Foster M, et al. Herpes simplex virus type 2 infection as a risk factor for human immunodeficiency virus acquisition in men who have sex with men. *J Infec Dis.* 2003;187:19–25.

100. Mole L, Ripich S, Margolis D, Holodniy M. The impact of active herpes simplex virus infection on human immunodeficiency virus load. *J Infec Dis.* 1997; 176:766–770.

101. Chang Y, Cesarman E, Pessin MS, et al. Identification of herpesvirus-like DNA sequences in AIDS-associated Kaposi's sarcoma. *Science.* 1994;266–1865–1869.

102. Beral V, Peterman TA, Berkelman RL, Jaffe HW. Kaposi's sarcoma among persons with AIDS: a sexually transmitted infection? *Lancet.* 1990;335:123–128.

103. Kedes DH, Operskalski E, Busch M, Kohn R, Flood J, Ganem D. The seroepidemiology of human herpesvirus 8 (Kaposi's sarcoma-associated herpesvirus): distribution of infection in KS risk groups and evidence for sexual transmission. *Nature Med.* 1996;2:918–924.

104. Casper C. Human Herpesvirus-8, Kaposi sarcoma, and AIDS associated neoplasms. HIV Insite Knowledge Base. August 2004. http://hivinsite.ucsf.edu/ InSite?page=kb-06–02–01. Accessed June 30, 2005.

105. Whitby D, Howard MR, Tenant-Flowers M, et al. Detection of Kaposi sarcoma associated herpesvirus in peripheral blood of HIV-infected individuals and progression to Kaposi's sarcoma. *Lancet.* 1995;346:799–802.

106. Gao, SJ, Kingsley L, Hoover DR, et al. Seroconversion to antibodies against Kaposi's sarcoma-associated herpesvirus-related latent nuclear antigens before the development of Kaposi's sarcoma. *N Engl J Med.* 1996;335:233–241.

107. Pellett PE, Wright EA, Engels DV, et al. Multicenter comparison of serologic assays and estimation of human herpesvirus 8 seroprevalence among US blood donors. *Transfusion.* 2003;43:1260–1268.

108. Lennette ET, Blackbourn DJ, Levy JA. Antibodies to human herpesvirus type 8 in the general population and in Kaposi's sarcoma patients. *Lancet.* 1996;348:858–861.

109. Simpson GR, Schulz TF, Whitby D, et al. Prevalence of Kaposi's sarcoma associated herpesvirus infection measured by antibodies to recombinant capsid protein and latent immunofluoresence antigen. *Lancet.* 1996;349:1133–1138.

110. Cannon MJ, Dollard SC, Smith DK, et al. Blood-borne and sexual transmission of human herpesvirus 8 in women with or at risk for human immunodeficiency virus infection. *N Engl J Med.* 2001;344:637–643.

111. Martin JN, Ganem DE, Osmond DH, Page-Shafer KA, Macrae D, Kedes DH. Sexual transmisison and natural history of human herpesvirus 8 infection. *N Engl J Med.* 1998;338:948–954.

112. Blackbourn DJ, Osmond D, Levy JA, Lennette ET. Increased human herpesvirus 8 seroprevalence in young homosexual men who have multiple sex contacts with different partners. *J Infec Dis.* 1999;179:237–239.

113. O'Brien TR, Kedes D, Ganem D, et al. Evidence for concurrent epidemics of human herpesvirus 8 and human immunodeficiency virus type 1 in US homosexual men: rates, risk factors, and relationship to Kaposi's sarcoma. *J Infec Dis.* 1999;180:1010–1017.

114. Dukers HN, Renwick N, Prins M, et al. Risk factors for human herpesvirus 8 seropositivity and seroconversion in a cohort of homosexual men. *Am J Epidemiol.* 2000;151:213–224.

115. Osmond DH, Buchbinder S, Cheng A, et al. Prevalence of Kaposi sarcoma-associated herpesvirus infection in homosexual men at beginning of and during the HIV epidemic. *JAMA.* 2002;287:221–225.

116. Diamond C, Thiede H, Perdue T, et al. Seroepidemiology of human herpesvirus 8 among young men who have sex with men. *Sex Trans Dis.* 2001;28:176–182.

117. Casper C, Wald A, Pauk J, Tabet SR, Corey L, Celum CL. Correlates of prevalent and incident Kaposi's sarcoma-associated herpesvirus infection in men who have sex with men. *J Infec Dis.* 2002;185:990–993.

118. Pauk J, Huang ML, Brodie SJ et al. Mucosal shedding of human herpesvirus 8 in men. *N Engl J Med.* 2000;343:1369–1377.

119. Eltom MA, Jemal A, Mbulaiteye SM, Devesa SS, Biggar RJ. Trends in Kaposi's sarcoma and non-Hodgkin's lymphoma incidence in the United States from 1973 through 1998. *J Natl Cancer Inst.* 2002;94:1204–1210.

120. Bader M, Pedersen AH, Williams R, Spearman J, Anderson H. Venereal transmission of shigellosis in Seattle-King County. *Sex Trans Dis.* 1977;4:89–91.

121. Tauxe RV, McDonald RC, Hargrett-Bean N, Blake PA. The persistence of *Shigella flexneri* in the United States: increasing role of adult males. *Am J Public Health.* 1988;78:1432–1435.

122. Centers for Disease Control and Prevention. *Shigella sonnei* outbreak among men who have sex with men—San Francisco, California, 2000–2001. *MMWR.* 2001;50: 922–926.

123. Reller ME, Olsen SJ, Kressel AM, et al. Sexual transmisison of typhoid fever: a multistate outbreak among men who have sex with men. *Clin Infec Dis.* 2003;37:141–144.

124. Meyers JD, Kuharic HA, Holmes KK. *Giardia lamblia* infection in homosexual men. *Br J Vener Dis.* 1977;53:54–55.

125. Schmerin MJ, Jones TC, Klein H. Giardiasis: association with homosexuality. *Ann Inter Med.* 1978;88:801–803.

126. Schmerin MJ, Geltson A, Jones TC. Amebiasis: an increasing problem among homosexuals in New York City. *JAMA.* 1977;1386–1387.

127. Pomerantz BM, Marr JS, Goldman WD. Amebiasis in New York City, 1958–1978: identification of the male homosexual high risk population. *Bull NY Acad Med.* 1980;56:232–244.

128. William DC, Shookhoff HB, Felman YM, DeRamos SW. High rates of enteric protozoal infections in selected homosexual men attending a venereal disease clinic. *Sex Trans Dis.* 1978;5:155–157.

129. Phillips SC, Mildvan D, William DC, Gelb AM, White MC. Sexual transmission of enteric protozoa and helminths in a venereal-disease-clinic population. *N Engl J Med.* 1981;305:603–606.

130. Quinn TC, Stamm WE, Goodell SE, et al. The polymicrobial origin of intestinal infections in homosexual men. *N Engl J Med.* 1983;309:576–582.

131. Ortega HB, Borchardt KA, Hamilton R, Ortega P, Mahood J. Enteric pathogenic protozoa in homosexual men from San Francisco. *Sex Trans Dis.* 1984; 11:59–63.

132. Baer JT, Vugia DJ, Reingold AL, Aragon T, Angulo FJ, Bradford WZ. HIV infection as a risk factor for shigellosis. *Emerg Infect Dis.* 1999;5:820–823.

133. Gupta A, Polyak CS, Bishop RD, Sobel J, Mintz ED. Laboratory-confirmed shigellosis in the Unites States, 1989–2002: epidemiologic trends and patterns. *Clin Infect Dis.* 2004;38:1372–1377.

134. Henderson R. Improving sexually transmitted disease health services for gays: a national prospective. *Sex Trans Dis.* 1977;4:58–62.

135. William DC. Sexually transmitted diseases in gay men: an insider's view. *Sex Trans Dis.* 1979;6:278–280.

136. Friedman RC, Downey JI. Homosexuality. *N Engl J Med.* 1994;331:923–930.

137. Billy JQ, Tanfer K, Grady WR, Klepinger DH. The sexual behavior of men in the United States. *Fam Planning Persp.* 1993;25:52–60.
138. Black D, Gates G, Sanders S, Taylor L. Demographics of the gay and lesbian population in the United States: evidence from available systematic data sources. *Demography.* 2000;37:139–154.
139. Eisenberg M. Differences in sexual risk behaviors between college students with same-sex and opposite-sex experience: results from a national survey. *Arch Sex Behav.* 2001;30:575–589.
140. Anderson JE, Stall R. Increased reporting of male-to-male sexual activity in a national survey. *Sex Trans Dis.* 2002;29:643–646.
141. Ostrow DG, Altman NL. Sexually transmitted diseases and homosexuality. *Sex Trans Dis.* 1983;10:208–215.
142. Dee, TS. Forsaking all others? The effects of "gay marriage" on risky sex. National Bureau of Economic Research. May 2005. www.nber.org/papers/w11327 Accessed June 30, 2005.
143. Immerman RS, Mackey WC. The societal dilemma of multiple sexual partners: the costs of the loss of pair-bonding. *Marriage Fam Rev.* 1999;29:3–19.
144. Schmitt DP. Universal sex differences in the desire for sexual variety: tests from 52 nations, 6 continents and 13 islands. *J Personality Soc Psychol.* 2003;85:85–104.
145. Johnson DK. *The Lavender Scare: The Cold War Persecution of Gays and Lesbians in the Federal Government.* Chicago, IL: University of Chicago Press; 2004.
146. Humphreys L. *Tearoom Trade: Impersonal Sex in Public Places.* Hawthorne, NY: Aldine de Gruyter; 1970.
147. Binson D, Woods WJ, Pollack L, Paul J, Stall R, Catania JA. Differential HIV risk in bathhouses and public cruising areas. *Am J Public Health.* 2001;91:1482–1486.
148. Berube A. The history of gay bathhouses. *J Homosex.* 2003;44:33–53.
149. Van Beneden CA, O'Brien K, Modesitt S, Yusem S, Rose A, Fleming D. Sexual behaviors in an urban bathhouse 15 years into the HIV epidemic. *J Acquir Immune Defic Syndr.* 2002; 30:522–526.
150. Smith LV, Aynalem G, Bemis C, et al. Commercial sex venues: a closer look at their impact on the syphilis epidemics among men who have sex with men (MSM) in Los Angeles. Abstract C05A; 2004 National STD Prevention Conference, Philadelphia, PA.
151. Collins B, Alvarez A, Katchy E, Pendleton B. Anonymous sex venues for MSM: implementing outreach screening for syphilis and HIV at adult bookstores. Abstract C05C; 2004 National STD Prevention Conference, Philadelphia, PA.
152. Doherty IA, Padian NS, Marlow C, Aral SO. Determinants and consequences of sexual networks as they affect the spread of sexually transmitted infections. *J Infec Dis.* 2005;191:S42-S54.
153. Klausner JD, Wolf W, Fischer-Ponce L, Zolt I, Katz, MH. Tracing a syphilis outbreak through cyberspace. *JAMA.* 2000;284:447–449.
154. Bull SS, McFarlane M, Rietmeijer C. HIV and sexually transmitted infection risk behaviors among men seeking sex with men on-line. *Am J Public Health.* 2001; 91:988–989.
155. Bull SS, McFarlane M, Lloyd L, Rietmeijer C. The process of seeking sex partners online and implications for STD/HIV prevention. *AIDS Care.* 2004;16:1012–1020.
156. Benotsch EG, Kalichman S, Cage M. Men who have met sex partners via the Internet: prevalence, predictors, and implications for HIV prevention. *Arch Sex. Behavior.* 2002;31:177–183.

157. Haraldsdottir S, Gupta S, Anderson RM. Preliminary studies of sexual networks in a male homosexual community in Iceland. *Acquir Immune Defic Syndr.* 1992; 5:374–381.

158. Laumann EO, Youm Y. Racial/ethnic differences in the prevalence of sexually transmitted diseases in the United States: a network explanation. *Sex Trans Dis.* 1999;26:250–261.

159. Bingham TA, Harawa NT, Johnson DF, Secura GM, MacKellar DA, Valleroy LA. The effect of partner characteristics on HIV infection among African American men who have sex with men in the Young Men's Survey, Los Angeles, 1999–2000. *AIDS Educ Prev.* 2003;15(Suppl A):39–52.

160. Harawa NT, Greenland S, Bingham TA, et al. Associations of race/ethnicity with HIV prevalence and HIV-related behaviors among young men who have sex with men in 7 urban centers in the United States. *J Acquir Immune Defic Syndr.* 2004;35:526–536.

161. Wohlfeiler D, Potterat JJ. Using gay men's sexual networks to reduce sexually transmitted disease (STD)/human immunodeficiency virus (HIV) Transmission. *Sex Trans Dis.* 2005;32:S48-S52.

162. Resnick MD, Bearman PS, Blum RW, et al. Protecting adolescents from harm: findings from the National Longitudinal Study on Adolescent Health. *JAMA.* 1997;278:823–832.

163. Rosario M, Meyer-Bahlburg HF, Hunter J, Gwadz M. Sexual risk behavior of gay, lesbian, and bisexual youths in New York City: prevalence and correlates. *AIDS Educ Prev.* 1999;11:476–496.

164. Stokes JP, Peterson JL. Homophobia, self-esteem, and risk for HIV among African American Men who have sex with men. *AIDS Educ Prev.* 1998;10:278–292.

165. Diaz RM, Ayala G, Bein E, Henne J, Marin BV. The impact of homophobia, poverty, and racism on the mental health of gay and bisexual Latino men: findings from 3 US cities. *Am J Public Health* 2001;91:927–932.

166. Choi KH, Han CS, Hudes ES, Kegeles S. Unprotected sex and associated risk factors among young Asian and Pacific Islander men who have sex with men. *AIDS Educ Prev.* 2002;14:472–481.

167. Fisher J, Jurgens R, Vassal A, Hughes R. *The Impact of Stigma and Discrimination.* Montreal: Canadian HIV/AIDS Legal Network; 1998.

168. Lenderking WR, Wold C, Mayer KH, Goldstein R, Losina E, Seage GR. Childhood sexual abuse among homosexual men: prevalence and association with unsafe sex. *J Gen Intern Med.* 1997;12:250–253.

169. Paul JP, Catania J, Pollack L, Stall R. Understanding childhood sexual abuse as a predictor of sexual risk-taking among men who have sex with men: The Urban Men's Health Study. *Child Abuse & Neglect.* 2001;25:557–584.

170. Specter M. Higher risk: crystal meth, the Internet, and dangerous choices about AIDS. *New Yorker.* March 23, 2005;81:38–45.

171. Halkitis PN, Shrem MT, Martin FW. Sexual behavior patterns of methamphetamine-using gay and bisexual men. *Substance Use & Misuse.* 2005;40:703–719.

172. Patterson TL, Semple SJ, Zians JK, Strathdee SA. Methamphetamine-using HIV positive men who have sex with men: correlates of polydrug use. *J Urban Health.* 2005;82 (Suppl. 1):120–126.

173. Kurtz SP. Post-circuit blues: motivations and consequences of crystal meth use among gay men in Miami. *AIDS Behav.* 2005;9:63–72.

174. Wong W, Chaw JK, Kent CK, Klausner JD. Risk factors for early syphilis among gay and bisexual men seen in an STD clinic: San Francisco, 2002–2003. *Sex Trans Dis.* 2005;32:458–463.

175. Thiede H, Valleroy L, MacKellar DA, et al. Regional patterns and correlates of substance use among young men who have sex with men in 7 US urban areas. *Am J Public Health.* 2003;93:1915–1921.

176. Hirshfield S, Remien RH, Humberstone M, Walavalkar I, Chiasson MA. Substance use and high-risk sex among men who have sex with men: a national online study in the USA. *AIDS Care.* 2004;16:1036–1047.

177. Strathdee SA, Hogg RS, Martindale SL, et al. Determinants of sexual risk-taking among young HIV-negative gay and bisexual men. *J Acquir Immune Defic Syndr.* 1998;19:61–66.

178. Colfax G, Coates TH, Husnik MJ, et al. Longitudinal patterns of methamphetamine, popper (amyl nitrite), and cocaine use and high-risk sexual behavior among a cohort of San Francisco men who have sex with men. *J Urban Health.* 2005;82 (Suppl. 1):62–70.

179. Stueve A, O'Donnell L, Duran R, et al. Being high and taking sexual risks: findings from a multisite survey of urban young men who have sex with men. *AIDS Educ Prev.* 2002;14:482–495.

180. Colfax GN, Mansergh G, Guzman R, et al. Drug use and sexual risk behavior among gay and bisexual men who attend circuit parties: a venue-based comparison. *J Acquir Immune Defic Syndr. 2001*;28:373–379.

181. Koblin BA, Chesney MA, Husnik MJ, et al. High-risk behaviors among men who have sex with men in 6 US cities: baseline data from the explore study. *Am J Public Health.* 2003;93:926–932.

182. Vanable PA, McKirnan DJ, Buchbinder SP, et al. Alcohol use and high-risk sexual behavior among men who have sex with men: the effects of consumption level and partner type. *Health Psychol.* 2004;23:525–532.

183. Ostrow DG. The role of drugs in the sexual lives of men who have sex with men: continuing barriers to researching this question. *AIDS Behav.* 2000;4:205–219.

184. Stall R, Purcell DW. Intertwining Epidemics: A review of research on substance use among men who have sex with men and its connection to the AIDS epidemic. *AIDS Behav.* 2000;4:181–192.

185. Gay and Lesbian Medical Association. *Healthy People 2010: Companion Document for Lesbian, Gay, Bisexual, and Transgender (LGBT) Health.* San Francisco, CA: Gay and Lesbian Medical Association; April 2001.

186. Douglas J. Dear Colleague Letter. Atlanta, GA: Division of STD Prevention and Treatment, U.S. Centers for Disease Control and Prevention; March 8, 2005.

187. Centers for Disease Control and Prevention. Human immunodeficiency virus (HIV) risk, prevention, and testing behaviors—United States, National HIV Behavioral Surveillance System: Men Who Have Sex With Men, November 2003-April 2005. Surveillance Summaries, July 7, 2006. *MMWR.* 2006;55:(No SS-6).

188. MacKellar DA, Valleroy LA, Secura GM, et al. Unrecognized HIV Infection, Risk Behavior, and Perceptions of Risk Among Young Men who Have Sex with Men. J Acquir Immune Defic Syndr. 2005;38:603–614.

189. Douglas JM, Peterman TA, Fenton KA. Syphilis among men who have sex with men: challenges to syphilis elimination in the United States. *Sex Trans Dis.* 2005; 32:S80-S83.

190. Chen JL, Bovee MC, Kerndt PR. Sexually transmitted disease surveillance among incarcerated men who have sex with men—an opportunity for HIV prevention. *AIDS Educ Prev* 2003;15:117–126.

191. Tao G, Irwin KL, Kassler WJ. Missed opportunities to assess sexually transmitted diseases in US adults during routine medical checkups. *Am J Prev Med.* 2000; 18:109–114.

192. Kurth AE, Holmes KK, Hawkins R, Golden RM. A national survey of clinic sexual histories for sexually transmitted infection and HIV screening. *Sex Trans Dis.* 2005;32:370–376.

193. Catallozzi M, Rudy BJ. Lesbian, gay, biseuxal, transgendered, and questioning youth: the importance of a sensitive and confidential sexual history in identifying the risk and implementing treatment for sexually transmitted diseases. *Adolesc Med.* 2004;15:353–367.

194. Public Health, Seattle and King County. Sexually transmitted disease and HIV screening guidelines for men who have sex with men. *Sex Trans Dis.* 2001;28:457–459.

195. Centers for Disease Control and Prevention. Sexually Transmitted Diseases Treatment Guidelines, 2006. *MMWR.* 2006;55(RR-10):1–94.

196. Taylor MM, McClain T, Javanbakht M, et al. Sexually transmitted disease testing protocols, sexually transmitted disease testing, and discussion of sexual behaviors in HIV clinics in Los Angeles County. *Sex Trans Dis.* 2005;32:341–345.

197. Allison JJ, Kiefe CI, Wall T, et al. Multicomponent Internet continuing medical education to promote chlamydia screening. *Am J Prev Med.* 2005;28:285–290.

198. Taylor M, Prescott L, Brown J, et al. Activities to increase provider awareness of early syphilis in men who have sex with men in 8 cities, 2000–2004. *Sex Trans Dis.* 2005;32:S24-S29.

199. Hogben M, Paffel J, Broussard D, et al. Syphilis partner notification with men who have sex with men: a review and commentary. *Sex Trans Dis.* 2005;32:S43-S47.

200. Golden MR, Manhart LE. Innovative approaches to the prevention and control of bacterial sexually transmitted infections. *Infect Dis Clin N Am.* 2005;19:513–540.

201. Judson FN, Miller KG, Schaffnit TR. Screening for gonorrhea and syphilis in the gay baths—Denver, Colorado. *Am J Public Health.* 1977;67:740–742.

202. Merino HI, Judson FN, Bennett D, Schaffnit TR. Screening for gonorrhea and syphilis in gay bathhouses in Denver and Los Angeles. *Public Health Rep.* 1979:94;376–379.

203. Wolf FC, Judson FN. Intensive screening for gonorrhea, syphilis, and hepatitis b in a gay bathhouse does not lower prevalence of infection. *Sex Trans Dis.* 1980; 7:49–52.

204. Woods WJ, Binson D, Mayne TJ, Gore LR, Rebchook GM. Facilities and HIV prevention in bathhouse and sex club environments. *J Sex Research.* 2001;38:68–74.

205. Buchacz KA, Siller JE, Bandy DW, et al. HIV and syphilis testing among men who have sex with men attending sex clubs and adult bookstores—San Francisco, 2003. *J Acquir Immune Defic Syndr.* 2004;1324–1326.

206. Ciesielski C, Kahn RH, Taylor M, Gallagher K, Prescott LJ, Arrowsmith S. Control of syphilis outbreaks in men who have sex with men: the role of screening in nonmedical settings. *Sex Trans Dis.* 2005;32:S37–S42.

207. Centers for Disease Control and Prevention. Using the Internet for partner notification of sexually transmitted diseases—Los Angeles County, California, 2003. *MMWR.* 2004; 53:129–131.

208. Levine DK, Scott KC, Klausner JD. Online syphilis testing—confidential and convenient. *Sex Trans Dis.* 2005;32:139–141.

209. McCright J, Strona F, Diosdado I, Kent CK, Klausner JD. In and out screening: feasibility and positivity of pharyngeal and self-collected rectal specimens obtained from men who have sex with men at street fairs, San Francisco, July-October 2005. Abstract A1b; 2006 National STD Prevention Conference, Jacksonville, FL.

210. Henry J. Kaiser Family Foundation. *National Survey of Adolescents and Young Adults: Sexual Health Knowledge, Attitudes and Experiences.* Menlo Park, CA: Henry J. Kaiser Family Foundation; 2003.

211. Ma J, Wang UY, Stafford RS. U.S. Adolescents receive suboptimal preventive counseling during ambulatory care. *J Adoles Health.* 2005;36:441.e1–41.e7.

212. Tao G, Branson BM, Anderson LA, Irwin KL. Do physicians provide counseling with HIV and STD testing at physician offices or hospital outpatient departments? *AIDS.* 2003;17:1243–1247.

213. Kamb ML, Fishbein M, Douglas JM, et al. Efficacy of risk reduction counseling to prevent human immunodeficiency virus and sexually transmitted diseases. *JAMA.* 1998;280:1161–1167.

214. Manhart LE, Holmes KK. Randomized controlled trials of individual-level, population-level, and multilevel interventions for preventing sexually transmitted infections: what has worked? *J Infec Dis.* 2005;191:S7-S24.

215. Yarnall KS, Pollak KI, Ostbye T, Krause KM, Michener JL. Primary care: is there enough time for prevention? *Am J Public Health.* 2003;93:635–641.

216. Kottke TE, Brekke ML, Solberg LI. Making "time" for preventive services. *Mayo Clin Proc.* 1993; 68:785–791.

217. Klausner JD, Levine DK, Kent CK. Internet-based site-specific interventions for syphilis prevention among gay and bisexual men. *AIDS Care.* 2004;16:964–970.

218. Anderton JA, Valdiserri RO. Combatting syphilis and HIV among users of Internet chatrooms. *J Health Educ.* 2005;10:665–671.

219. Rhodes SD. Hookups or health promotion? an exploratory study of a chat room-based HIV prevention intervention for men who have sex with men. *AIDS Educ Prev.* 2004;16:315–327.

220. Blake SM, Ledsky R, Lehman T, Goodenow C, Sawyer R, Hack T. Preventing sexual risk behaviors among gay, lesbian, and bisexual adolescents: the benefits of gay-sensitive HIV instruction in schools. *Am J Public Health.* 2001;91:940–946.

221. Woods WJ, Binson D, Pollack LM, Wohlfeiler D, Stall RD, Catania JA. Public policy regulating private and public space in gay bathhouses. *J Acquir Immune Defic Syndr.* 2003;32:417–423.

222. Shoptaw S, Reback CJ, Peck JA, et al. Behavioral treatment approaches for methamphetamine dependence and HIV-related sexual risk behaviors among urban gay and bisexual men. *Drug Alcohol Depend.* 2005;78:125–134.

223. Vega MY, Roland EL. Social marketing techniques for public health communication: a review of syphilis awareness campaigns in 8 US cities. *Sex Trans Dis.* 2005;32:S30-S36.

224. Haviland ML. The enduring myth of power to the people: community participation in public health. *Curr Issues Public Health.* 1995;1:156–159.

225. Montoya JA, Kent CK, Rotblatt H, McCright J, Kerndt PR, Klausner JD. Social marketing campaign significantly associated with increases in syphilis testing among gay and bisexual men in San Francisco. *Sex Trans Dis.* 2005;32:395–399.

226. MSM HIV/STD Prevention Task Force. A community manifesto: a new response to HIV and STDs. www.metrokc.gov/health/apu/taksforce/manifesto.htm. Accessed October 7, 2003.
227. World Health Organization. Preamble to the Constitution of the World Health Organization. www.who.int/about/definition/en/print.htm. Accessed February 11, 2006.

7

Hepatitis A, B, and C Virus Infections among Men Who Have Sex with Men in the United States: Transmission, Epidemiology, and Intervention

Scott D. Rhodes and Leland J. Yee

Introduction to Hepatitis A, B, and C

Simply defined, hepatitis is a gastroenterological disease, characterized by inflammation of the liver. Although the signs and symptoms of hepatitis have been recognized for centuries, with references to epidemic jaundice recorded in many historical writings,[1] only relatively recently has an appreciation emerged for the specific viruses that may cause hepatitis. Hepatitis is most commonly attributed to a specific set of hepatotropic viral infections; however, other causes may include infection with other microorganisms (including nonhepatotropic viruses), excessive alcohol use, intake of hepatotoxic illicit drugs, consumption of medications that have a harmful effect on the liver, environmental toxin exposure, and some autoimmune diseases in which the liver is the primary organ affected.

A number of viral infections also may affect the liver and cause hepatitis, such as cytomegalovirus (CMV) infection, measles, rubella, and mumps. However, several viruses with primary hepatotropic effects are known collectively as the hepatitis viruses: *hepatitis A virus* (HAV), *hepatitis B virus* (HBV), *hepatitis C virus* (HCV), *hepatitis delta virus* (HDV), and *hepatitis E virus* (HEV). HDV is a "satellite" virus that may occur as a coinfection or superinfection with HBV, and HEV is currently endemic in regions of the world outside the United States. For these reasons, HDV and HEV are not addressed in this chapter. Instead, this chapter focuses on HAV, HBV, and HCV infections, which are important with respect to the health of men who have sex with men (MSM) in the United States.

Both HAV and HBV may be transmitted by sexual contact, and MSM are considered to be at increased risk for HAV and HBV through sexual behavior,[2,3] as evidenced through outbreaks and the presence of serological markers that reflect exposure as well as infection.[4–22]

Recently, HCV has become an increasing public health concern. Although the risk of sexual transmission of HCV is considered to be low,[23–26] HCV is a particularly important health issue for MSM who inject drugs or who are co-infected with HIV. Furthermore, in contrast to HAV and HBV, no vaccine for the prevention of HCV currently exists.

This chapter describes HAV, HBV, and HCV, including the routes of transmission; examines the epidemiology of hepatitis through available data within the general US male population and within samples of MSM; outlines the extent to which evidence of disparities exists by sexual orientation; explores existing responses; and proposes new approaches to reducing the burden of viral hepatitis among MSM.

Hepatitis A Virus Infection

HAV continues to be the one of the most frequently reported vaccine-preventable diseases in the United States.[27] Even with the availability of an HAV vaccine, the overall infection rate in 2004 was 1.9 per 100,000.[28] HAV is spread through fecal-oral contact, generally from person to person, or via contaminated food or water. Sexual transmission may occur via direct oral-anal contact (i.e., "rimming") or by oral contact with fingers, sex toys, or condoms that have been in or near the anus of an infected person and thus are contaminated by feces containing the virus. Infection with HAV does not become chronic (persistent) and rarely results in death. Signs and symptoms of infection with HAV include abdominal pain, fever, fatigue, lack of appetite, nausea, jaundice, dark urine, and weakness and malaise that may be debilitating.[29]

Clinical manifestations of HAV infection are age-related, with infection among older individuals being associated with more severe clinical presentation. For example, the frequency of jaundice, the occurrence of severe, debilitating symptoms, and fulminant hepatic failure increases with age,[27,30,31] with jaundice occurring in over 70% of adult infections, for example.[32]

In addition to clinical morbidity, HAV exerts an important economic burden. Medical care and lost wages associated with HAV in the United States have been estimated at more than $300 million annually.[33–35] Adults who become ill lose an average of 27 days of work, and estimates suggest that up to 22% of HAV-infected individuals become hospitalized. The average costs (including lost wages and medical and health department costs) associated with HAV infection range from $1,817 to $2,894 per case for adults.[35,36] In a single, common-source, HAV outbreak in the United States among 43 individuals, the estimated total societal cost was approximately $800,000.[37]

An effective two-dose vaccine exists for HAV, and MSM have been identified as a group to target for vaccination.[36] The HAV vaccine induces protective immunity in over 90% of individuals vaccinated.[38] Although the vaccine has the potential to reduce the morbidity and mortality associated with HAV, data suggest that currently a majority of MSM remain unvaccinated against HAV.[9,39,40] The limited available studies that explore HAV vaccination rates among MSM in the United States suggest that from 15% to 40% have been vaccinated against HAV.[10,12,41,42] Many studies of HAV vaccination uptake have been based on self-report, and therefore must be interpreted with caution. Furthermore, why some MSM seek vaccination and others do not is not well understood.[39,40] Similarly, how other groups for whom the vaccine is indicated compare to MSM in vaccination uptake and series completion remains predominately unexplored.

Hepatitis B Virus Infection

Another commonly reported and vaccine-preventable disease, HBV is blood borne, transmitted sexually, and may be acquired by both percutaneous as well as permucosal exposure to an infected person. Individuals with HBV may present with varied manifestations, ranging from asymptomatic presentation to jaundice, fever, and malaise. In approximately 10% of those infected with HBV, chronic infection develops. Possible sequelae from chronic HBV infection include outcomes such as cirrhosis of the liver and liver cancer. In the United States, 1.25 million individuals are estimated to be chronically infected with HBV; 240,000 new cases of HBV are identified annually, and 6,000 deaths are believed to occur each year from complications of HBV.[31,43,44]

The economic impact of HBV within the United States has not been well documented, and estimating the economic burden of HBV is complicated by its various stages of disease. Excluding post-transplantation care, Lee and colleagues have estimated that treatment for an HBV chronic carrier may be as high as $90,000 per liver transplantation (in US dollars in the year 2000).[45]

Since the early 1980s an effective multidose vaccine has been available for the prevention of HBV infection. Vaccine effectiveness has been rigorously documented: 95% of children and 90% of adults receiving the full three-dose series develop protective antibodies.[1,46,47] The US Centers for Disease Control and Prevention (CDC) has identified MSM, among others, as a target population for vaccination.[48] Yet, despite over two decades of vaccine licensure, seroprevalence surveys continue to find low rates of vaccination uptake among MSM.[49–52] The limited available studies that explore HBV vaccination rates among MSM in the United States suggest that between 11% and 48% have been vaccinated against HBV.[11,53–56] Many studies of HBV vaccination uptake have been based on self-report, and therefore must be interpreted with caution. Future studies will need to include objective serologic markers of infection and vaccination to validate self-reported behaviors as well as compare uptake and series completion by groups for whom vaccination is indicated.

Hepatitis C Virus Infection

Identified in 1989 as the major cause of non-A, non-B hepatitis,[57] HCV infection is currently recognized as the most common blood-borne infection and the leading indication for a liver transplantation in the United States.[58,59]

Chronic infection develops in the majority of individuals exposed to HCV. Approximately 4 million Americans and an estimated 200 million persons globally have been infected with HCV. Among these, approximately 80% have persistent or chronic infections.[60–64]

The major route of HCV transmission is via contact with infected blood, most commonly through the sharing of injecting-drug use equipment or receipt of contaminated blood or blood products. However, due to the implementation of effective screening for HCV shortly after its discovery in 1989, blood and blood products are quite safe in the developed world. Permucosal transmission and, in particular, the degree of risk of sexual transmission of HCV continues to be debated.[24,26] In a recent population-based study of HCV, a number of individuals reported sexual behavior as the sole risk factor for HCV infection.[58] Several case reports also suggest sexual transmission.[65,66] These studies document HCV transmission in individuals at risk in temporal relationships with an HCV-infected partner. High levels of viral sequence homology in some of the studies also suggest sexual transmission.[65,66]

In contrast, another study examined 18 heterosexual couples (36 persons) recruited from 430 HCV-infected persons.[67] After screening for risk factors, all but one reported exposure to parenteral risk factors. In half of the couples, sexual transmission within the dyad was ruled out because the couples were infected with different HCV viral genotypes. In the remaining individuals, analysis of the viral sequences suggested that transmission could have occurred in only one couple, and this couple also shared equipment for injecting-drug use.[67]

The sexual transmission of HCV most likely occurs with a very low frequency, and this low frequency has contributed to making it difficult to quantify the risk of sexual transmission and, in particular, the differential risks of different sexual acts. In addition, sexual transmission in the presence of other risk factors (e.g., needle sharing), has made it difficult to fully eliminate these other confounding factors. Further research is needed to accurately quantify the risk of the sexual transmission of HCV. The risk of sexual transmission of HCV among MSM and the role of coinfection with HIV, which has been identified as potentially enhancing sexual transmission of HCV, possibly by elevating levels of HCV viremia,[68–70] need further elucidation.

HCV is often asymptomatic and is therefore considered an insidious disease. Frequently, individuals are diagnosed decades after infection. The majority of individuals infected with HCV develop chronic infection, with only 14% to 46% able to naturally clear the virus.[71–75] Chronic infection exhibits a variability in progression. Why some individuals have only mild or moderately progressive liver disease, while others develop cirrhosis of the liver or liver cancer, is not well understood. HCV-associated end-stage liver disease is the leading indication for liver transplantation in the United States and the developed Western world. In fact, an estimated 8,000–10,000 deaths are estimated to occur as a result of HCV annually in the United States.[58]

As existing cases progress, HCV is expected to impose an immense burden on the US healthcare system in the near future. Over the next two decades,

HCV is expected to account for a 180% increase in liver-related deaths in United States,[59] result in more than 1.83 million years of life lost among individuals under 65 years of age, and cost more than $10.7 billion in direct medical expenditures.[76,77]

Currently, a vaccine against HCV does not exist, but the implementation of routine screening for HCV in the US blood supply has resulted in a decline of the number of incident HCV cases. Combination therapy, using pegylated interferon-α and ribavirin, is the current treatment for individuals with chronic HCV, and is effective in approximately 40% to 46% of those infected with genotype-1 HCV infection, and approximately 76% to 80% in those with non-1 genotype HCV infections.[78,79] Unfortunately, the more resilient genotype-1 virus is the most prevalent genotype of HCV in the United States, and significant racial disparities exist. African Americans have an approximate twofold higher prevalence of HCV compared to Caucasians,[58] and have a significantly lower treatment response rate compared to Caucasians (19% to 26% for African Americans vs. 39% to 52% for Caucasians).[80–83] The mechanisms accounting for the lack of response to therapy, as well as the mechanisms behind the observed racial disparities, are not understood.

Descriptive Epidemiology

Methods

With the goal of examining the burden of HAV, HBV, and HCV borne by MSM, a systematic review was performed of English-language publications pertaining to the prevalence of hepatitis using Medline and Web of Science databases, 1966 through August 2005, and ERIC, CINAHL, PubMed, and EMBASE, 1980 through August 2005, to identify empirical and peer-reviewed research related to the transmission, prevalence, and prevention of HAV, HBV, and HCV among MSM. A series of keyword and subject searches were conducted, first, to identify papers concerning the prevalence of each type of hepatitis (i.e., HAV, HBV, and HCV) separately, and then to identify papers including MSM. Subsequently, combinations of the search results were used to identify papers specifically addressing prevalence of HAV, HBV, and HCV among MSM. In addition, citations from the bibliographies of these papers were analyzed, and relevant citations were selected for review. Analyses were restricted to MSM in the United States.

For each type of hepatitis, estimates and 95% confidence intervals (CI) of the prevalence of hepatitis among adult men in the United States are provided, based on the Third National Health and Nutrition Examination Survey (NHANES III). NHANES III was used because it provides data from a representative sample of the civilian noninstitutionalized US population, collected between 1988 and 1994. Estimates and 95% CI, when available, of the prevalence of hepatitis among samples of MSM in United States are provided.

Hepatitis A

Fortunately, improvements in sanitation over the past several decades have brought a concomitant decrease in the number of incident cases of HAV infection; however, this decrease remains heterogeneous across demographics, geographic location, socioeconomic status, and risk behavior.[27] Approximately one-third of the US population has serologic evidence of previous HAV infection, and approximately 100 HAV cases result in death each year in the United States.[31 36] During the 1980s and 1990s, an average of 26,000 HAV cases were reported annually to US public health agencies. Taking asymptomatic infections without jaundice (anicteric) into account, it is estimated that 270,000 HAV infections occur yearly in the United States.[84] MSM are considered to be an important target group for HAV prevention, along with other groups such as household contacts of infected individuals, sexual partners of infected individuals, travelers to countries where HAV is endemic, and injecting-drug users.

Table 7-1 presents a summary of studies, documenting the prevalence of HAV among various samples of men. NHANES III data ($n = 40,000$), which were collected between 1988 and 1994, found over one-third (37.2%, 95% CI: 34.5–40.0) of all men in the United States, ages 20–59 years, had antibodies against HAV. Four studies of the prevalence of HAV within samples of MSM were identified. Key demographic descriptors differed most notably by mean age in years. Prevalence levels ranged from 14% among younger MSM[10] to 30% among MSM, ages 18–58.[85]

Corey and Holmes offered the first US study to establish a significant difference in HAV prevalence between MSM and heterosexual men.[85] Their study, which took place prior to the existence of a vaccine against HAV, collected serologic markers and self-reported sexual behaviors among 102 MSM and 57 heterosexual men visiting an STD clinic in Seattle, Washington. At baseline, prevalence of HAV was significantly different: 30% among MSM and 12% among heterosexual men ($p < .01$). After over 6 months follow-up, the incidence of HAV in susceptible (seronegative) MSM was 22%, whereas no heterosexual men in their sample acquired HAV during the period.

Although MSM appeared to have higher prevalence compared to heterosexual men, the differences found by Corey and Holmes may have been affected by the slightly older age of the MSM because of cumulative exposures to HAV over their lifespan.[85] Furthermore, other ways in which these men may have differed were not well explored, especially in terms of their other risk factors. Finally, in retrospect, it appears that a localized gay community outbreak may have been occurring during their study period because the number of incident HAV infections declined after the study period (1977–1979).

A recent Canadian review of HAV examined seroprevalence among a variety of population subgroups and concluded that when compared to heterosexuals, MSM had only marginally higher HAV seroprevalence (adjusted odds ratio: 2.4; 95% CI: 0.9–6.1).[86] Although current available data do not

Table 7-1. Estimated prevalence of HAV among samples of men in the United States

Study Period	Study Site	Sampling Strategy	Sample Size	Key Demographic Descriptors	Prevalence (95% CI)	Measurement	References
1988–1994	US	Multi-stage, probability cluster design	15,580	Men, ages 20–59 years	37.2% (34.5%–40.0%)	Anti-HAV	139
1997–2000	King County, Washington	Time-space sampling	833	MSM, ages 15–29 years	14.0%	HAV IgG+ without vaccination	10
1993–1994	Baltimore	Cohort	294	Homosexual men	27.3%	Anti-HAV	116
1992–1993	San Francisco and Berkeley	Public venue outreach	411	Homosexual and bisexual men, ages 17–22 years	28.0% (23.7%–32.6%)	Anti-HAV	41
1977–1979	Seattle	STD Clinic	129	Homosexual men, ages 18–58 years	30.0%	Anti-HAV	85

consistently show evidence of disproportionate HAV infection burden among MSM, several important considerations require elaboration. First, available aggregate data may obscure the increased prevalence within specific communities of MSM. In their study in San Francisco and Berkeley, California, Katz and colleagues recruited men in 26 public venues "frequented by young homosexual and bisexual men" and found an HAV seroprevalence of 28% (95% CI: 23.7–32.6) among MSM, ages 17–22 years.[41] The prevalence among a broader age group of MSM may have been even higher within this community, potentially surpassing the prevalence identified for men by NHANES III, because as individuals age the potential for exposure increases.

Moreover, periodic outbreaks of HAV among susceptible groups, including MSM, occur and pose significant public health problems, both within the United States[9,12,13,15,87] and internationally.[4,6,16,18–21] During a 1997 outbreak of HAV infection in Atlanta, Georgia, incidence among MSM increased by 730%. In the first eight months of the outbreak, 222 cases of HAV were documented, compared to a prior average of about 27 cases per year. About 75% of the men infected self-identified as MSM, and nearly all cases were diagnosed at medical practices predominantly serving MSM.[88] Although outbreaks may not provide evidence of disproportionate burden borne by MSM, outbreaks are clearly important considerations in the appreciation of the burden borne by subgroups within MSM communities. Although available data on the prevalence of HAV among MSM and heterosexual men appear to be comparable, social and sexual networks and modes of transmission may be affected disproportionately.

Finally, NHANES III data were collected prior to the existence of a vaccine against HAV. Given the success of infant and childhood vaccination strategies, HAV infection through non-gay or household contact and the child-care industry is declining and thus changing the epidemiologic profile of HAV, increasing the potential for disproportionate burden among MSM in the short term. Over time, however, as those who are vaccinated against HAV as children and adolescents age, HAV will become less prevalent for all groups currently identified to be at increased risk or targeted for vaccination.[89,90]

Hepatitis B

In the United States, it is estimated that approximately 1.25 million individuals have chronic HBV infection.[46 91] Up to 6,000 deaths occur each year from acute or chronic HBV.[43,92] Population-based estimates from NHANES suggests that 323,462 incident HBV infections occurred annually during 1976–1980, while 334,863 incident infections occurred annually between 1988–1994.[46,91] MSM are considered to be at increased risk for HBV infection, along with individuals with multiple sex partners, persons who have a history of STDs, sex partners of infected individuals, injection-drug users, household contacts of chronically infected individuals, health care and public safety workers, and hemodialysis patients.

Table 7-2 presents a summary of studies documenting the prevalence of HBV among various samples of men. According to NHANES III data, 4.9% (95% CI: 4.3–5.6) of the US population has evidence of past exposure to HBV.[91] Among men, prevalence was 6.5% (95% CI: 5.6–7.6), and among MSM, the prevalence of HBV was 26.8% (95% CI: 18.4–39.2), providing evidence for disproportionate HBV infection among MSM within the same NHANES III sample.

Twelve studies of the prevalence of HBV within samples of MSM were identified. Key demographic descriptors differed by age in years and race/ethnicity. Prevalence ranged from 5.0% among MSM ages 15–17 years[93] to 81.0% among MSM ages 22–61 years.[94] All studies that included a broad range of ages reported a high prevalence among MSM.

In a study initiated in 1995, Tabet and colleagues found the prevalence of HBV was 34.8% (95% CI: 30.2–39.6) among 578 HIV-negative MSM, ages 18–71 years, in Seattle, Washington.[95] In a more narrowly defined study population, the San Francisco Bay Area Young Men's Survey II ($n = 619$) found an HBV prevalence of 14.1% among MSM, ages 18–22 years.[93] A multisite study of young MSM ($n = 3432$) in seven major U.S. metropolitan areas found overall prevalence for markers for HBV to be over 10% overall, ranging from 2% among 15-year-olds to 17% among 22-year-olds.[17]

In their sample of Asian and Pacific Islander MSM, age 18–29 years, Choi and colleagues (2005) found 28% prevalence for HBV.[8] Although this study sampled a relatively young group, the prevalence was within the range identified by NHANES III for MSM. In general, Asian and Pacific Islanders tend to have higher levels of HBV than other ethnic groups, and the high levels of HBV reported among MSM in this study may have been affected by the ethnicity of the cohort.[46]

Extremely high levels of exposure to HBV among MSM (>60%) have been reported in several published studies.[96–98] A variety of factors may contribute to the high prevalence reported. First, many of the studies were conducted within cohorts at high risk for the acquisition of HBV via sexual transmission; for example, men from a gay bathhouse[98] and men who have presented themselves to an STD clinic seeking care for non-hepatitis-related screening and medical treatment.[96] Therefore, it is important to consider the populations from which the various study samples were drawn. Furthermore, some studies were undertaken prior to the existence of a vaccine against HBV. Prevalence levels might be lower if the study were replicated today.

Hepatitis C

Population-based estimates from the NHANES III study suggest that approximately 4 million individuals in the United States have evidence of past exposure to HCV. Among these individuals, an estimated 2.7 million (~75%) have chronic HCV infection.[58] Table 7-3 presents a summary of studies documenting the prevalence of HCV among various samples of men.

Table 7-2. Estimated prevalence of HBV among samples of men in the United States

Study Period	Study Site	Sampling Strategy	Sample Size	Key Demographic Descriptors	Prevalence (95% CI)	Measurement	References
1988–1994	US	Multi-stage, probability cluster design	10,624	Men, ages 20–59	6.5% (5.6%–7.6%)	AntiHBc	139
1988–1994	US	Multi-stage, probability cluster design	80	MSM, ages 17–59 years	26.8% (18.4%–39.2%)	Anti-HBc	91
2000–2001	San Francisco	Time-space sampling	489	Asian/Pacific Islander MSM, ages 18–29 years	28.0%	Anti-HBc	8
1997–2000	King County, Washington	Time-space sampling	833	MSM, ages 15–29 years	14.4%	Anti-HBc	10
1998	San Diego STD Clinic	Convenience	66	Non-IDU MSM	37%	Anti-HBc	99
1994–1998	7 US metropolitan areas	Time-space sampling	3,432	MSM, ages 15–22 years	10.4%	Anti-HBc	17
1994–1995	San Francisco Bay Area	Time-space sampling	100	MSM, ages 15–17 years	5.0%	Anti-HBc	93
1994–1995	San Francisco Bay Area	Time-space sampling	619	MSM, ages 18–22 years	14.1%	Anti-HBc	93
1995	Seattle, Washington	Outreach	578	HIV-negative MSM, ages 18–71 years	34.8% (30.2%–39.6%)	Anti-HBc	95

(continued)

Table 7-2. (continued)

Study Period	Study Site	Sampling Strategy	Sample Size	Key Demographic Descriptors	Prevalence (95% CI)	Measurement	References
1992–1994	Boston	Outreach	508	Gay and bisexual men, ages 18–29 years	12.9%	Anti-HBc	56
1984–1985 and 1987–1991	Multicenter AIDS Cohort Study	Cohort	5,293	Predominantly MSM	64.0%	HBsAG	97
1983–1984	San Francisco	Cohort	735	Homosexual and bisexual men, ages 22–61	81%	HBsAg	94
1978–1979	5 STD clinics	Convenience	3,816	MSM, ages ≥18 years	61.5%	HBsAG	96
1977	Denver bathhouse	Convenience	543	Adult men	60.9%	Anti-HBs or HBsAg	98

Table 7-3. Estimated prevalence of HCV among samples of men in the United States

Study Period	Study Site	Sampling Strategy	Sample size	Key Demographic Descriptors	Prevalence (95% CI)	Measurement	References
1988–1994	US	Multi-stage, probability cluster design	10,612	Men, ages 20–59	3.4% (2.6%–4.4%)	Anti-HCV	139
1998	San Diego STD Clinic	Convenience	66	Non-IDU MSM	0.0%	Anti-HBc	99
1984	Baltimore/Washington Multicenter AIDS Cohort Study	Cohort	926	Predominantly MSM	1.6%	Anti-HCV	140
1983–1984	San Francisco	Cohort	435	Homosexual men, ages 22–66 years	9.2%	Anti-HCV	100
1983–1984	San Francisco	Cohort	735	Homosexual and bisexual men, ages 22–61	4.6%	Anti-HCV	94

NHANES III reported a 3.4% (95% CI: 2.6–4.4) HCV prevalence among all men ages 20–59 years. Studies among MSM have found seroprevalence ranging from 0.0%[99] to 9.2%.[100]

Four studies of the prevalence of HCV within samples of MSM were identified. Key demographic descriptors differed mainly by whether the sample included injecting-drug users. Prevalence ranged from 0.0% among MSM who did not use injecting-drugs[99] to 9.2% among MSM, ages 22–61 years.[100] This high rate was primarily attributable to injecting-drug use and blood transfusions.[100]

Evidence is mounting to conclude that, although HCV is sexually transmissible, the efficiency of transmission via this mode may be far less than other blood-borne viruses such as hepatitis B or HIV.[25,65,101–104] In a recent longitudinal cohort study of MSM, HCV prevalence at entry was 2.9%, and was strongly associated with injecting-drug use. Only one HCV seroconversion was detected in 2653 person-years of follow-up (incidence rate = 0.038 per 100 person-years), and the man who seroconverted was an active injecting-drug user who reported needle sharing.[23]

Other studies also have suggested low levels of sexual transmission of HCV.[65,66,102] However, it may be that sexual transmission of HCV among MSM is facilitated by other risk factors such as coinfection with HIV[7,25,68,70,105–107] or other STDs,[108,109] increased number of sexual partners,[25,110,111] and high-risk sexual practices (including "fisting" and other activities that may lead to trauma to anal tissue).[25,103,108,111–114] The challenge is to eliminate confounding risk factors such as unrecognized (or undisclosed) parenteral transmission due to sharing of items that might carry infected blood, such as toothbrushes, razors, needles, and syringes. These risk factors may be either easily overlooked or stigmatizing and thus may be undocumented.[104,115,116]

Furthermore, all sexual behaviors may not carry the same level of risk, and future studies should examine potential differences in the risk conferred by different sexual behaviors. For example, studies have identified increased number of partners, bleeding during anal intercourse, and "fisting" among the potential contributors to HCV transmission.[103,112–114] In addition, it will be important to document the role of coinfections such as HIV in facilitating HCV transmission through sexual contact.

For MSM who use injecting drugs, HCV clearly poses an important health risk. Current recommendations are for individuals who have risk factors, such as injecting-drug use, to be tested for HCV. Although scant data exist pertaining to HCV testing among MSM, an Internet-recruited study of HCV testing among MSM found only 39% of MSM reported ever having been tested for HCV.[115] Excluding MSM behavior, over 95% reported having at least one other risk factor for HCV, which included sharing injecting-drug needles or "works," sharing straws to snort cocaine or other drugs, body piercing, tattooing, and increased number of sexual partners.[115]

The Extent to Which Disparities Exist

Accurate population-based assessment of the public health impact of hepatitis virus infection among MSM has been hindered, at least in part, by the lack of systematic measurement of sexual orientation. Only recently have some population-based epidemiologic studies attempted to incorporate measures (both direct or, more often, proxy measures) of sexual orientation among study participants.[117] Without data on sexual orientation, accurate assessment of the health needs of MSM remains problematic.

The available data for HAV suggest that MSM may have higher rates of infection, when comparing heterosexual men of comparable ages. However, data from the same sampling frame currently are not available to confirm this supposition. Nevertheless, the disproportionate burden of HBV among MSM is clearly evident. Comparable US data were available from the same data source, the NHANES III, showing that the HBV prevalence for MSM was four times that of men in general. The existence of disparities in HCV infection among MSM is not likely, but the current data are inadequate.

Promising Responses to Resolving Disparities in Hepatitis Infection among MSM

HAV and HBV

Documented barriers to HAV and HBV vaccination among MSM include living in rural communities, having less knowledge about hepatitis, inadequate access to health care, lack of openness about one's sexual orientation, limited provider communication about MSM behavior, and negative attitudes about vaccination.[22,39,42,51,118–121] A variety of strategies have been either used or proposed to reduce the hepatitis disease burden borne by MSM. Three promising approaches that have been evaluated include: (1) a social marketing approach to HAV vaccination,[12] (2) a targeted HAV and HBV series adherence intervention that involved clinician recommendation and telephone follow-up,[122] and (3) combined dosing of vaccines against HAV and HBV.[123]

"*Girlfriend, yellow is not your color*" was a campaign that included a targeted, culturally appropriate advertising campaign sponsored by the Georgia Division of Public Health and AID Atlanta. The campaign was designed to educate gay and bisexual men about their risk of hepatitis A and B infection, to increase hepatitis A and B vaccination rates within the Atlanta, Goergia, community, and to encourage public and private health care providers to incorporate hepatitis A and B education and vaccination in their standard of care for MSM. The Atlanta-based campaign reflected the humor of the local MSM community by featuring three popular local "drag queens." The advertisements playfully focused on the potential effects of hepatitis infection, addressed sexual risk behaviors, and promoted vaccination. Advertisements were sequentially placed over a four-month period in five publications that target the local gay community in Atlanta. In addition, during the Atlanta Gay and Lesbian Pride Festival, nearly 10,000 hepatitis awareness fans featuring the drag queens were distributed along the parade route.

Evaluation of this social marketing campaign suggested that increased exposure to vaccination-promotion messages was associated with self-reported vaccination acceptance and uptake; vaccine coverage rates among MSM increased linearly as the number of information exposures increased ($p <$ .0001).[12] Furthermore, this campaign suggested that the local gay print media is an effective mode to distribute health-related information to MSM.[12] This social marketing intervention was conducted during a period of transition in media use; the Internet has become much more frequently used. This increasing use of the Internet may create new challenges—and opportunities—for marketing health campaigns to MSM communities.

Another intervention of note is a clinic-based intervention that offered routine HAV and HBV screening and free vaccination during routine STD clinic visits.[122] This intervention was implemented by the Los Angeles Gay and Lesbian Center in collaboration with the Los Angeles County Health Department and the CDC in 1999. The intervention included the use of telephone reminders to improve series completion. The success of this intervention was mixed: nearly a third of eligible participants obtained full vaccination against HAV and HBV, and nearly two-thirds received at least one dose of both vaccines. Reminder telephone calls were potentially important for boosting vaccine series completion, but disconnected telephone numbers or incorrect numbers were identified as challenges in this study.[122] The increased use of mobile telephones would further affect this type of intervention.

A third approach to increasing vaccination among MSM is combining vaccines and/or changing vaccination series intervals. In 2001, the Food and Drug Administration (FDA) licensed a combined hepatitis A and B vaccine (Twinrix®) for use in persons aged 18 years and older.[124] Twinrix is made of the antigenic components used in Havrix® and Engerix-B® (GlaxoSmithKline). The antigenic components in Twinrix® have been used routinely in separate single antigen vaccines in the United States since 1989 and 1995 as HBV and HAV vaccines, respectively. Combining vaccines reduces the number of injections required, resulting in greater convenience for the patient and the health care provider, increased compliance with the vaccination schedule, less discomfort for the patient, and reduced costs, medical waste, workload, and number of medical visits required.[123]

Preliminary evidence suggests that accelerated vaccination schedules for combined vaccines may provide effective protection while improving uptake and series completion. The current combined HAV and HBV vaccination schedule for Twinrix®, for example, is three vaccinations at 0, 1, and 6 months. An accelerated vaccination schedule of combined HAV/HBV vaccines at 0, 7, and 21 days has been shown to provide over 90% protective immunity at month 12.[125] If found to be consistently effective in providing sufficient protective immunity and safe in replication studies, an accelerated vaccination schedule could improve series completion because after three weeks (i.e., the final vaccination) no additional visits would be required.

These three highlighted interventions identify important approaches to vaccinating MSM in the United States against HAV and HBV. Yet, further research on vaccination access and uptake among MSM is needed to offer new insights into potential solutions to disease burden. Although a variety of vaccination strategies have been proposed to increase vaccination rates among MSM, few have been implemented, and fewer still have been evaluated to measure the effectiveness of these efforts.

Next Steps in Reducing the Burden of Hepatitis among MSM

This section explores potential intervention strategies to reduce hepatitis risk behaviors and increase HAV and HBV vaccination rates. To increase vaccination among MSM, multiple-level strategies must be developed, implemented, and evaluated. This will require the use of complimentary approaches that target multiple levels within a socio-ecological framework because addressing hepatitis disparities through a single strategy is not likely to sufficiently affect the infection rates among MSM. This section provides an overview of potentially useful strategies.

First, at the individual level, MSM need increased awareness and information about hepatitis. Although knowledge does not guarantee behavior change, in order for action-orientated health promotion and disease prevention messages to be placed in context, MSM must have a basic understanding of the facts around hepatitis. Studies have shown that MSM in the United States do not have an adequate understanding of either hepatitis or hepatitis vaccination—including the indicated vaccination series required to provide sufficient immunity and the process of vaccination (e.g., where to get vaccinated, the costs of vaccination, etc.).[55,119,121,126]

Innovative "sex-positive" and "gay-positive" approaches to disseminating information about hepatitis and hepatitis vaccination must be explored and tested to determine whether they can positively influence vaccination rates among MSM. Messages must be well tailored to attract the attention of the intended audience and provide practical information about local resources for vaccination. The social marketing campaign *"Girlfriend, yellow is not your color"* is an example of such an approach. Other campaigns exist; unfortunately, evaluation of these campaigns is quite limited.

It is important to note, too, that no one approach will meet the prevention needs of all segments of the MSM community. *"Girlfriend, yellow is not your color"* may not resonate with all members of the MSM community or necessarily be successfully transferable to other communities of MSM. In any successful health education effort, effort must be paid to (1) identifying those at risk, (2) defining them narrowly, and (3) selecting appropriate strategies given the narrowly defined target based on their risk, the ability to reach them, and the potential to effect change. Often, these early phases are not sufficiently explored, resulting in incorrect assumptions about the target group and ineffective interventions.

At the interpersonal level, trust between health care providers and MSM must be increased. Because MSM need to feel comfortable to discuss stigmatized behaviors, providers—in either public or private clinical settings—must create environments that are conducive to accurate risk disclosure so as to gain the necessary information that will direct appropriate vaccination recommendations. Computer-based delivery of patient education that provides theory-based "cues to action" for patients to discuss risks with providers may assist in prompting accurate risk disclosure. Although this approach for MSM has not been explored in the literature, a similar approach has been used within other populations for other health risks.[127,128]

Interventions targeting providers also may increase HAV and HBV vaccination rates. Providers must be comfortable with assessing risk among MSM patients, including refraining from the assumption that all patients are heterosexual. They must inform their at-risk patients about the efficacy and safety of vaccines to encourage vaccination.[39,55] Paramount to communicating with patients about risk and vaccine efficacy and safety, a provider must build trust. Patient trust in the medical establishment has been found to be positively associated with accessing health and medical care services and accepting and following provider recommendations.[129] Research has suggested that distrust of the medical establishment is a salient concern of some African American MSM in particular[119]; thus, enhancing patient trust must remain a priority. Chapter 13 further addresses issues of trust in the medical establishment.

Providers who hope to correctly assess risk and encourage hepatitis risk reduction will need thorough training in (1) developing and maintaining nonhomophobic assumptions and attitudes, (2) distinguishing patients' sexual behaviors from identities, (3) communicating clearly and sensitively, (4) using gender-neutral terms when referring to sexual partners, and (5) being attuned to how personal provider attitudes affect clinical judgments.[117,130]

The opinions and recommendations of "important others" and peers also have been found to be crucial to the acceptance and uptake of vaccination against HAV and HBV.[131] This finding has at least two implications. First, for MSM, efforts to influence vaccination behavior could involve a peer education or peer leadership approach. Unfortunately, despite the success of a peer-based approach with condom promotion and the reduction of partners to protect against HIV,[132] the use of peer opinion leaders, such as bartenders, has not been well-utilized and well-tested to promote other health-promoting behaviors among MSM, such as vaccination against HAV and HBV.

Second, success of using peers in HIV prevention illustrates the importance of understanding the diversity within MSM communities. Just as "*Girlfriend, yellow is not your color*" may not resonate with all MSM communities, effective strategies to promote vaccination acceptance and uptake may be more successful when built on what is important to MSM. In many cases, what is

important to MSM, as with other communities of identification, is their connection to social networks and communities.[133] This is a basic principle of
health promotion and must be adhered to as strategies to affect hepatitis
behaviors are developed.

At the institutional level, providing vaccination services in untraditional
locations, such as bars and clubs, bathhouses, bookstores, "circuit parties,"
coffee shops, gyms, house parties, and parks, may reach MSM who have or
perceive a variety of barriers to vaccination services in traditional settings.
Strategies of vaccinating MSM against hepatitis in locations where MSM meet
have not been commonly implemented or evaluated, however. Moreover, the
provision of free vaccination services in these untraditional outreach sites may
further encourage vaccination and thus prevent the morbidity and mortality
associated with HAV and HBV. Despite the vaccination setting, to minimize
the number of visits required for vaccination, screening to identify those with
natural immunity or chronic infection could occur at first dose.

HCV

HCV poses a different set of challenges given that there is no available vaccine.
Therefore, any approach to preventing HCV must be targeted to the behaviors that put MSM at risk for HCV, especially injecting-drug use. Additional
empirical evidence will be needed to clarify the relative contribution of specific sexual behaviors (e.g., "fisting") to sexual transmission of HCV and
whether a disparity in HCV exists for MSM. Because injecting-drug use is
clearly associated with HCV transmission, effective interventions for injecting
drug-using MSM, including drug treatment, should be developed, implemented, and evaluated.

Vision for the Future

Much of the current public health dialogue in the United States conceptu-
alizes health disparities in terms of biological sex and race and ethnicity.[134–136]
Less discussion has focused on health disparities that exist by sexual
orientation—except for the notable exception of HIV infection rates by sexual
orientation.[117] In part, this is because the data that identify health outcomes
and their associated behaviors by sexual orientation and behavior are extremely limited and inexact. In most behavioral and epidemiologic studies,
including those studies that are population based, measures of sexual orientation are not routinely included.[3,117,137,138] Without data on sexual orientation, assessing the impact of HAV, HBV, and HCV among MSM is difficult.

Thus, future research should include: (1) epidemiologic studies that collect
biological markers to compliment behavior data in order to determine whether specific health disparities exist among MSM and to what extent; (2) comprehensive surveillance and ongoing data collection to document the prevalence of associated health-promoting and health-compromising behaviors and

hepatitis outcomes among MSM of all ages; and (3) the development, implementation, and evaluation of creative yet scientifically sound interventions to increase vaccination against HAV and HBV and reduce risk behaviors for HCV among MSM. These interventions must reflect multiple-level ecological strategies that target not only the individual but his social and sexual networks, his sense of community, provider attitudes, patient-provider communication, access to care and services, and service delivery.

Finally, given the impact and the economic outcomes resulting from HCV infections in the United States, research must work toward both improved management of the disease and the development and distribution of an effective and safe vaccine.

References

1. Keeffe EB. Clinical approach to viral hepatitis in homosexual men. *Med Clin North Am.* 1986;70:567–586.
2. Centers for Disease Control and Prevention. Sexually transmitted diseases treatment guidelines. *MMWR Morb Mortal Wkly Rep* 2002;RR-6:59–63.
3. Gay and Lesbian Medical Association. *Healthy People 2010: Companion Document for Lesbian, Gay, Bisexual, and Transgender (LGBT) Health.* San Francisco, CA: Gay and Lesbian Medical Association; 2001.
4. Allard R, Beauchemin J, Bedard L, Dion R, Tremblay M, Carsley J. Hepatitis A vaccination during an outbreak among gay men in Montreal, Canada, 1995–1997. *J Epidemiol Community Health.* 2001;55:251–256.
5. Atkins M, Nolan M. Sexual transmission of hepatitis B. *Curr Opin Infect Dis.* 2005;18:67–72.
6. Bell A, Ncube F, Hansell A, Davison KL, Young Y, Gilson R, et al. An outbreak of hepatitis A among young men associated with having sex in public venues. *Commun Dis Public Health.* 2001;4:163–170.
7. Brook MG. Sexually acquired hepatitis. *Sex Transm Infect.* 2002;78:235–240.
8. Choi KH, McFarland W, Neilands TB, Nguyen S, Secura G, Behel S, et al. High level of hepatitis B infection and ongoing risk among Asian/Pacific Islander men who have sex with men, San Francisco, 2000–2001. *Sex Transm Dis.* 2005;32:44–48.
9. Cotter SM, Sansom S, Long T, et al. Outbreak of hepatitis A among men who have sex with men: implications for hepatitis A vaccination strategies. *J Infect Dis.* 2003;187:1235–1240.
10. Diamond C, Thiede H, Perdue T, et al. Viral hepatitis among young men who have sex with men: prevalence of infection, risk behaviors, and vaccination. *Sex Transm Dis.* 2003;30:425–432.
11. Dufour A, Remis RS, Alary M, Otis J, Masse B, Turmel B, et al. Factors associated with hepatitis B vaccination among men having sexual relations with men in Montreal, Quebec, Canada. Omega Study Group. *Sex Transm Dis.* 1999;26:317–324.
12. Friedman MS, Blake PA, Koehler JE, Hutwagner LC, Toomey KE. Factors influencing a communitywide campaign to administer hepatitis A vaccine to men who have sex with men. *Am J Public Health.* 2000;90:1942–1946.
13. Henning KJ, Bell E, Braun J, Barker ND. A community-wide outbreak of hepatitis A: risk factors for infection among homosexual and bisexual men. *Am J Med.* 1995;99:132–136.

14. Kahn J. Preventing hepatitis A and hepatitis B virus infections among men who have sex with men. *Clin Infect Dis.* 2002;35:1382–1387.

15. Kosatsky T, Middaugh JP. Linked outbreaks of hepatitis A in homosexual men and in food service patrons and employees. *West J Med.* 1986;144:307–310.

16. Leentvaar-Kuijpers A, Kool JL, Veugelers PJ, Coutinho RA, van Griensven GJ. An outbreak of hepatitis A among homosexual men in Amsterdam, 1991–1993. *Int J Epidemiol.* 1995;24:218–222.

17. MacKellar DA, Valleroy LA, Secura GM, et al. Two decades after vaccine license: hepatitis B immunization and infection among young men who have sex with men. *Am J Public Health.* 2001;91:965–971.

18. Mazick A, Howitz M, Rex S, Jensen I, Weis N, Katzenstein T, et al. Hepatitis A outbreak among MSM linked to casual sex and gay saunas in Copenhagen, Denmark. *Euro Surveill.* 2005;10:111–114.

19. Reintjes R, Bosman A, de Zwart O, Stevens M, van der Knaap L, van den Hoek K. Outbreak of hepatitis A in Rotterdam associated with visits to 'darkrooms' in gay bars. *Commun Dis Public Health.* 1999;2:43–46.

20. Stene-Johansen K, Jenum PA, Hoel T, Blystad H, Sunde H, Skaug K. An outbreak of hepatitis A among homosexuals linked to a family outbreak. *Epidemiol Infect.* 2002;129:113–117.

21. Stewart T, Crofts N. An outbreak of hepatitis A among homosexual men in Melbourne. *Med J Aust.* 1993;158:519–521.

22. Yee LJ, Rhodes SD. Understanding correlates of hepatitis B virus vaccination in men who have sex with men: what have we learned? *Sex Transm Infect.* 2002; 78:374–377.

23. Alary M, Joly JR, Vincelette J, Lavoie R, Turmel B, Remis RS. Lack of evidence of sexual transmission of hepatitis C virus in a prospective cohort study of men who have sex with men. *Am J Public Health.* 2005;95:502–505.

24. Osella AR, Massa MA, Joekes S, et al. Hepatitis B and C virus sexual transmission among homosexual men. *Am J Gastroenterol.* 1998;93:49–52.

25. Terrault NA. Sexual activity as a risk factor for hepatitis C. *Hepatology.* 2002;36(5 Suppl 1):S99–S105.

26. Weinstock HS, Bolan G, Reingold AL, Polish LB. Hepatitis C virus infection among patients attending a clinic for sexually transmitted diseases. *JAMA.* 1993;269:392–394.

27. Bell BP, Shapiro CN, Alter MJ, et al. The diverse patterns of hepatitis A epidemiology in the United States: implications for vaccination strategies. *J Infect Dis.* 1998;178:1579–1584.

28. Wasley A, Fiore A, Bell BP. Hepatitis A in the era of vaccination. *Epidemiol Rev.* 2006;28:101–111.

29. Zachoval R, Deinhardt F. Natural history and experimental models. In: Zuckerman A, Thomas HC, eds. *Viral Hepatitis.* 2nd ed. London: Churchill Livingstone; 1998:43–57.

30. Gingrich GA, Hadler SC, Elder HA, Ash KO. Serologic investigation of an outbreak of hepatitis A in a rural day-care center. *Am J Public Health.* 1983;73:1190–1193.

31. Koff RS. Hepatitis A. *Lancet.* 1998;351:1643–1649.

32. Lednar WM, Lemon SM, Kirkpatrick JW, Redfield RR, Fields ML, Kelley PW. Frequency of illness associated with epidemic hepatitis A virus infections in adults. *Am J Epidemiol.* 1985;122:226–233.

33. Berge JJ, Drennan DP, Jacobs RJ, et al. The cost of hepatitis A infections in American adolescents and adults in 1997. *Hepatology.* 2000;31:469–473.

34. Hadler S. Global impact of hepatitis A virus infection: Changing patterns. In: Hollinger F, Lemon S, Margolis H, eds. *Viral Hepatitis and Liver Diseases.* Baltimore, MD: Williams and Wilkins; 1991:14–20.

35. Sansom SL, Cotter SM, Smith F, et al. Costs of a hepatitis A outbreak affecting homosexual men: Franklin County, Ohio, 1999. *Am J Prev Med.* 2003;25:343–346.

36. Centers for Disease Control and Prevention. Prevention of hepatitis A through active or passive immunization: recommendations of the Advisory Committee on Immunization Practices (ACIP). *MMWR Morb Mortal Wkly Rep.* 1999;48(RR12): 1–37.

37. Dalton CB, Haddix A, Hoffman RE, Mast EE. The cost of a food-borne outbreak of hepatitis A in Denver, Colo. *Arch Intern Med.* 1996;156:1013–1016.

38. Orr N, Klement E, Gillis D, et al. Long-term immunity in young adults after a single dose of inactivated Hepatitis A vaccines. *Vaccine.* 2006;24:4328–4332.

39. Rhodes SD, Yee LJ, Hergenrather KC. Hepatitis A vaccination among young African American men who have sex with men in the Deep South: psychosocial predictors. *J Natl Med Assoc.* 2003;95(4 Suppl):31S-36S.

40. Rhodes SD, Arceo R. Developing and testing measures predictive of hepatitis A vaccination in a sample of men who have sex with men. *Health Educ Res.* 2004; 19:272–283.

41. Katz MH, Hsu L, Wong E, Liska S, Anderson L, Janssen RS. Seroprevalence of and risk factors for hepatitis A infection among young homosexual and bisexual men. *J Infect Dis.* 1997;175:1225–1229.

42. Rhodes SD, Hergenrather KC. Using an integrated approach to understand vaccination behavior among young men who have sex with men: stages of change, the health belief model, and self-efficacy. *J Community Health.* 2003;28:347–362.

43. Schafer DF, Sorrell MF. Hepatocellular carcinoma. *Lancet.* 1999;353:1253–1257.

44. van Leeuwen DJ, Dadrat A. Viral hepatitis and its imitators. In: Blackwell RE, ed. *Women's Medical Text.* Boston, MA: Blackwell Science; 1996:324–338.

45. Lee TA, Veenstra DL, Iloeje UH, Sullivan SD. Cost of chronic hepatitis B infection in the United States. *J Clin Gastroenterol.* 2004;38(10 Suppl):S144–S147.

46. Coleman PJ, McQuillan GM, Moyer LA, Lambert SB, Margolis HS. Incidence of hepatitis B virus infection in the United States, 1976–1994: estimates from the National Health and Nutrition Examination Surveys. *J Infect Dis.* 1998;178:954–959.

47. Hadler SC, Francis DP, Maynard JE, et al. Long-term immunogenicity and efficacy of hepatitis B vaccine in homosexual men. *N Engl J Med.* 1986;315:209–214.

48. Centers for Disease Control and Prevention. Update on adult immunization recommendations of the Immunization Practices Advisory Committee (ACIP). *MMWR Morb Mortal Wkly Rep.* 1991;40(RR-12):1–52.

49. Goldberg D, McMenamin J. The United Kingdom's hepatitis B immunisation strategy—where now? *Commun Dis Public Health.* 1998;1:79–83.

50. Remis RS, Dufour A, Alary M, et al. Association of hepatitis B virus infection with other sexually transmitted infections in homosexual men. Omega Study Group. *Am J Public Health.* 2000;90:1570–1574.

51. Rhodes SD, Hergenrather KC. Attitudes and beliefs about hepatitis B vaccination among men who have sex with men: The Birmingham Measurement Study. *Journal of Homosexuality.* In press.

52. Silvestre AJ, Kingsley LA, Wehman P, Dappen R, Ho M, Rinaldo CR. Changes in HIV rates and sexual behavior among homosexual men, 1984 to 1988/92. *Am J Public Health.* 1993;83:578–580.

53. Kane M. Epidemiology of hepatitis B infection in North America. *Vaccine.* 1995;13 Suppl 1:S16–17.

54. Neighbors K, Oraka C, Shih L, Lurie P. Awareness and utilization of the hepatitis B vaccine among young men in the Ann Arbor area who have sex with men. *J Am Coll Health.* 1999;47:173–178.

55. Rhodes SD, DiClemente RJ, Yee LJ, Hergenrather KC. Correlates of hepatitis B vaccination in a high-risk population: an Internet sample. *Am J Med.* 2001;110: 628–632.

56. Seage GR, III, Mayer KH, Lenderking WR, et al. HIV and hepatitis B infection and risk behavior in young gay and bisexual men. *Public Health Rep.* 1997;112: 158–167.

57. Choo QL, Kuo G, Weiner AJ, Overby LR, Bradley DW, Houghton M. Isolation of a cDNA clone derived from a blood-borne non-A, non-B viral hepatitis genome. *Science.* 1989;244:359–362.

58. Alter MJ, Kruszon-Moran D, Nainan OV, et al. The prevalence of hepatitis C virus infection in the United States, 1988 through 1994. *N Engl J Med.* 1999;341:556–562.

59. Davis GL, Albright JE, Cook SF, Rosenberg DM. Projecting future complications of chronic hepatitis C in the United States. *Liver Transpl.* 2003;9:331–338.

60. Alter MJ, Margolis HS, Krawczynski K, Judson FN, Mares A, Alexander WJ, et al. The natural history of community-acquired hepatitis C in the United States. The Sentinel Counties Chronic non-A, non-B Hepatitis Study Team. *N Engl J Med.* 1992;327:1899–1905.

61. Kenny-Walsh E. Clinical outcomes after hepatitis C infection from contaminated anti-D immune globulin. Irish Hepatology Research Group. *N Engl J Med.* 1999; 340:1228–1233.

62. Seeff LB, Hollinger FB, Alter HJ, et al. Long-term mortality and morbidity of transfusion-associated non-A, non-B, and type C hepatitis: a National Heart, Lung, and Blood Institute collaborative study. *Hepatology.* 2001;33:455–463.

63. Thomas DL, Astemborski J, Rai RM, et al. The natural history of hepatitis C virus infection: host, viral, and environmental factors. *JAMA.* 2000;284:450–456.

64. Wiese M, Berr F, Lafrenz M, Porst H, Oesen U. Low frequency of cirrhosis in a hepatitis C (genotype 1b) single-source outbreak in germany: a 20-year multi-center study. *Hepatology.* 2000;32:91–96.

65. Capelli C, Prati D, Bosoni P, et al. Sexual transmission of hepatitis C virus to a repeat blood donor. *Transfusion.* 1997;37:436–440.

66. Halfon P, Riflet H, Renou C, Quentin Y, Cacoub P. Molecular evidence of male-to-female sexual transmission of hepatitis C virus after vaginal and anal inter-course. *J Clin Microbiol.* 2001;39:1204–1206.

67. Hollinger FB. Confounding factors in the study of HCV infection in couples. 10th international symposium on viral hepatitis and liver disease, Atlanta. International Medical Press; 2000.

68. Filippini P, Coppola N, Scolastico C, et al. Hepatitis viruses and HIV infection in the Naples area. *Infez Med.* 2003;11:139–145.

69. Filippini P, Coppola N, Scolastico C, et al. Does HIV infection favor the sexual transmission of hepatitis C? *Sex Transm Dis.* 2001;28:725–729.

70. Ndimbie OK, Kingsley LA, Nedjar S, Rinaldo CR. Hepatitis C virus infection in a male homosexual cohort: risk factor analysis. *Genitourin Med.* 1996;72:213–216.
71. Thomas DL, Seeff LB. Natural history of hepatitis C. *Clin Liver Dis.* 2005;9:383–398.
72. Rodger AJ, Roberts S, Lanigan A, Bowden S, Brown T, Crofts N. Assessment of long-term outcomes of community-acquired hepatitis C infection in a cohort with sera stored from 1971 to 1975. *Hepatology.* 2000;32:582–587.
73. Seeff LB. The natural history of chronic hepatitis C virus infection. *Clin Liver Dis.* 1997;1:587–602.
74. Strader DB, Seeff LB. Hepatitis C: a brief clinical overview. *ILAR J.* 2001;42:107–116.
75. Vogt M, Lang T, Frosner G, et al. Prevalence and clinical outcome of hepatitis C infection in children who underwent cardiac surgery before the implementation of blood-donor screening. *N Engl J Med.* 1999;341(12):866–870.
76. Davis GL. Chronic hepatitis C and liver transplantation. *Rev Gastroenterol Disord.* 2004;4:7–17.
77. Wong JB, McQuillan GM, McHutchison JG, Poynard T. Estimating future hepatitis C morbidity, mortality, and costs in the United States. *Am J Public Health.* 2000;90:1562–1569.
78. Dienstag JL, McHutchison JG. American Gastroenterological Association technical review on the management of hepatitis C. *Gastroenterology.* 2006;130:231–264.
79. Dienstag JL, McHutchison JG. American Gastroenterological Association medical position statement on the management of hepatitis C. *Gastroenterology.* 2006;130:225–230.
80. Conjeevaram HS, Fried MW, Jeffers LJ, et al. Peginterferon and ribavirin treatment in African American and Caucasian American patients with hepatitis C genotype 1. *Gastroenterology.* 2006;131:470–477.
81. Hepburn MJ, Hepburn LM, Cantu NS, Lapeer MG, Lawitz EJ. Differences in treatment outcome for hepatitis C among ethnic groups. *Am J Med.* 2004;117:163–168.
82. Jeffers LJ, Cassidy W, Howell CD, Hu S, Reddy KR. Peginterferon alfa-2a (40 kd) and ribavirin for black American patients with chronic HCV genotype 1. *Hepatology.* 2004;39:1702–1708.
83. Muir AJ, Bornstein JD, Killenberg PG. Peginterferon alfa-2b and ribavirin for the treatment of chronic hepatitis C in blacks and non-Hispanic whites. *N Engl J Med.* 2004;350:2265–2271.
84. Armstrong GL, Bell BP. Hepatitis A virus infections in the United States: model-based estimates and implications for childhood immunization. *Pediatrics.* 2002;109:839–845.
85. Corey L, Holmes KK. Sexual transmission of hepatitis A in homosexual men: incidence and mechanism. *N Engl J Med.* 1980;302:435–438.
86. Pham B, Duval B, De Serres G, et al. Seroprevalence of hepatitis A infection in a low endemicity country: a systematic review. *BMC Infect Dis.* 2005;5:56.
87. Fiore AE, Wasley A, Bell BP. Prevention of hepatitis A through active or passive immunization: recommendations of the Advisory Committee on Immunization Practices (ACIP). *MMWR Recomm Rep.* 2006;55(RR-7):1–23.
88. Centers for Disease Control and Prevention. Hepatitis A vaccination of men who have sex with men–Atlanta, Georgia, 1996–1997. *MMWR Morb Mortal Wkly Rep.* 1998;47:708–711.

89. Centers for Disease Control and Prevention. *Hepatitis Surveillance Report No. 59.* Atlanta, GA: US Department of Health and Human Services, 2004.

90. Wasley A, Samandari T, Bell BP. Incidence of hepatitis A in the United States in the era of vaccination. *JAMA.* 2005;294:194–201.

91. McQuillan GM, Coleman PJ, Kruszon-Moran D, Moyer LA, Lambert SB, Margolis HS. Prevalence of hepatitis B virus infection in the United States: the National Health and Nutrition Examination Surveys, 1976 through 1994. *Am J Public Health.* 1999;89:14–18.

92. Koff RS. Advances in the treatment of chronic viral hepatitis. *JAMA.* 1999;282: 511–512.

93. Waldo CR, McFarland W, Katz MH, MacKellar D, Valleroy LA. Very young gay and bisexual men are at risk for HIV infection: the San Francisco Bay Area Young Men's Survey II. *J Acquir Immune Defic Syndr.* 2000;24:168–174.

94. Osmond DH, Charlebois E, Sheppard HW, et al. Comparison of risk factors for hepatitis C and hepatitis B virus infection in homosexual men. *J Infect Dis.* 1993;167:66–71.

95. Tabet SR, Krone MR, Paradise MA, Corey L, Stamm WE, Celum CL. Incidence of HIV and sexually transmitted diseases (STD) in a cohort of HIV-negative men who have sex with men (MSM). *AIDS* 1998;12:2041–2048.

96. Schreeder MT, Thompson SE, Hadler SC, et al. Hepatitis B in homosexual men: prevalence of infection and factors related to transmission. *J Infect Dis.* 1982; 146:7–15.

97. Thio CL, Seaberg EC, Skolasky R, Jr., et al. HIV-1, hepatitis B virus, and risk of liver-related mortality in the Multicenter Cohort Study (MACS). *Lancet* 2002;360:1921–1926.

98. Wolf FC, Judson FN. Intensive screening for gonorrhea, syphilis, and hepatitis B in a gay bathhouse does not lower the prevalence infection. *Sex Transm Dis.* 1980;7: 49–52.

99. Gunn RA, Murray PJ, Brennan CH, Callahan DB, Alter MJ, Margolis HS. Evaluation of screening criteria to identify persons with hepatitis C virus infection among sexually transmitted disease clinic clients: results from the San Diego Viral Hepatitis Integration Project. *Sex Transm Dis.* 2003;30:340–344.

100. Buchbinder SP, Katz MH, Hessol NA, Liu J, O'Malley PM, Alter MJ. Hepatitis C virus infection in sexually active homosexual men. *J Infect.* 1994;29:263–269.

101. Clarke A, Kulasegaram R. Hepatitis C transmission—where are we now? *Int J STD AIDS.* 2006;17:74–80.

102. Tahan V, Karaca C, Yildirim B, et al. Sexual transmission of HCV between spouses. *Am J Gastroenterol.* 2005;100:821–824.

103. Turner JM, Rider AT, Imrie J, et al. Behavioural predictors of subsequent hepatitis C diagnosis in a UK clinic sample of HIV positive men who have sex with men. *Sex Transm Infect.* 2006;82:298–300.

104. Vandelli C, Renzo F, Romano L, Tisminetzky S, De Palma M, Stroffolini T, et al. Lack of evidence of sexual transmission of hepatitis C among monogamous couples: results of a 10-year prospective follow-up study. *Am J Gastroenterol.* 2004; 99:855–859.

105. Clarke A, Kulasegaram R. Hepatitis C transmission—where are we now? *Int J STD AIDS* 2006;17:74–80.

106. Ghosn J, Pierre-Francois S, Thibault V, et al. Acute hepatitis C in HIV-infected men who have sex with men. *HIV Med.* 2004;5:303–306.

107. Hammer GP, Kellogg TA, McFarland WC, et al. Low incidence and prevalence of hepatitis C virus infection among sexually active non-intravenous drug-using adults, San Francisco, 1997–2000. *Sex Transm Dis.* 2003;30:919–924.
108. Serpaggi J, Chaix ML, Batisse D, et al. Sexually transmitted acute infection with a clustered genotype 4 hepatitis C virus in HIV-1-infected men and inefficacy of early antiviral therapy. *AIDS.* 2006;20:233–240.
109. Thomas DL, Zenilman JM, Alter HJ, et al. Sexual transmission of hepatitis C virus among patients attending sexually transmitted diseases clinics in Baltimore—an analysis of 309 sex partnerships. *J Infect Dis.* 1995;171:768–775.
110. Melbye M, Biggar RJ, Wantzin P, Krogsgaard K, Ebbesen P, Becker NG. Sexual transmission of hepatitis C virus: cohort study (1981–9) among European homosexual men. *BMJ.* 1990;301:210–212.
111. Tedder RS, Gilson RJ, Briggs M, et al. Hepatitis C virus: evidence for sexual transmission. *BMJ.* 1991;302:1299–1302.
112. Browne R, Asboe D, Gilleece Y, et al. Increased numbers of acute hepatitis C infections in HIV positive homosexual men; is sexual transmission feeding the increase? *Sex Transm Infect.* 2004;80:326–327.
113. Gambotti L, Batisse D, Colin-de-Verdiere N, et al. Acute hepatitis C infection in HIV positive men who have sex with men in Paris, France, 2001–2004. *Euro Surveill.* 2005;10:115–117.
114. Gotz HM, van Doornum G, Niesters HG, den Hollander JG, Thio HB, de Zwart O. A cluster of acute hepatitis C virus infection among men who have sex with men—results from contact tracing and public health implications. *AIDS.* 2005; 19:969–974.
115. Rhodes SD, DiClemente RJ, Yee LJ, Hergenrather KC. Factors associated with testing for hepatitis C in an internet-recruited sample of men who have sex with men. *Sex Transm Dis.* 2001;28:515–520.
116. Villano SA, Nelson KE, Vlahov D, Purcell RH, Saah AJ, Thomas DL. Hepatitis A among homosexual men and injection drug users: more evidence for vaccination. *Clin Infect Dis.* 1997;25:726–728.
117. Rhodes SD, Yee LJ. Public health and gay and bisexual men: a primer for practitioners, clinicians, and researchers. In: Shankle M, ed. *The Handbook of Lesbian, Gay, Bisexual, and Transgender Public Health: A Practitioner's Guide to Service.* Binghamton, NY: Haworth; 2006:119–143.
118. Rhodes SD, Grimley DM, Hergenrather KC. Integrating behavioral theory to understand hepatitis B vaccination among men who have sex with men. *Am J Health Behav.* 2003;27:291–300.
119. Rhodes SD, Hergenrather KC. Exploring hepatitis B vaccination acceptance among young men who have sex with men: facilitators and barriers. *Prev Med.* 2002;35:128–134.
120. Rhodes SD, Hergenrather KC, Yee LJ. Increasing hepatitis B vaccination among young African-American men who have sex with men: simple answers and difficult solutions. *AIDS Patient Care STDS.* 2002;16:519–525.
121. Rhodes SD, DiClemente RJ, Yee LJ, Hergenrather KC. Hepatitis B vaccination in a high risk MSM population: the need for vaccine education. *Sex Transm Infect.* 2000;76:408–409.
122. Sansom S, Rudy E, Strine T, Douglas W. Hepatitis A and B vaccination in a sexually transmitted disease clinic for men who have sex with men. *Sex Transm Dis.* 2003; 30:685–688.

123. Van Damme P, Van Herck K. A review of the efficacy, immunogenicity and tolerability of a combined hepatitis A and B vaccine. *Expert Rev Vaccines.* 2004;3:249–267.

124. Centers for Disease Control and Prevention. Notice to readers: FDA approval for a combined Hepatitis A and B vaccine. *MMWR Morb Mortal Wkly Rep.* 2001;50:806–807.

125. Nothdurft HD, Dietrich M, Zuckerman JN, et al. A new accelerated vaccination schedule for rapid protection against hepatitis A and B. *Vaccine.* 2002;20:1157–1162.

126. McCusker J, Hill EM, Mayer KH. Awareness and use of hepatitis B vaccine among homosexual male clients of a Boston community health center. *Public Health Rep.* 1990;105:59–64.

127. Bellis JM, Grimley DM, Alexander LR. Feasibility of a tailored intervention targeting STD-related behaviors. *Am J Health Behav.* 2002;26:378–85.

128. Manning T. Interactive environments for promoting health. In: Street RL, Gold WR, Manning T, eds. *Health Promotion and Interactive Technology: Theoretical Applications and Future Directions.* Mahwah, NJ; Lawrence Erlbaum, 1997:67–78.

129. Freimuth VS, Quinn SC, Thomas SB, Cole G, Zook E, Duncan T. African Americans' views on research and the Tuskegee Syphilis Study. *Soc Sci Med.* 2001;52:797–808.

130. Harrison AE, Silenzio VM. Comprehensive care of lesbian and gay patients and families. *Prim Care.* 1996;23:31–46.

131. Schutten M, de Wit JB, van Steenbergen JE. Why do gay men want to be vaccinated against hepatitis B? An assessment of psychosocial determinants of vaccination intention. *Int J STD AIDS.* 2002;13:86–90.

132. Kelly JA, St Lawrence JS, Stevenson LY, Hauth AC, Kalichman SC, Diaz YE, et al. Community AIDS/HIV risk reduction: the effects of endorsements by popular people in three cities. *Am J Public Health.* 1992;82:1483–1489.

133. Eng E, Salmon M, Mullan F. Community empowerment: the critical base for primary care. *J Family Community Health.* 1992;15:1–12.

134. Amaro H, de la Torre A. Future health needs of women of color: public health needs and scientific opportunities in research on Latinas. *Am J Public Health.* 2002;92:525–529.

135. Treadwell HM, Ro M. Poverty, race, and the invisible men. *Am J Public Health.* 2003;93:705–707.

136. Courtenay WH. Constructions of masculinity and their influence on men's well-being: a theory of gender and health. *Soc Sci Med.* 2000;50:1385–1401.

137. Greenwood GL, Paul JP, Pollack LM, et al. Tobacco use and cessation among a household-based sample of US urban men who have sex with men. *Am J Public Health.* 2005;95:145–151.

138. Sell RL, Becker JB. Sexual orientation data collection and progress toward Healthy People 2010. *Am J Public Health.* 2001;91:876–882.

139. Kruszon-Moran D, McQuillan GM. Seroprevalence of six infectious diseases among adults in the United States by race/ethnicity: data from the third national health and nutrition examination survey, 1988–94. *Adv Data.* 2005:1–9.

140. Donahue JG, Nelson KE, Munoz A, et al. Antibody to hepatitis C virus among cardiac surgery patients, homosexual men, and intravenous drug users in Baltimore, Maryland. *Am J Epidemiol.* 1991;134:1206–1211.

8

HIV Infection among Gay
and Bisexual Men

Patrick S. Sullivan and Richard J. Wolitski

HIV infection and AIDS have been a devastating epidemic in the United States since the early 1980s. By 2005, over 550,000 persons in the United States had died with HIV infection[1]—more than 8 times the number of American soldiers who died in the Vietnam War. More than half of these deaths— 300,669—have been among men who have sex with men (MSM). As of the end of 2004, over a million persons in the United States were living with HIV infection.[2] In the mid-1990s, HIV infection was the leading cause of death among Americans aged 25–44.[3] Since 1996, when highly active antiretroviral therapy became increasingly available, HIV infection decreased in prominence as a cause of death among Americans: among persons aged 25–44, it was ranked as the fifth leading cause of death during 1997–2000, and as the sixth leading cause during 2001–2002.[4] The impact of HIV infection on mortality varies among racial and ethnic groups: in 2003, the HIV death rate for African American men was 7.5 times greater than the HIV death rate for white men.[5] Despite the impact of effective therapy on the survival of persons living with HIV, over 7,000 men who had acquired HIV through male-male sex died in 2005.[1]

Gay and bisexual men constitute the US demographic group that has been most severely impacted since the beginning of the HIV epidemic. The first cases of HIV-related opportunistic illnesses were recognized among gay men in Los Angeles, San Francisco, and New York.[6,7] Gay men are at particular risk for HIV infection from sexual transmission because the virus is transmitted more efficiently by anal intercourse than by vaginal intercourse.[8] The per-episode risk of transmission from receptive anal intercourse is five times greater than the risk from receptive vaginal intercourse.

In the early years of the epidemic, large numbers of sex partners among a group of transmitters of sexually transmitted diseases (STDs)[9,10] and generally high levels of STDs among gay men[11] further increased risk (see Chapter 6 in this volume) because the presence of other STDs increases the risk for HIV transmission.[12] Many infections have undoubtedly been prevented by better understanding of transmission risks, outreach to and education of at-risk men, and declines in concurrent STDs. However, new diagnoses of HIV infection and AIDS continue to be most common among MSM: of the AIDS cases diagnosed in 2005, for example, 17,230 were attributed to male-male sex, and 12,388 were attributed to male-female sex.[1]

Descriptive Epidemiology

HIV Case Surveillance Data

The most systematic source of data on HIV infections among MSM in the United States is HIV and AIDS case reporting.[13] All US states use consistent methods to collect information on persons diagnosed with AIDS. Although all US states collect surveillance information on persons with HIV infection (not AIDS), the reporting methods vary: as of September 2006, 45 US states used the recommended name-based methods,[14–16] and 5 states used code-based systems.

Through 2005, a total of 517,992 cases of AIDS had been diagnosed among MSM in the United States, and an estimated 217,323 MSM were living with AIDS.[1] In 2005, diagnoses for MSM represented 46% of all new diagnoses of AIDS.[1] Of these new AIDS cases reported in MSM, 46% were reported among white men, 32% were reported among black men, and 19% were reported among Hispanic men. Although the proportion of AIDS cases diagnosed among MSM has decreased from about 65% in 1985, MSM continue to constitute the highest proportion of newly diagnosed HIV and AIDS cases in the US (see Figure 8-1).

Prevalence Estimates

Estimating the prevalence of HIV infection among MSM is complicated, in part, because of the lack of reliable data on the number of MSM in the United States. Therefore, HIV prevalence has been estimated for specific subgroups of gay men, but with full realization of the limitations of these estimates. At the time of this writing, the most robust estimates of HIV prevalence among MSM come from HIV testing conducted in conjunction with the National HIV Behavioral Surveillance (NHBS) survey of the Centers for Disease Control and Prevention (CDC). NHBS data from 1767 MSM in five large US cities from 2004–2005 documented an overall prevalence of HIV infection of 25%. In this survey, men were recruited in diverse settings, such as bars, dance clubs, cafes and retail stores, social organizations, gyms, and parks.

Considering data from publicly funded HIV counseling and testing sites in the United States, the proportion of positive test results for MSM during 1999–2004 (i.e., the prevalence of infection among those seeking testing)

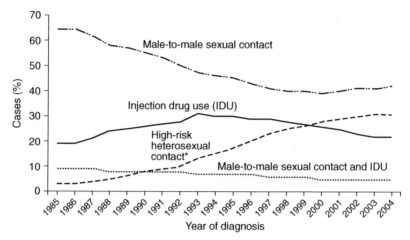

Figure 8-1. Proportion of AIDS Cases Among Adults and Adolescents, by Transmission Category and Year of Diagnosis, 1985–2004—United States. Data adjusted for reporting delays and cases without risk factor information were proportionally redistributed.

*Heterosexual contact with a person known to have or at high risk for HIV infection.

decreased from 5.7% in 1999 to 5.0% in 2004[17]; these figures significantly underestimate the prevalence among MSM because men who are aware that they are HIV infected would be unlikely to present for HIV testing in these settings.

Various surveys of MSM have revealed clear, consistent correlates in the prevalence of HIV infection of MSM (see Table 8-1). In the seven-city Young Men's Survey conducted from 1994–2000, HIV seropositivity was higher among young MSM who were black, of mixed race, of Hispanic ethnicity, who had ever had anal sex with a man, or who had had sex with 20 or more men in their lifetime.[18] In the NHBS data from June 2004 through April 2005, the prevalence of HIV infection among black respondents was more than twice the prevalence among white respondent and Hispanic respondents.[19] Age is also related to the prevalence of HIV infection: in the NHBS survey, the prevalence of HIV infection ranged from 14% among respondents aged 18–24 years to 37% among those aged 40–49.[19] HIV prevalence among MSM has also been associated with injection drug use, less education, recreational drug use during sex, unprotected anal intercourse, more sex partners, and history of STDs other than HIV (see Table 8-1).

HIV Incidence

HIV incidence can be measured directly, through cohort studies in which MSM who are not infected are enrolled and observed over time, or indirectly,

Table 8-1. Demographic, behavioral, and clinical correlates of HIV prevalence, HIV incidence, and high-risk sexual behavior for men who have sex with men—United States

Factor	References
Factors associated with HIV prevalence:	
Demographic	
Black race	18–22
Hispanic ethnicity	18, 21–23
Less education	20, 23, 24
Older age	20, 21, 25
Behavioral	
Higher numbers of sex partners	18, 22, 26
Injection drug use	18, 20, 21, 23, 27
Recreational drug use during sex	21, 23, 28, 29
Unprotected anal intercourse	18, 21, 24, 26, 29, 30
Clinical	
History of sexually transmitted disease	18, 22, 24, 29
Factors associated with HIV incidence:	
Demographic	
Black race	31
Younger age	31–34
Behavioral	
Heavy alcohol use	35
Higher numbers of sex partners	26, 34, 35
Inhalant nitrite (popper) use	29, 31, 34
Methamphetamine use	31, 35, 36
Unprotected anal intercourse	26, 29, 34, 35
Clinical	
Lack of circumcision	34
Recent sexually transmitted disease	31, 35, 37
*Factors associated with high-risk sexual behavior**	
Demographic	
Lower education	38, 39
Younger age	23, 38, 40–47
Behavioral	
Higher number of sex partners	38, 41, 47–49
Methamphetamine use	27, 47, 50–54
Nitrite inhalant (popper) use	39, 47, 48
Alcohol use	27
Use of Internet to meet sex partners	54–57
Sex in commercial environments	47, 48
Treatment optimism	58–63
Viagra use	47, 51, 64

*Typically defined as unprotected anal intercourse, acquisition of a bacterial sexually transmitted disease, or multiple sex partners.

through serologic assays that estimate recent HIV infection.[65] In the 1980s, HIV incidence among MSM peaked, depending on the report, at 5% to 20% per year.[66] Estimates of HIV incidence since the 1990s suggest that HIV incidence among MSM is currently lower, but it remains at 1% to 4% per year in various subgroups of MSM. During 1998–2002, in the phase III clinical trial of a candidate HIV vaccine (AIDSVAX), the annual incidence of HIV infection among 4697 participants who were MSM at high risk was 2.8% per year.[31] In the NHBS five-city survey (2004–2005), in which the sample included both MSM at high risk and MSM at low risk, city-specific incidence estimates were 1.2% to 8.0% per year.[19] In New York City, in 2001, HIV incidence among MSM was estimated at 2.5% per year.[67] In San Francisco, from 1995–1997, HIV incidence was estimated at 1.6%[34]; in 2001, incidence was estimated at 2.8%.[68]

A recent systematic review of available data on HIV incidence among MSM suggests that incidence estimates cluster at about 2% per year.[69] Despite the variance of incidence in specific subpopulations, this annual incidence has been predicted to lead to very high prevalence rates among MSM, if incidence is not decreased through prevention programs.[69]

The incidence of HIV infection also has important correlates among MSM. In a project conducted from 1994 through 2000 in seven US cities, CDC and local health departments measured HIV incidence among MSM aged 18–29. Overall incidence among MSM aged 18–22 was 2.6% per year; incidence among men aged 23–29 was 4.4%.[70] In similar age groups, incidence was higher among African American men (4.0% among men aged 18–24 and 14.7% among those aged 25–29) than among white men. Among MSM recruited for the AIDSVAX phase III vaccine trial because of their high risk for HIV infection, incidence decreased with age group: annual HIV incidence was 3.8%, 2.9%, 2.0%, and 1.7% among MSM aged 18–30, 31–40, 41–50, and 51–64, respectively.[31] Of note, the observed incidence among AIDSVAX participants aged 18–30 was between the estimates from the seven-city study for MSM aged 18–22 and those aged 23–29. The finding of increased HIV incidence among younger MSM is supported by numerous studies that have found higher levels of high risk sexual behaviors among younger, compared to older, MSM (see Table 8-1).[45,71]

HIV incidence is also associated with specific behaviors. For example, higher numbers of sex partners,[26,34,72] unprotected anal intercourse,[26,29,34] use of nitrite inhalants,[29,34,72,73] lack of condom use,[74] and lack of circumcision[34] are associated with higher HIV incidence. More recently, methamphetamine use[53,54] and use of the Internet to meet sex partners[54–57] have been associated with higher numbers of sex partners, STD acquisition, and higher rates of unprotected anal intercourse. Studies have implicated methamphetamine use in increased HIV incidence,[31,35,36] and this emerging understanding of the intersecting epidemics of methamphetamine use and HIV among MSM is cause for concern.

Measuring the Extent of Disparity

The disproportionate burden of HIV infection among MSM can be demonstrated in several ways: through comparing estimates of HIV incidence, through case surveillance data, and through differences in HIV seropositivity rates among persons seeking HIV testing in certain settings.

Comparison of HIV incidence rates between MSM and other groups provides the strongest epidemiologic evidence of disparities in the distribution of the epidemic. At a national level, CDC estimates that approximately 40,000 new HIV infections occur annually[75,76]; this translates to a population incidence rate of approximately 0.01 per 100 person-years.[77] In contrast, HIV incidence among MSM in various settings is approximately 1% to 4%—over 100-fold the incidence in the general US population. Even this measure likely underestimates the disparity in incidence because incident MSM cases are included in the overall US incidence estimate. In a prison-based screening program that determined HIV incidence immediately before entry into prison, the HIV incidence among all men entering prison (a group generally recognized to have high risk for HIV infection) was 0.7% annually—a fraction of the annual incidence among MSM.[78]

HIV and AIDS case surveillance data illustrate the disproportionate impact of HIV infection on MSM. Data from 32 US states with reportable data on both HIV infection and AIDS from 2000 through 2004 illustrate that more reports of new cases of HIV infection were for MSM than for any other risk group (see Figure 8-2).[79] In 2004, 44% of the new HIV cases in these states were in MSM. The disparity is evident on its face, but is even more dramatic when one considers that this large number of infections is occurring in a subpopulation of men that likely constitute less than 10% of US men.

It is also possible to compare the rate of new positive HIV test results for persons seeking HIV testing at certain types of facilities. Publicly funded HIV testing sites (e.g., STD clinics, health department clinics, and certain community-based organizations) are important sources of data for this purpose because such sites collect consistent data about HIV risk behaviors and the results of HIV tests. Among persons tested at publicly funded counseling and testing sites during 1999–2004, the annual positivity rates for men with a history of male-male sex were 3.9–4.9 times the annual rates for women who had male partners only.[17] MSM seeking HIV testing at publicly funded sites may have higher positivity rates than those who seek HIV testing at their private physician's office and MSM who seek testing from community-based organizations affiliated with the gay community.

Although it is clear that MSM are disproportionately affected by the HIV epidemic, there are limitations that make it difficult to quantify these disparities more definitively or to examine trends in the disparities. The primary limitation is the lack of good information about the number of MSM in the United States. Ideally, rates of HIV infection should be calculated to express the annual number of new HIV infections per 100 MSM in the United States.

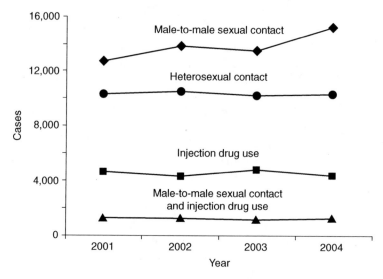

Figure 8-2. Cases of HIV infection (with or without AIDS) among persons age 13 or older, but year of diagnosis and transmission category, 2001–2004—33 US areas with confidential name-based HIV infection reporting.

Because the number of MSM is not known, rates are instead calculated as new infections per 100 *men*.[80] This method considerably underestimates the impact of the epidemic among MSM.

Temporal Trends in the HIV Epidemic among MSM

From the mid-1980s into the 1990s, many MSM rapidly adopted safer sex practices, including condom use and fewer partners, which likely contributed to declines in the numbers of new HIV infections through at least the late 1980s.[10,11,81–83] Data from behavioral surveys[83] and declining syphilis rates among MSM[84] bear witness to the adoption of protective behaviors from the mid-1980s through the mid-1990s. Also, HIV positivity rates among MSM tested at publicly funded counseling and testing centers decreased from 7.3% in 1995[85] to a low of 3.5% in 2002.[17]

In recent years, the estimated number of newly diagnosed HIV infections among MSM has increased in the 33 HIV surveillance areas with confidential name-based HIV reporting. Since 2001, when 12,750 cases were diagnosed, annual diagnoses have increased through 2004, when 15,294 cases were diagnosed (See Figure 8-2). Although increases in the number of new HIV diagnoses could result from increasing numbers of MSM who were tested[86], behavioral data from HIV testing surveys do not provide evidence of increased HIV testing from 2000 through 2002.[87–89] Increases in new HIV diagnoses during this period have occurred in concert with outbreaks of syphilis[12,90,91] and data from behavioral surveys that suggest decreases in protective behaviors.[92] Synthesis of these multiple data sources suggest a true increase in HIV risk behaviors and perhaps an increase in new HIV infections among MSM since 2000.

Although not the focus of this chapter, data from other industrialized countries where the epidemic among MSM is significant suggest that reported increases in high risk sexual activity and, possibly, HIV incidence are not unique to the United States. Data from Western Europe.[93] Rome,[94] the Netherlands,[95] and Spain[96] confirm high levels of STDs and ongoing HIV spread among MSM. Recent reports also document a significant HIV epidemic among MSM in Thailand and confirm high levels of risk behaviors.[51,97–99]

Challenges to HIV Prevention among MSM

Recent advances in HIV treatment, changes in how gay men perceive the threat of HIV infection, and the ongoing and evolving nature of the epidemic have presented new challenges to promoting and maintaining reduced risk behaviors and further reducing the rates of new HIV infections. Advances in treatment, while offering stunning improvements in the health and survival of persons living with HIV infection,[100] have also created new challenges for HIV prevention. Beliefs about HIV, specifically beliefs about susceptibility to infection[101,102] and the severity of HIV infection,[103] may influence the adoption of preventive behaviors. Since the advent of highly active antiretroviral therapy (HAART), attitudes in the gay community have changed substantially in terms of susceptibility to HIV and the consequences of becoming infected, and these changed attitudes bear directly on these two component beliefs.[104] For example, some men believe that HAART reduces the likelihood that an HIV-infected sex partner will transmit HIV, or they believe that the severity of HIV infection will be less because of the availability of HAART. Optimistic beliefs about HAART (*treatment optimism*) perhaps may be held by as many as 25% of MSM[58–60,101,105–108] and have been associated with higher risk sex behaviors in this population.[109]

In the early years of the epidemic, many believed that changes in sexual behavior would be required for a limited time, not for a lifetime. The fact that many MSM may be at risk of acquiring or transmitting HIV for much of their adult lives creates substantial challenges to maintaining behavioral changes throughout a lifetime. In surveys of HIV-related attitudes and practices, MSM have reported being "tired of always practicing safer sex,"[110] being "burned out thinking about HIV,"[111] and failing to take protective behaviors because they "are tired of being careful."[111] These beliefs are representative of *prevention burnout*, which is one important aspect of what many see as a rising complacency about HIV infection and AIDS among MSM in the United States.[104]

Beliefs about HAART and prevention burnout may have contributed to the emergence of "barebacking," intentional unprotected anal sex with casual partners, as a trend among MSM in the United States. Barebacking, although more common among MSM living with HIV than among HIV-seronegative MSM, has been reported by substantial proportions of urban MSM.[112,113] Some men who have bareback sex limit this activity to seroconcordant partners (a practice known as serosorting), but others have unprotected anal sex without regard to or knowledge of a partner's HIV serostatus. One study found that 57% of HIV-seropositive MSM who identified themselves as barebackers reported that they had bareback sex with partners who were HIV-seronegative or whose serostatus they did not know.[114] However, very few MSM report "bug chasing" (having unprotected anal sex in an effort to contract HIV). In an online survey of more than 2500 MSM, only 1.9% reported that they had ever had anal sex without a condom because they wanted to get HIV.[115]

Finally, sustained prevention efforts are challenged by the coming of age of new cohorts of young MSM who are establishing their sexual identifies and becoming sexually active and who may be placing themselves at risk for HIV infection. The urgent sense of threat that motivated behavioral changes within the MSM community during the mid-1980s does not necessarily exist for younger MSM, who may not have witnessed the destructive effects of the early years of the HIV epidemic. Emotional closeness to a person with HIV infection or AIDS has been an important correlate of the adoption of protective behaviors; younger MSM may be less likely to have personal experience with HIV-infected persons.[116] The challenge of HIV prevention in younger MSM is also clear from data on HIV prevalence and knowledge of serostatus: of MSM aged 18–29 in a recent multicity survey, 70% to 79% of young, HIV-infected MSM had not known that they were infected.[19] Thus, HIV prevention efforts must be ongoing, sustained, consistent, and diligent in reaching MSM as they become sexually active and enter the pool of those at high risk for HIV infection.

HIV Infection and African American MSM

The HIV epidemic in African American MSM bears special consideration: the national rate (including men and women) of HIV infection in 2003 was 73.9 per 100,000 persons among US blacks, and was 8.1 per 100,000 among US whites. Among black MSM, the prevalence of HIV in five large cities during 2004–2005 was 46%, and nearly two-thirds of those infected were not aware of their HIV infection.[19] In a multi-city survey of young MSM, the prevalence of HIV infection was nearly five times greater for blacks than for whites; however, this disparity in HIV infection serostatus was not associated with higher levels of risky sexual behaviors or drug use.[21]

The reasons for the higher prevalence of HIV among black MSM are not clear, although several hypotheses have been advanced.[117] The two best-substantiated hypotheses are that (1) HIV prevalence may be higher because STDs other than HIV are more common among blacks,[118,119] and coinfection with an STD may increase the risk of acquiring or transmitting HIV,[12] and (2) that the higher prevalence of unrecognized HIV among black men may lead to more instances of exposure to sex partners.[19,120] Other hypotheses are less clearly supported by the scientific literature. For example, black men are less likely than white men to be circumcised,[121] and being uncircumcised increases the risk for HIV infection.[34,122] Also, white men may be more likely to have protective genetic traits (e.g., CCR5 deletion mutations) that have been associated with a decreased risk for HIV infection.[123,124] Because 90% of sexual partnerships in the United States are between persons of concordant race,[125] the high prevalence of HIV infection among black MSM may also be self-perpetuating (i.e., black MSM who choose black male partners are choosing partners from a partner pool with higher HIV prevalence). Recent evidence also suggests that younger black MSM, despite having comparable levels of high risk sex behaviors, are more likely to choose older sex partners— again, reflecting selection of sex partners from a partner pool with higher HIV prevalence.[126]

Important aspects of sexual identification vary among races and ethnicities. For example, in a survey of 10,030 MSM living with HIV infection in 15 US states, black MSM who had sex only with men were more likely than white men to identify themselves as straight or bisexual.[127] For MSM, identifying themselves as gay may confer some increased access to HIV prevention messages and services directed toward MSM, and MSM who identify themselves as gay, compared to MSM who identify themselves as heterosexual, may more accurately identify their risk for HIV infection. Black MSM living with HIV are also more likely than are MSM of other races and ethnicites to be behaviorally bisexual.[128] Although behaviorally bisexual MSM who do not identify themselves as gay may have fewer behavioral risk factors than do MSM who identify themselves as gay,[117] HIV prevention efforts for MSM need to address the multiple sexual risks,[128–131] and interventions may need to be tailored to the prevention needs of subgroups of MSM.

Opportunities for Intervention

Efforts to promote HIV testing and motivate MSM to protect themselves from HIV have proven successful. On the whole, behavioral interventions that have been evaluated in experimental trials have reduced the risk of HIV transmission from MSM at high risk.[132,133] According to a review of data from nine intervention trials that were available through June 1998, participation in these interventions was associated with a 26% reduction in the proportion of men reporting unprotected anal sex (odds ratio [OR] 0.69; 95% confidence interval [CI] 0.56–0.86).[132] A more recent meta-analysis of 33 studies that used data available as of July 2003 (and included most of the studies in the earlier review) confirmed that behavioral interventions reduced HIV risk behavior among MSM. The behavioral interventions included in this review led to significant decreases in self-reported unprotected anal intercourse (OR 0.77;

95% CI 0.65–0.92) and number of sex partners (OR 0.85; 95% CI 0.61–0.92) as well as a significant increase in self-reported condom use during anal intercourse (OR 1.61; 95% CI 1.16–2.22).[133] These conclusions were supported by an independent meta-analysis that also found significant reductions in the behaviors of MSM following intervention.[134]

Not only have HIV interventions reduced risk among MSM, several behavioral interventions for MSM have been shown to be cost-effective when compared with medical interventions used in the treatment and prevention of other health problems.[135–137] Evaluations of two community-level interventions found these programs to be cost-saving.[135,136] That is, the costs of these programs were substantially less than the cost of treating the new cases of HIV infection that were predicted to have occurred in the intervention communities if the intervention had not been provided.

Although the overall efficacy and cost-effectiveness of behavioral interventions for MSM at risk for HIV infection have been clearly demonstrated, all interventions for MSM are not equally effective, and some interventions do not lead to significant behavior change. Meta-analyses have been conducted to identify intervention characteristics associated with intervention efficacy. Efficacious interventions have the following characteristics: they (1) have a theoretical basis, (2) use four or more strategies to deliver intervention content, (3) provide training in interpersonal skills such as negotiation of condom use, and (4) have greater intervention intensity and duration as measured by number of sessions, hours of exposure to the intervention, and number of days the intervention was conducted.[133]

One might assume that distinguishing efficacious interventions from those that are not would be easy, but this is not always true. Limitations in the design or implementation of some trials make it difficult to reliably assess whether an intervention did or did not work. These limitations include: (1) the lack of an appropriate comparison group, (2) potentially biased assignment to condition, (3) short recall periods that do not allow the evaluation of intermediate and long-term effects, (4) poor retention at follow-up assessments, and (5) failure to analyze data according to the originally assigned condition, or other analytical problems.[138]

As a result, many interventions lack sufficient evidence of efficacy, and relatively few interventions for MSM at high risk for HIV infection have been recommended by federal funding agencies for use in local HIV prevention programs. Of 42 efficacious interventions identified by CDC's Prevention Research Synthesis project, only 7 (17%) were targeted to MSM at high risk.[138,139] These interventions represent a range of prevention strategies that include individual, small-group, and community-level interventions that are delivered by specially trained professionals or peers in office or community settings that took place during a single contact or over the course of 10 or more sessions (see Table 8-2).

Despite the potential challenges, a growing number of interventions have reduced HIV transmission risk behavior among MSM and other persons living

Table 8-2. Effective behavioral interventions designed exclusively for men who have sex with men identified by the HIV Prevention Research Synthesis Project of the Centers for Disease Control and Prevention

Author (Year)	Sample	Intervention Description	Design	Main Outcome
Dilley, Woods, Sabatino, et al., (2002)[140]	248 MSM retesting for HIV	Individual 1-session counseling intervention focused on selfjustifications plus standard HIV counseling and testing. Conducted by trained mental health counselors.	RCT	Reduction in UAI with non-primary partners of discordant/unknown HIV status
Koblin, Chesney, Coates (2004)[141]	4,295 HIV-negative MSM	EXPLORE: Individual 10-session counseling intervention with booster sessions every 3 months and HIV counseling and testing every 6 months. Intervention sessions focused on individual, interpersonal, and contextual factors associated with HIV risk. Conducted by trained counselors.	RCT	Reduction in UAI and URAI with partners of serodiscordant or unknown serostatus
Kegeles, Hays, Coates (1996)[142]	800 young MSM	Mpowerment: Community-level peer-led intervention including outreach, small groups, community mobilization, and publicity campaign.	RCT	Reduction in UAI
Kelly, St. Lawrence, Hood, Brasfield (1989)[143]	104 MSM	Project ARIES: 12-session small-group intervention including risk reduction information, cognitive-behavioral self-management, sexual assertion training, and development of relationship skills.	RCT	Increase in condom use during AI and reduction in UAI

(continued)

Table 8-2. (*continued*)

Author (Year)	Sample	Intervention Description	Design	Main Outcome
Kelly, St. Lawrence, Stevenson, et al. (1992)[144-146]	1,469 MSM attending gay bars	Popular Opinion Leader: Community-level intervention using environmental cues and popular peers to initiate discussions about HIV risk reduction.	Quasi-experimental	Reduction in UAI
Valdiserri, Lyter, Leviton, et al. (1989)[147]	584 MSM	AIDS Prevention Project: 2-session small-group intervention with informational and skills-building components.	RCT	Increase in condom use during AI
Wolitski, Gomez, Parsons, and the SUMIT Study Group (2005)[148]	811 HIV-positive MSM	SUMIT: 6-session group intervention with large-group and small-group activities conducted during 6 sessions led by HIV-positive peers. Activities addressed knowledge, personal responsibility for protecting others, assumptions about serostatus, substance use, mental health, communication, and disclosure of HIV serostatus.	RCT	Reduction in URAI with partners of HIV-negative or unknown serostatus

with HIV.[158] A meta-analysis of 12 trials of interventions for people living with HIV (all of which met strict criteria for methodological rigor) found that these interventions significantly reduced unprotected sex (OR 0.57; 95% CI 0.40, 0.82) and the incidence of STDs (OR 0.20; CI .05, 0.73)—reductions that are comparable to the effects of interventions for persons who are at risk.[158] However, few of these interventions were tested with MSM. In only 4 of these 12 trials did MSM constitute two-thirds or more of the participants. When the studies were stratified by target population, the significant intervention effects that were observed in the overall meta-analysis were not observed for studies conducted with MSM only or with any other population because of the small number of studies in each stratum.

In addition to behavioral interventions, biomedical interventions are becoming increasingly available. Clinical guidelines now exist for post-exposure prophylaxis, in which medications are given immediately after a risky sexual exposure, in hopes of averting HIV infection.[159] Pre-exposure prophylaxis, in which antiretroviral drugs are given before risky sexual exposures, shows promise in primate models,[160] and is being evaluated in clinical trials in the United States, Africa, and Asia.[161,162] In Africa, circumcision has recently been demonstrated to reduce HIV acquisition by men who have female sex partners[163,164]; the findings of this trial do not have direct implications for reducing HIV transmission through male-male sex in the United States.[165] However, the evidence of a protective effect of circumcision in MSM in a vaccine preparedness cohort suggests that circumcision may have potential as an HIV prevention strategy in the United States and should be rigorously evaluated.[34]

Other biomedical interventions that are currently in clinical trials may be important elements of a comprehensive approach to HIV prevention among MSM in the future. At the time of this writing, five efficacy trials of microbicides are in progress; although they are focused on vaginal use of microbicides, a microbicide of proven effectiveness might also have value in rectal application. Finally, substantial resources have been committed to the development of the international capacity to evaluate candidate HIV vaccines,[166] and a health pipeline of candidate vaccines using novel approaches exists.[167]

Critical Gaps

To reduce the disparities in the impact of HIV on gay and bisexual men, especially among MSM of color, we must address critical gaps in knowledge about how to best curb the epidemic among MSM. Sadly, critical gaps in knowledge abound, and much remains to be learned about the evolving nature of MSM's sexual relationships and practices and how to best prevent further HIV transmissions. MSM are increasingly adopting HIV risk-reduction strategies that do not depend solely on using condoms every time with every

partner. These strategies include not using condoms in serocondordant relationships with a long-term primary partner but consistently using condoms
with all other partners (negotiated safety),[168,169] not using condoms with
seroconcordant partners (serosorting),[168,170,171] and selectively engaging in
unprotected insertive or receptive anal sex depending on the HIV serostatus
of the partner (strategic positioning).[170,172]

Research is needed on the effectiveness of these strategies, which heavily
depend on the ability of MSM to know their own HIV serostatus, truthfully
disclose it to their partners, and for their partners to do the same. Data
showing that many MSM who have tested HIV-seropositive had not known
they were infected raise concerns about the relative effectiveness of these
strategies. Of MSM tested in five cities from 2004–2005, 48% of those who
tested HIV-positive incorrectly believed that they were not infected, underscoring the critical importance of at least annual HIV testing among at risk
MSM.[19]

As HIV infections continue to occur among MSM at a rate at least 100 times
higher than that in the general population, there is an urgent need to pri-
oritize and assess prevention activities for MSM at the local and national levels.
This assessment should address the allocation of HIV prevention resources
with regard to effectiveness of strategies as well as the characteristics of persons receiving prevention services. To be maximally effective, prevention resources need to be invested in the most effective strategies, and must take into
account the disparities in rates between risk groups, and between subgroups
of MSM.

Additional research is needed to increase the number of effective interventions for MSM. The current numbers of proven interventions for HIV-
seronegative and HIV-seropositive MSM are insufficient given the diversity of
the MSM community and the multitude of issues that affect HIV risk. Of major
concern is the relative lack of proven interventions specifically designed for
African American or Latino MSM. Rigorous trials of interventions developed
specifically for these populations are urgently needed. Until such interventions are available, research is needed to evaluate the effectiveness of interventions that were originally tested with white MSM and that have been tailored and adapted for MSM of color. The results of the evaluation of a
community-level intervention that was adapted for African American MSM in
North Carolina indicate that such interventions can be acceptable to the
target population and can reduce HIV risk behavior.[173] Additional prevention
interventions are also needed to meet the diverse needs of other subgroups of
MSM, including MSM who use methamphetamine and other substances, seek
sex partners via the Internet, are living with HIV, engage in barebacking, or do
not identify themselves as gay.

It is important to recognize that interventions that worked 10 years ago may
not be comparably effective today. Thus, the effectiveness of these interventions should be monitored continually. Behavioral interventions may need to
be changed or updated to incorporate new scientific information, respond to

changes in community perceptions and norms, and avoid prevention fatigue (i.e., overexposure to a limited number of prevention messages).

In addition to the need to review and strengthen prevention efforts for MSM, there is a critical need to facilitate the transfer of proven interventions for MSM and to move beyond strategies that promote behavior change at the individual level. Resource limitations and other barriers make it difficult for many community-based organizations to adopt approaches to HIV prevention that are based on the best available prevention research.[174–177] Addressing these barriers will require sustained technology transfer efforts and a long-term commitment on the part of the government, universities, and private foundations to building the capacity of community-based organizations to provide science-based interventions to MSM.

Historically, the data for systematically characterizing, over time, the risk behaviors among MSM in the United States have been limited. In 2003, the National HIV Behavioral Surveillance System was implemented by the health departments in 25 US cities.[178] In 2006, the first data from the system, representing the risk behaviors, use of prevention services, and use of HIV testing by MSM, were reported.[127] A similar behavioral surveillance system—of persons receiving medical care for HIV infection—scheduled for 2007 will allow the ongoing evaluation of the HIV transmission risk-behaviors of MSM living with HIV infection.[179] These systems will fill critical gaps in our ability to monitor the behaviors of HIV-seronegative and HIV-seropositive MSM on a national basis.

The health disparities related to risk for HIV infection and other health disparities for MSM described in this volume do not stand in isolation. For some time now, researchers and prevention providers have understood that MSM who are at greatest risk for HIV infection are also those who are most likely to experience other health-related problems such as substance use, physical and sexual abuse, and STDs.[93,180,181] Achieving sustainable long-term gains in HIV prevention efforts for MSM may require a more holistic approach to the health and well-being of MSM, one that recognizes the inter-relationship of these problems. Many of the health threats and disparities that MSM face may be exacerbated by the homophobia, stigma, and discrimination that MSM in the United States continue to experience.[182,183] Addressing these interconnections and the broader effects of stigma and homophobia will require a more ecological approach to HIV prevention—one that emphasizes individual treatment of substance abuse, mental health problems, and other underlying disorders, as well as efforts to intervene at the community, structural, and policy levels.[93,184,185] These prevention challenges represent the convergence of health disparities among MSM, who may have multiple needs for prevention and health promotion. A comprehensive multilevel approach may be what is ultimately needed to stop what has become an entrenched epidemic that continues to threaten the well-being of future generations of MSM.

Authors' Note

The findings and conclusions in this chapter are those of the authors and do not necessarily represent the views of the Centers for Disease Control and Prevention.

References

1. Centers for Disease Control and Prevention. *HIV/AIDS Surveillance Report, 2005.* Vol. 17. Rev ed. Atlanta, GA: US Department of Health and Human Services, Centers for Disease Control and Prevention; 2007:1–46. Also available at: http://www.cdc.gov/hiv/topics/surveillance/resources/reports.htm.
2. Glynn M, Rhodes P. Estimated HIV prevalence in the United States at the end of 2003. National HIV Prevention Conference, Atlanta, GA, June 2005. Abstract T1-B1-B1101.
3. Centers for Disease Control and Prevention. HIV mortality slide set. http://www.cdc.gov/hiv/graphics/mortalit.htm. Accessed August 18, 2005.
4. Anderson RN, Smith BL. Deaths: Leading causes for 2002. National Vital Statistics Reports; vol 53, no 17. Hyattsville, MD: National Center for Health Statistics; 2005. Annual reports on leading causes of mortality for earlier years are available at: http://www.cdc.gov/nchs/deaths.htm.
5. National Center for Health Statistics. *Health, United States, 2006 with Chartbook on Trends in the Health of Americans.* Hyattsville, MD: 2004; p. 220.
6. Centers for Disease Control and Prevention. *Pneumocystis* Pneumonia—Los Angeles. *Morb Mortal Wkly Rep.* 1981;30:1–3.
7. Centers for Disease Control and Prevention. Kaposi's sarcoma and *Pneumocystis* pneumonia among homosexual men—New York City and California. *MMWR* 1981;30:306–308.
8. Varghese B, Maher JE, Peterman TA, et al. Reducing the risk of sexual HIV transmission: quantifying the per-act risk for HIV on the basis of choice of partner, sex act, and condom use. *Sex Transm Dis.* 2002;29:38–43.
9. Ostrow DG, DiFranceisco WJ, Chmiel JS, et al. A case-control study of human immunodeficiency virus type 1 seroconversion and risk-related behaviors in the Chicago MACS/CCS Cohort, 1984–1992. Multicenter AIDS Cohort Study. Coping and Change Study. *Am J Epidemiol.* 1995;142:875–883.
10. McKusick L, Wiley JA, Coates TJ, et al. Reported changes in the sexual behavior of men at risk for AIDS, San Francisco, 1982–84—the AIDS Behavioral Research Project. *Public Health Rep.* 1985;100:622–629.
11. Schwarcz S, Kellogg T, McFarland W, et al. Differences in the temporal trends of HIV seroincidence and seroprevalence among sexually transmitted disease clinic patients, 1989–1998: application of the serologic testing algorithm for recent HIV seroconversion. *Am J Epidemiol.* 2001;153:925–934.
12. Ciesielski CA. Sexually transmitted diseases in men who have sex with men: an epidemiologic review. *Curr Infect Dis Rep.* 2003;5:145–152.
13. Nakashima AK, Fleming PL. HIV/AIDS surveillance in the United States, 1981–2001. *J Acquir Immune Defic Syndr.* 2003;32 Suppl 1:S68-S85.
14. Centers for Disease Control and Prevention. Guidelines for national human immunodeficiency virus case surveillance, including monitoring for human

immunodeficiency virus infection and acquired immunodeficiency syndrome. *MMWR* 1999;48(No. RR-13):1–36.

15. Glynn MK, Lee LM, McKenna MT. The status of national HIV case surveillance, United States 2006. *Pub Health Rep* 2007;122 (Supp 1):63–72.

16. Gerberding, JL. "Dear Colleague" letter recommending HIV infection reporting by name. July 5, 2005. http://www.cdc.gov/hiv/PUBS/070505_dearcolleague _gerberding.pdf. Accessed August 22, 2007.

17. Centers for Disease Control and Prevention. HIV Counseling and Testing at CDC supported sites—United States, 1999–2004. 2006:1–33. Available at: http:// www.cdc.gov/hiv/topics/reports.htm.

18. Valleroy LA, MacKellar DA, Karon JM, et al. HIV prevalence and associated risks in young men who have sex with men. Young Men's Survey Study Group. *JAMA.* 2000;284:198–204.

19. Centers for Disease Control and Prevention. HIV prevalence, unrecognized infection, and HIV testing among men who have sex with men—five U.S. cities, June 2004-April 2005. *MMWR Morb Mortal Wkly Rep.* 2005;52:597–601.

20. Catania JA, Osmond D, Stall RD, et al. The continuing HIV epidemic among men who have sex with men. *Am J Public Health.* 2001;91:907–914.

21. Harawa NT, Greenland S, Bingham TA, et al. Associations of race/ethnicity with HIV prevalence and HIV-related behaviors among young men who have sex with men in 7 urban centers in the United States. *J Acquir Immune Defic Syndr.* 2004;35:526–536.

22. Celentano DD, Sifakis F, Hylton J, et al. Race/ethnic differences in HIV prevalence and risks among adolescent and young adult men who have sex with men. *J Urban Health.* 2005;82:610–621.

23. Xia Q, Osmond DH, Tholandi M, et al. HIV prevalence and sexual risk behaviors among men who have sex with men: results from a statewide population-based survey in California. *J Acquir Immune Defic Syndr.* 2006;41:238–245.

24. Chmiel JS, Detels R, Kaslow RA, et al. Factors associated with prevalent human immunodeficiency virus (HIV) infection in the Multicenter AIDS Cohort Study. *Am J Epidemiol.* 1987;126:568–577.

25. Buchacz KA, Siller JE, Bandy DW, et al. HIV and syphilis testing among men who have sex with men attending sex clubs and adult bookstores—San Francisco, 2003. *J Acquir Immune Defic Syndr.* 2004;37:1324–1326.

26. Samuel MC, Hessol N, Shiboski S, et al. Factors associated with human immunodeficiency virus seroconversion in homosexual men in three San Francisco cohort studies, 1984–1989. *J Acquir Immune Defic Syndr.* 1993;6:303–312.

27. Celentano DD, Valleroy LA, Sifakis F, et al. Associations between substance use and sexual risk among very young men who have sex with men. *Sex Transm Dis.* 2006;33:265–271.

28. Ostrow DG, DiFranceisco WJ, Chmiel JS, et al. A case-control study of human immunodeficiency virus type 1 seroconversion and risk-related behaviors in the Chicago MACS/CCS Cohort, 1984–1992. Multicenter AIDS Cohort Study. Coping and Change Study. *Am J Epidemiol.* 1995;142:875–883.

29. Seage GR, III, Mayer KH, Horsburgh CR, Jr., et al. The relation between nitrite inhalants, unprotected receptive anal intercourse, and the risk of human immunodeficiency virus infection. *Am J Epidemiol.* 1992;135:1–11.

30. Williamson LM, Hart GJ. HIV prevalence and undiagnosed infection among a community sample of gay men in Scotland. *J Acquir Immune Defic Syndr* 2007; 45:224–230.

31. Ackers M, Greenbery A, Lin C, Batholow B, Hirsch A, Longhi M, Gurwith M. High HIV incidence among men who have sex with men participating in an HIV vaccine efficacy trial, United States, 1998–2002. 11th Conference on Retroviruses and Opportunistic Infections, San Francisco, CA, February 2003. Abstract 857.

32. Schechter MT, Boyko WJ, Douglas B, et al. The Vancouver Lymphadenopathy-AIDS Study: 6. HIV seroconversion in a cohort of homosexual men. *CMAJ.* 1986;135:1355–1360.

33. Penkower L, Dew MA, Kingsley L, et al. Behavioral, health and psychosocial factors and risk for HIV infection among sexually active homosexual men: the Multicenter AIDS Cohort Study. *Am J Public Health.* 1991;81:194–196.

34. Buchbinder SP, Vittinghoff E, Heagerty PJ, et al. Sexual risk, nitrite inhalant use, and lack of circumcision associated with HIV seroconversion in men who have sex with men in the United States. *J Acquir Immune Defic Syndr.* 2005;39:82–89.

35. Koblin BA, Husnik MJ, Colfax G, et al. Risk factors for HIV infection among men who have sex with men. *AIDS.* 2006;20:731–739.

36. Buchacz K, McFarland W, Kellogg TA, et al. Amphetamine use is associated with increased HIV incidence among men who have sex with men in San Francisco. *AIDS.* 2005;19:1423–1424.

37. Hanson J, Posner S, Hassig S, et al. Assessment of sexually transmitted diseases as risk factors for HIV seroconversion in a New Orleans sexually transmitted disease clinic, 1990–1998. *Ann Epidemiol.* 2005;15:13–20.

38. Kelly JA, Murphy DA, Roffman RA, et al. Acquired immunodeficiency syndrome/human immunodeficiency virus risk behavior among gay men in small cities. Findings of a 16-city national sample. *Arch Intern Med.* 1992;152:2293–2297.

39. Choi KH, Operario D, Gregorich SE, et al. Substance use, substance choice, and unprotected anal intercourse among young Asian American and Pacific Islander men who have sex with men. *AIDS Educ Prev.* 2005;17:418–429.

40. Richwald GA, Morisky DE, Kyle GR, et al. Sexual activities in bathhouses in Los Angeles County: implications for AIDS prevention education. *J Sex Res.* 1988; 25:169–180.

41. Ekstrand ML, Coates TJ. Maintenance of safer sexual behaviors and predictors of risky sex: the San Francisco Men's Health Study. *Am J Public Health.* 1990;80:973–977.

42. McKusick L, Coates TJ, Morin SF, et al. Longitudinal predictors of reductions in unprotected anal intercourse among gay men in San Francisco: the AIDS Behavioral Research Project. *Am J Public Health.* 1990;80:978–983.

43. Kelly JA, Kalichman SC, Kauth MR, et al. Situational factors associated with AIDS risk behavior lapses and coping strategies used by gay men who successfully avoid lapses. *Am J Public Health.* 1991;81:1335–1338.

44. Stall R, Barrett D, Bye L, et al. A comparison of younger and older gay men's HIV risk-taking behaviors: the Communication Technologies 1989 Cross-Sectional Survey. *J Acquir Immune Defic Syndr.* 1992;5:682–687.

45. Mansergh G, Marks G. Age and risk of HIV infection in men who have sex with men. *AIDS.* 1998;12:1119–1128.

46. Bartholow BN, Buchbinder S, Celum C, et al. HIV sexual risk behavior over 36 months of follow-up in the world's first HIV vaccine efficacy trial. *J Acquir Immune Defic Syndr.* 2005;39:90–101.

47. Brewer DD, Golden MR, Handsfield HH. Unsafe sexual behavior and correlates of risk in a probability sample of men who have sex with men in the era of highly active antiretroviral therapy. *Sex Transm Dis.* 2006;33:250–255.
48. Ekstrand ML, Stall RD, Paul JP, et al. Gay men report high rates of unprotected anal sex with partners of unknown or discordant HIV status. *AIDS.* 1999;13:1525–1533.
49. Marcus U, Bremer V, Hamouda O, et al. Understanding recent increases in the incidence of sexually transmitted infections in men having sex with men: changes in risk behavior from risk avoidance to risk reduction. *Sex Transm Dis.* 2006;33:11–17.
50. Shoptaw S. Methamphetamine use in urban gay and bisexual populations. *Top HIV Med.* 2006;14:84–87.
51. Mansergh G, Shouse RL, Marks G, et al. Methamphetamine and sildenafil (Viagra) use are linked to unprotected receptive and insertive anal sex, respectively, in a sample of men who have sex with men. *Sex Transm Infect.* 2006;82:131–134.
52. Drake AJ, Mansergh G, Sullivan PS. Methamphetamine and amphetamine use and sexual risk among men who have sex with men: findings from the CDC National HIV Behavioral Surveillance System. Presented at XVI International AIDS Conference, Toronto, August 13–18, 2006.
53. Morin SF, Steward WT, Charlebois ED, et al. Predicting HIV transmission risk among hiv-infected men who have sex with men: findings from the Healthy Living Project. *J Acquir Immune Defic Syndr.* 2005;40:226–235.
54. Wong W, Chaw JK, Kent CK, et al. Risk factors for early syphilis among gay and bisexual men seen in an STD clinic: San Francisco, 2002–2003. *Sex Transm Dis.* 2005;32:458–463.
55. Liau A, Millett G, Marks G. Meta-analytic examination of online sex-seeking and sexual risk behavior among men who have sex with men. *Sex Transm Dis.* 2006; 33:576–584.
56. Benotsch EG, Kalichman S, Cage M. Men who have met sex partners via the Internet: prevalence, predictors, and implications for HIV prevention. *Arch Sex Behav.* 2002;31:177–183.
57. Centers for Disease Control and Prevention. Internet use and early syphilis infection among men who have sex with men—San Francisco, California, 1999–2003. *MMWR Morb Mortal Wkly Rep.* 2003;19;52:1229–1232.
58. Sullivan PS, Drake AJ, Sanchez TH. Prevalence of treatment optimism-related risk behavior and associated factors among men who have sex with men in 11 states, 2000–2001. *AIDS Behav.* 2006;11:123–129.
59. Kelly JA, Hoffman RG, Rompa D, et al. Protease inhibitor combination therapies and perceptions of gay men regarding AIDS severity and the need to maintain safer sex. *AIDS.* 1998;12:F91–F95.
60. Remien RH, Wagner G, Carballo-Dieguez A, et al. Who may be engaging in high-risk sex due to medical treatment advances? *AIDS.* 1998;12:1560–1561.
61. Stolte IG, Dukers NH, Geskus RB, et al. Homosexual men change to risky sex when perceiving less threat of HIV/AIDS since availability of highly active antiretroviral therapy: a longitudinal study. *AIDS.* 2004;18:303–309.
62. International Collaboration on HIV Optimism. HIV treatments optimism among gay men: an international perspective. *J Acquir Immune Defic Syndr.* 2003;32:545–550.

63. Huebner DM, Rebchook GM, Kegeles SM. A longitudinal study of the association between treatment optimism and sexual risk behavior in young adult gay and bisexual men. *J Acquir Immune Defic Syndr.* 2004;37:1514–1519.

64. Sanchez TH, Gallagher KM. Factors associated with recent sildenafil (Viagra) use among men who have sex with men in the United States. *J Acquir Immune Defic Syndr.* 2006;42:95–100.

65. Janssen RS, Satten GA, Stramer SL, et al. New testing strategy to detect early HIV-1 infection for use in incidence estimates and for clinical and prevention purposes. *JAMA.* 1998;280:42–48.

66. Vu MQ, Steketee RW, Valleroy L, et al. HIV incidence in the United States, 1978–1999. *J Acquir Immune Defic Syndr.* 2002;31:188–201.

67. Nash D, Bennani Y, Ramaswamy C, et al. Estimates of HIV incidence among persons testing for HIV using the sensitive/less sensitive enzyme immunoassy, New York City, 2001. *J Acquir Immune Defic Syndr.* 2005;39:102–111.

68. Centers for Disease Control and Prevention. Trends in primary and secondary syphilis and HIV infections in men who have sex with men—San Francisco and Los Angeles, California, 1998–2002. *MMWR Morb Mortal Wkly Rep.* 2004;53:575–578.

69. Stall RD. Re-emerging HIV epidemics among MSM in the United States and other industrialized nations: Evidence and insight. XVI International AIDS Conference, Toronto, Canada, August 13–18, 2006. Abstract THBS0202.

70. Centers for Disease Control and Prevention. HIV incidence among young men who have sex with men—seven U.S. cities, 1994–2000. *MMWR Morb Mortal Wkly Rep.* 2001;50:440–444.

71. Crepaz N, Marks G, Mansergh G, et al. Age-related risk for HIV infection in men who have sex with men: examination of behavioral, relationship, and serostatus variables. *AIDS Educ Prev.* 2000;12:405–415.

72. Read TR, Hocking J, Sinnott V, Hellard M. Risk factors for incident HIV infection in men having sex with men: a case-control study. *Sex Health* 2007; 4:35–39.

73. Rawstone P, Digiusto E, Worth H, Zablotska I. Associations between crystal methamphetamine use and potentially unsafe sexual activity among gay men in Australia. *Arch Sex Behav* 2007; [Epub ahead of print: August 10, 2007].

74. Rhodes SD, Hergenrather KC, Yee LJ, Knipper E, Wilkin AM, Omli MR. Characteristics of a sample of men who have sex with men, recruited from gay bars and internet chat rooms, who report methamphetamine use. *AIDS Patient Care STD* 2007; 21:575–583.

75. Janssen RS, Holtgrave DR, Valdiserri RO, et al. The Serostatus Approach to Fighting the HIV Epidemic: prevention strategies for infected individuals. *Am J Public Health.* 2001;91:1019–1024.

76. Centers for Disease Control and Prevention. Advancing HIV prevention: new strategies for a changing epidemic—United States, 2003. *MMWR Morb Mortal Wkly Rep.* 2003;52:329–332.

77. United States Census Bureau. US Census, 2000. www.census.gov. Accessed September 30, 2005.

78. Wang L, Sabin K, Wright LN, Smith PF, Sahakyan L, Glebatis D. HIV seroprevalence and seroincidence among inmates entering New York State Department of Correctional Services. Presented at 9th Annual Conference on

Retroviruses and Opportunistic Infections, Seattle Washington, February 24–28, 2002.

79. Centers for Disease Control and Prevention. Diagnoses of HIV/AIDS—32 States, 2000–2003. *MMWR Morb Mortal Wkly Rep.* 2004;53:1106–1110.

80. Sullivan PS, Chu SY, Fleming PL, et al. Changes in AIDS incidence for men who have sex with men, United States 1990–1995. *AIDS.* 1997;11:1641–1646.

81. Martin JL. The impact of AIDS on gay male sexual behavior patterns in New York City. *Am J Public Health.* 1987;77:578–581.

82. Schechter MT, Craib KJ, Willoughby B, et al. Patterns of sexual behavior and condom use in a cohort of homosexual men. *Am J Public Health.* 1988;78:1535–1538.

83. Stall RD, Coates TJ, Hoff C. Behavioral risk reduction for HIV infection among gay and bisexual men: a review of results from the United States. *Am Psychol.* 1988;43:878–885.

84. Nakashima AK, Rolfs RT, Flock ML, et al. Epidemiology of syphilis in the United States, 1941–1993. *Sex Transm Dis.* 1996;23:16–23.

85. Centers for Disease Control and Prevention. HIV counseling and testing in publicly funded sites: 1995 summary report. Atlanta, GA: US Department of Health and Human Services. Centers for Disease Control and Prevention, September 1997.

86. Dougan S, Elford J, Chadborn TR, et al. Does the recent increase in HIV diagnoses among men who have sex with men in the UK reflect a rise in HIV incidence or increased uptake of HIV testing? *Sex Transm Infect.* 2007;86:120–125.

87. Centers for Disease Control and Prevention. *HIV Testing Survey, 2002.* Atlanta, GA: U.S. Department of Health and Human Services, Centers for Disease Control and Prevention; 2004:1–28. HIV/AIDS Special Surveillance Report 5. Also available at http://www.cdc.gov/hiv/stats/hasrsupp.htm.

88. Centers for Disease Control and Prevention. *HIV Testing Survey, 2001.* Atlanta, GA: U.S. Department of Health and Human Services, Centers for Disease Control and Prevention; 2004; Special Surveillance Report Number 1:1–28.

89. Centers for Disease Control and Prevention. *HIV/AIDS Special Surveillance Report,* 2003; Vol 1(No. 1):1–27. http://www.cdc.gov/hiv/stats/special-reportVol1No1 .htm. Accessed August 25, 2005.

90. Chen JL, Kodagoda D, Lawrence AM, et al. Rapid public health interventions in response to an outbreak of syphilis in Los Angeles. *Sex Transm Dis.* 2002;29:277–284.

91. Williams LA, Klausner JD, Whittington WL, et al. Elimination and reintroduction of primary and secondary syphilis. *Am J Public Health.* 1999;89:1093–1097.

92. Wolitski RJ, Valdiserri RO, Denning PH, et al. Are we headed for a resurgence of the HIV epidemic among men who have sex with men? *Am J Public Health.* 2001;91:883–888.

93. Fenton KA, Imrie J. Increasing rates of sexually transmitted diseases in homosexual men in Western Europe and the United States: why? *Infect Dis Clin North Am.* 2005;19:311–331.

94. Giuliani M, Di CA, Palamara G, et al. Increased HIV incidence among men who have sex with men in Rome. *AIDS.* 2005;19:1429–1431.

95. van der Snoek EM, de Wit JB, Gotz HM, et al. Incidence of sexually transmitted diseases and HIV infection in men who have sex with men related to knowledge, perceived susceptibility, and perceived severity of sexually transmitted diseases and HIV infection: Dutch MSM-Cohort Study. *Sex Transm Dis.* 2006;33:193–198.

96. Hurtado I, Alastrue I, Ferreros I, et al. Trends in HIV testing, serial HIV prevalence and HIV incidence among persons attending a Center for AIDS Prevention from 1988 to 2003; increases in HIV incidence in men who have sex with men in recent years? *Sex Transm Infect.* 2007;83:23–28.

97. Beyrer C, Sripaipan T, Tovanabutra S, et al. High HIV, hepatitis C and sexual risks among drug-using men who have sex with men in northern Thailand. *AIDS.* 2005;19:1535–1540.

98. van Griensven F, Thanprasertsuk S, Jommaroeng R, et al. Evidence of a previously undocumented epidemic of HIV infection among men who have sex with men in Bangkok, Thailand. *AIDS.* 2005;19:521–526.

99. Centers for Disease Control and Prevention. HIV prevalence among populations of men who have sex with men–Thailand, 2003 and 2005. *MMWR Morb Mortal Wkly Rep.* 2006;55:844–848.

100. Palella FJ, Jr., Delaney KM, Moorman AC, et al. Declining morbidity and mortality among patients with advanced human immunodeficiency virus infection. HIV Outpatient Study Investigators. *N Engl J Med.* 1998;338:853–860.

101. Halkitis PN, Zade DD, Shrem M, et al. Beliefs about HIV non-infection and risky sexual behavior among MSM. *AIDS Educ Prev.* 2004;16:448–458.

102. Catania JA, Kegeles SM, Coates TJ. Towards an understanding of risk behavior: an AIDS risk reduction model (ARRM). *Health Educ Q.* 1990;17:53–72.

103. Morin SF, Vernon K, Harcourt JJ, et al. Why HIV infections have increased among men who have sex with men and what to do about it: findings from California focus groups. *AIDS Behav.* 2003;7:353–362.

104. Valdiserri RO. Mapping the roots of HIV/AIDS complacency: implications for program and policy development. *AIDS Educ Prev.* 2004;16:426–439.

105. Vanable PA, Ostrow DG, McKirnan DJ, et al. Impact of combination therapies on HIV risk perceptions and sexual risk among HIV-positive and HIV-negative gay and bisexual men. *Health Psychol.* 2000;19:134–145.

106. Elford J, Bolding G, Sherr L. High-risk sexual behaviour increases among London gay men between 1998 and 2001: what is the role of HIV optimism? *AIDS.* 2002;16:1537–1544.

107. Koblin BA, Perdue T, Ren L, et al. Attitudes about combination HIV therapies: the next generation of gay men at risk. *J Urban Health.* 2003;80:510–519.

108. Williamson LM, Hart GJ. HIV optimism does not explain increases in high-risk sexual behaviour among gay men in Scotland. *AIDS.* 2004;18:834–835.

109. Crepaz N, Hart TA, Marks G. Highly active antiretroviral therapy and sexual risk behavior: a meta-analytic review. *JAMA.* 2004;292:224–236.

110. Ostrow DE, Fox KJ, Chmiel JS, et al. Attitudes towards highly active antiretroviral therapy are associated with sexual risk taking among HIV-infected and uninfected homosexual men. *AIDS.* 2002;16:775–780.

111. Stockman JK, Schwarcz SK, Butler LM, et al. HIV prevention fatigue among high-risk populations in San Francisco. *J Acquir Immune Defic Syndr.* 2004;35:432–434.

112. Halkitis PN, Parsons JT, Wilton L. Barebacking among gay and bisexual men in New York City: explanations for the emergence of intentional unsafe behavior. *Arch Sex Behav.* 2003;32:351–357.

113. Mansergh G, Marks G, Colfax GN, et al. "Barebacking" in a diverse sample of men who have sex with men. *AIDS.* 2002;16:653–659.

114. Halkitis PN, Wilton L, Wolitski RJ, et al. Barebacking identity among HIV-positive gay and bisexual men: demographic, psychological, and behavioral correlates. *AIDS.* 2005;19 (Suppl 1):S27–35.:S27-S35.

115. Wolitski RJ, Chiasson MA, Hirshfield S, Humberstone M, Remien RH, Wasserman JL, Wong T. Is "bug chasing" real? An online study of HIV seeking among men who have sex with men (MSM). Paper presented at the 2005 National HIV Prevention Conference, Atlanta, GA. 2005.

116. Mansergh G, Marks G, Miller L, et al. Is 'knowing people with HIV/AIDS' associated with safer sex in men who have sex with men? *AIDS.* 2000;14:1845–1851.

117. Millett GA, Peterson JL, Wolitski RJ, et al. Greater risk for hiv infection of black men who have sex with men: a critical literature review. *Am J Public Health.* 2006;96:1007–1019.

118. Centers for Disease Control and Prevention. Primary and secondary syphilis—United States, 2003–2004. *MMWR Morb Mortal Wkly Rep.* 2006;55:269–273.

119. Centers for Disease Control and Prevention. *Sexually Transmitted Disease Surveillance, 2004.* Atlanta, GA: U.S. Department of Health and Human Services, September 2005.

120. MacKellar DA, Valleroy LA, Behel S, et al. Unintentional HIV exposures from young men who have sex with men who disclose being HIV-negative. *AIDS.* 2006;20:1637–1644.

121. Laumann EO, Youm Y. Racial/ethnic group differences in the prevalence of sexually transmitted diseases in the United States: a network explanation. *Sex Transm Dis.* 1999;26:250–261.

122. Weiss HA, Quigley MA, Hayes RJ. Male circumcision and risk of HIV infection in sub-Saharan Africa: a systematic review and meta-analysis. *AIDS.* 2000;14:2361–2370.

123. Samson M, Libert F, Doranz BJ, et al. Resistance to HIV-1 infection in Caucasian individuals bearing mutant alleles of the CCR-5 chemokine receptor gene. *Nature.* 1996;382:722–725.

124. Marmor M, Sheppard HW, Donnell D, et al. Homozygous and heterozygous CCR5-Delta32 genotypes are associated with resistance to HIV infection. *J Acquir Immune Defic Syndr.* 2001;27:472–481.

125. Michael RT, Gagnon JH, Laumann EO, Kolata G. *Sex in America: A Definitive Survey.* Boston: Little, Brown and Company; 1994.

126. Berry M, Raymond HF, Behel S, Sanchez T, McFarland W. Sexual networks and risk behaviors among racial/ethnic groups of men who have sex with men. Presented at XVI International AIDS Conference, Toronto, Canada, August 2006. Abstract TUPE0617.

127. Sanchez T, Finlayson T, Drake A, et al. Human immunodeficiency virus (HIV) risk, prevention, and testing behaviors–United States, National HIV Behavioral Surveillance System: men who have sex with men, November 2003-April 2005. *MMWR Surveill Summ.* 2006;55:1–16.

128. Montgomery JP, Mokotoff ED, Gentry AC, et al. The extent of bisexual behaviour in HIV-infected men and implications for transmission to their female sex partners. *AIDS Care.* 2003;15:829–837.

129. Goldbaum G, Perdue T, Wolitski RJ, et al. Differences in risk behavior and sources of AIDS information among gay, bisexual, and straight-identified men who have sex with men. *AIDS Behav.* 1998;2:13–21.

130. Doll LS, Petersen LR, White CR. Homosexually and nonhomosexually identified men who have sex with men: a behavioral comparison. *J Sex Res.* 1992;29: 1–14.

131. Millett G, Malebranche D, Mason B, et al. Focusing "down low": bisexual black men, HIV risk and heterosexual transmission. *J Natl Med Assoc.* 2005;97:52S-59S.

132. Johnson WD, Hedges LV, Ramirez G, et al. HIV prevention research for men who have sex with men: a systematic review and meta-analysis. *J Acquir Immune Defic Syndr.* 2002;30 Suppl 1:S118–29.:S118-S129.

133. Herbst JH, Sherba RT, Crepaz N, et al. A meta-analytic review of HIV behavioral interventions for reducing sexual risk behavior of men who have sex with men. *J Acquir Immune Defic Syndr.* 2005;39:228–241.

134. Johnson WD, Holtgrave DR, McClellan WM, et al. HIV intervention research for men who have sex with men: a 7-year update. *AIDS Educ Prev.* 2005;17:568–589.

135. Kahn JG, Kegeles SM, Hays R, et al. Cost-effectiveness of the Mpowerment Project, a community-level intervention for young gay men. *J Acquir Immune Defic Syndr.* 2001;27:482–491.

136. Pinkerton SD, Holtgrave DR, DiFranceisco WJ, et al. Cost-effectiveness of a community-level HIV risk reduction intervention. *Am J Public Health.* 1998;88: 1239–1242.

137. Tao G, Remafedi G. Economic evaluation of an HIV prevention intervention for gay and bisexual male adolescents. *J Acquir Immune Defic Syndr Hum Retrovirol.* 1998;17:83–90.

138. Lyles CM, Kay LS, Crepaz N, et al. Best evidence interentions: findings from systematic review of HIV behavioral interventions for U.S. populations at high risk, 2000–2004. *Am J Public Health.* 2007;97:133–143.

139. Centers for Disease Control and Prevention. Compendium of HIV prevention interventions with evidence of effectiveness. November 1999; revised Augsut 2001. http://www.cdc.gov/hiv/pubs/hivcompendium/hivcompendium.htm. Accessed November 14, 2006.

140. Dilley JW, Woods WJ, Sabatino J, et al. Changing sexual behavior among gay male repeat testers for HIV: a randomized, controlled trial of a single-session intervention. *J Acquir Immune Defic Syndr.* 2002;30:177–186.

141. Koblin B, Chesney M, Coates T. Effects of a behavioural intervention to reduce acquisition of HIV infection among men who have sex with men: the EXPLORE randomised controlled study. *Lancet.* 2004;364:41–50.

142. Kegeles SM, Hays RB, Coates TJ. The Mpowerment Project: a community-level HIV prevention intervention for young gay men. *Am J Public Health.* 1996;86:1129–1136.

143. Kelly JA, St Lawrence JS, Hood HV, et al. Behavioral intervention to reduce AIDS risk activities. *J Consult Clin Psychol.* 1989;57:60–67.

144. Kelly JA, St Lawrence JS, Stevenson LY, et al. Community AIDS/HIV risk reduction: the effects of endorsements by popular people in three cities. *Am J Public Health.* 1992;82:1483–1489.

145. Kelly JA, St Lawrence JS, Diaz YE, et al. HIV risk behavior reduction following intervention with key opinion leaders of population: an experimental analysis. *Am J Public Health.* 1991;81:168–171.

146. St Lawrence JS, Brasfield TL, Diaz YE, et al. Three-year follow-up of an HIV risk-reduction intervention that used popular peers. *Am J Public Health.* 1994;84: 2027–2028.

147. Valdiserri RO, Lyter DW, Leviton LC, et al. AIDS prevention in homosexual and bisexual men: results of a randomized trial evaluating two risk reduction interventions. *AIDS*. 1989;3:21–26.

148. Wolitski RJ, Gomez CA, Parsons JT. Effects of a peer-led behavioral intervention to reduce HIV transmission and promote serostatus disclosure among HIV-seropositive gay and bisexual men. *AIDS*. 2005;19 (Suppl 1):S99–109.:S99–109.

149. Schwartz DJ, Bailey CJ. Between the sheets and between the ears: sexual practices and risk beliefs of HIV-positive gay and bisexual men. In Halkitis P, Gómez C, and Wolitski RJ, eds. *HIV+ Sex: The Psychological and Interpersonal Dynamics of HIV-Seropositive Gay and Bisexual Men's Relationships*. Washington, DC: American Psychological Association; 2005:55–72.

150. Wolitski RJ, Bailey CJ, O'Leary A, et al. Self-perceived responsibility of HIV-seropositive men who have sex with men for preventing HIV transmission. *AIDS Behav*. 2003;7:363–372.

151. Gold RS, Skinner M, Ross MW. Unprotected anal intercourse in HIV-infected and non-HIV-infected gay men. *J Sex Res*. 1994;31:59–77.

152. Díaz RM. HIV stigmatization and mental health outcomes in Latino gay men. Society for Community Research and Action Biennial Meeting. Las Vegas, NV, June 2003.

153. Courtenay-Quirk C, Wolitski RJ, Parsons JT, et al. Is HIV/AIDS stigma dividing the gay community? Perceptions of HIV-positive men who have sex with men. *AIDS Educ Prev*. 2006;18:56–67.

154. Weinhardt LS. HIV diagnosis and risk behavior. In: Kalichman SC, ed. *Positive Prevention: Reducing HIV Transmission Among People Living with HIV/AIDS*. New York: Kluwer Academic/Plenum Publishers; 2005:29–63.

155. Higgins DL, Galavotti C, O'Reilly KR, et al. Evidence for the effects of HIV antibody counseling and testing on risk behaviors. *JAMA*. 1991;266:2419–2429.

156. Wolitski RJ, MacGowan RJ, Higgins DL, et al. The effects of HIV counseling and testing on risk-related practices and help-seeking behavior. *AIDS Educ Prev*. 1997;9:52–67.

157. McGowan JP, Shah SS, Ganea CE, et al. Risk behavior for transmission of human immunodeficiency virus (HIV) among HIV-seropositive individuals in an urban setting. *Clin Infect Dis*. 2004;38:122–127.

158. Crepaz N, Lyles CM, Wolitski RJ, et al. Do prevention interventions reduce HIV risk behaviours among people living with HIV? A meta-analytic review of controlled trials. *AIDS*. 2006;20:143–157.

159. Centers for Disease Control and Prevention. Antiretroviral postexposure prophylaxis after sexual, injection-drug use, or other nonoccupational exposure to HIV in the United States: recommendations from the U.S. Department of Health and Human Services. *MMWR* 2005;54(No. RR-2):1–28.

160. Garcia-Lerma J, Otten R, Qari S, Jackson E, Luo W, Monsour M, Schinazi R, Janssen R, Folks T, Heneine W. Prevention of rectal SHIV transmission in macaques by Tenofovir/FTC combination. Presented at 13th Conference on Retroviruses and Opportunistic Infections, February 2006. Abstract 32LB.

161. Singh JA, Mills EJ. The abandoned trials of pre-exposure prophylaxis for HIV: what went wrong? *PLoS Med*. 2005;2:e234.

162. Lange JM. We must not let protestors derail trials of pre-exposure prophylaxis for HIV. *PLoS Med*. 2005;2:e248.

163. Auvert B, Taljaard D, Lagarde E, et al. Randomized, controlled intervention trial of male circumcision for reduction of HIV infection risk: the ANRS 1265 Trial. *PLoS Med.* 2005;2:e298.

164. Bailey RC, Moses S, Parker CB, et al. Male circumcision for HIV prevention in young men in Kisumu, Kenya: a randomised controlled trial. *Lancet* 2007; 369:643–656.

165. Sullivan PS, Kilmarx PH, Peterman TA, et al. Male circumcision for prevention of HIV infection: what the new data mean for HIV prevention in the United States. *PLoS Med* 4:e223.

166. Klausner RD, Fauci AS, Corey L, et al. The need for a global HIV vaccine enterprise. *Science.* 2003;300:2036–2039.

167. Duerr A, Wasserheit JN, Corey L. HIV vaccines: new frontiers in vaccine development. *Clin Infect Dis.* 2006;43:500–511.

168. Kippax S, Race K. Sustaining safe practice: twenty years on. *Soc Sci Med.* 2003;57:1–12.

169. Kippax S, Noble J, Prestage G, et al. Sexual negotiation in the AIDS era: negotiated safety revisited. *AIDS.* 1997;11:191–197.

170. Parsons JT, Schrimshaw EW, Wolitski RJ, et al. Sexual harm reduction practices of HIV-seropositive gay and bisexual men: serosorting, strategic positioning, and withdrawal before ejaculation. *AIDS.* 2005;19 Suppl 1:S13–25:S13–S25.

171. Suarez TP, Kelly JA, Pinkerton SD, et al. Influence of a partner's HIV serostatus, use of highly active antiretroviral therapy, and viral load on perceptions of sexual risk behavior in a community sample of men who have sex with men. *J Acquir Immune Defic Syndr.* 2001;28:471–477.

172. Van de Ven P, Kippax S, Crawford J, et al. In a minority of gay men, sexual risk practice indicates strategic positioning for perceived risk reduction rather than unbridled sex. *AIDS Care.* 2002;14:471–480.

173. Jones K, Gray P, Wang T, Johnson W, Foust E, Dunbar E. Evaluation of a community-level peer-based HIV prevention intervention adapted for young black men who have sex with men (MSM). Presented at XVI International AIDS, August 2006. Abstract MOAC0103.

174. Somlai AM, Kelly JA, Otto-Salaj L, et al. Current HIV prevention activities for women and gay men among 77 ASOs. *J Public Health Manag Pract.* 1999;5:23–33.

175. Goldstein E, Wrubel J, Faigeles B, et al. Sources of information for HIV prevention program managers: a national survey. *AIDS Educ Prev.* 1998;10:63–74.

176. Kraft JM, Mezoff JS, Sogolow ED, et al. A technology transfer model for effective HIV/AIDS interventions: science and practice. *AIDS Educ Prev.* 2000;12:7–20.

177. Valdiserri RO. Technology transfer: achieving the promise of HIV prevention. In: Peterson J, DiClemente R, eds. *Handbook of HIV Prevention.* New York, NY: Klewer Academic/Plenum; 2000:267–283.

178. Gallagher K, Sullivan PS, Lansky A. Behavioral surveillance among persons at risk for HIV infection in the US: The National HIV Behavioral Surveillance System. *Public Health Rep.* 2007;122 (Supp 1):32–38.

179. Sullivan PS, McKenna MT, Janssen R. Progress towards implementation of integrated systems for surveillance of HIV infection and morbidity in the US. *Public Health Rep.* 2007;122 (Supp 1):1–3.

180. Stall R, Purcell DW. Intertwining epidemics: A review of research on substance use among men who have sex with men and its connection to the AIDS epidemic. *AIDS Behav.* 2000;4:181–192.

181. Stall R, Mills TC, Williamson J, et al. Association of co-occurring psychosocial health problems and increased vulnerability to HIV/AIDS among urban men who have sex with men. *Am J Public Health.* 2003;93:939–942.
182. Meyer IH. Minority stress and mental health in gay men. *J Health Soc Behav.* 1995;36:38–56.
183. Stokes JP, Peterson JL. Homophobia, self-esteem, and risk for HIV among African American men who have sex with men. *AIDS Educ Prev.* 1998;10:278–292.
184. Marks G, Burris S, Peterman TA. Reducing sexual transmission of HIV from those who know they are infected: the need for personal and collective responsibility. *AIDS.* 1999;13:297–306.
185. Wohlfeiler D. Structural and environmental HIV prevention for gay and bisexual men. *AIDS.* 2000;14 Suppl 1:S52–6.:S52-S56.

Part III

Cross-Cutting Issues

9

Interacting Epidemics and Gay Men's Health: A Theory of Syndemic Production among Urban Gay Men

Ron Stall, Mark Friedman, and Joseph A. Catania

As discussed in prior chapters in this volume, American men who have sex with men (MSM) suffer from a number of different health disparities, among them far greater prevalence rates of greater drug use[1-6] greater rates of HIV and STI infections,[7,8] and greater rates of clinical depression[1,4,9-12] than do comparison samples of American men who have sex only with women. This state of affairs is surprising in view of the often rather advantaged social position (in particular, regarding educational attainment) that gay men report in many of the same studies that have yielded evidence for health disparities. The remarkably consistent body of findings based on these samples raises an interesting epidemiological question: how could it be possible that a group of men with a rather advantaged social demographic profile have such a disadvantaged health profile?

This chapter will argue that one answer to this perplexing epidemiological puzzle is that urban gay male communities are suffering from the effects of a syndemic, or a set of mutually interacting epidemics that are functioning to make each other worse. Syndemics are a set of mutually reinforcing epidemics that together lower the overall health profile of a population more than each epidemic by itself might be expected to do. Although there is an empirical literature stretching back for at least 20 years that documents high levels of substance use, as well as what we now call sexual risk taking and depression, among American MSM, relatively few studies have investigated the possibility that these epidemics are mutually reinforcing and function together to lower the health profile of urban American MSM.

The evidence base for mutually reinforcing epidemics among MSM also has a history at least two decades old, as some of the earliest papers on the behavioral epidemiology of AIDS described the associations between substance use and high risk sexual behavior. However, the term *syndemics* was coined in connection with the groundbreaking work of Merrill Singer and colleagues to explain the very low health profiles of substance-using Puerto Ricans in the Northeastern region of the United States.[13,14] Singer's work pointed out that the interconnections between substance use, poverty, violence, racism, and HIV had a powerful effect in lowering health profiles. Singer's central hypothesis was that class and cultural marginalization dynamics work to create syndemic situations among ethnic minority, impoverished populations in the American Northeast. In short, Singer argued that syndemics were culturally produced, and resulted from the intersection of cultural marginalization and poverty. This chapter will extend Singer's analysis to argue that cultural marginalization alone is sufficient to produce a syndemic among American MSM. Although this chapter will focus on the deleterious health effects of cultural marginalization among American MSM, it should not be taken to mean that we are arguing the effects of race and class are negligible or that syndemics among MSM are unique to Americans. The chapter explicitly argues that MSM who are drawn from lower socioeconomic status (SES) and/or culturally marginalized ethnic groups are especially likely to be vulnerable to syndemic situations. This chapter will present evidence that syndemics exist among American MSM, will propose a theory of syndemic production among American MSM, and will suggest a set of health promotion activities that could be designed to raise levels of health among American MSM based on syndemic theory.

Evidence for Syndemic Situations among American MSM

As previously noted, the intersections between different epidemics among American gay men have been documented for as long as 20 years, starting with the interconnections between substance use and HIV infection,[6,15–20] but also including a sizable set of papers on depression and HIV risk,[21–24] childhood sexual abuse and HIV risk,[25–28] as well as other interconnecting epidemics. The published literature tends to reflect the funding priorities of "single issue" granting agencies whose mission is to further research on substance use, HIV infection, mental health functioning, or violence, separately; this approach, in practice, discouraged a more holistic investigation of the intersections of all of these epidemics. Hence, to date, there is only a small evidence base that describes the interrelationships of epidemics among American gay men.

An exception to this generalization is the body of work based on the Urban Men's Health Study, a household-based sample of MSM who resided in some of America's largest cities who were interviewed in the late 1990s.[6,11,29–39] That study investigated a wide set of health conditions among American MSM in large urban settings (among them HIV risk, substance abuse, depression, partner violence, suicidality), and it became apparent as these analyses were pursued that many of the most prevalent and deadly health conditions that afflict MSM are interconnected. Stall and other members of the UMHS team investigated the question of whether these intersecting conditions drove HIV risk and infection among these men. Their analysis of the UMHS data set concluded that there are at least four different epidemics operating among American MSM, that all are interconnected, and that each makes the others worse. As described by Stall and colleagues[39]:

> Notable . . . is the extent to which each of these psychosocial health conditions appears as an independent correlate of the others in the multivariable models. For example, childhood sexual abuse is independently associated with depression and partner violence; depression is independently associated with childhood sexual abuse, polydrug use and partner violence; polydrug use is independently associated with depression and partner violence, and partner violence is independently associated with childhood sexual abuse; depression and polydrug use. Each of these associations is in the expected positive direction.

Furthermore, men who scored higher on a numerical count of measures for any one of these health problems were at higher risk for HIV transmission and for HIV infection itself. These relationships still held after controlling for background demographic and behavioral variables that might modify these relationships.[39] This analysis shows, in one important household-based sample of MSM, that syndemic processes are at work and that they drive AIDS risk among American MSM. However, the Stall et al.[39] paper did not attempt to theorize the creation of syndemics or to show how they might emerge in the specific case of urban gay men.

It is important to note that the vast majority of the men in the Urban Men's Health study could not be characterized as being caught up in a syndemic. Only a minority of men in the sample (18%) reported positive scores for two or more psychosocial health conditions.[39] Accounting for the high degree of resilience to syndemics among contemporary urban gay men in this study needs to be part of any theoretical explanation of syndemics. Nonetheless, enough men appear to be caught up in syndemic conditions to help account for the higher overall prevalence rates of psychosocial health problems among gay men compared to their heterosexual male counterparts.

Numerous epidemiological surveys have described elevated rates of depression,[1,4,9,10,12] suicidality,[9,12,40] substance abuse,[2,5,41] and HIV infection[8,30,42,43] among men who have sex with other men, compared to heterosexual controls. One notable aspect of the epidemiology of these problems among gay men is their early onset among gay men, in that a disproportionate number of adolescent and young adult MSM report high prevalence levels of depression and anxiety, substance abuse, and HIV.[8,44–52] The early onset of this cluster of psychosocial health problems suggests that some phenomenon that occurs during childhood and/or adolescence shapes experiences of health problems in adulthood. Any theory of syndemic production must then incorporate the experiences of gay men during childhood and adolescence.

Towards a Theory of Syndemic Production among Urban Gay Men

The theory of syndemic development outlined in this chapter rests on a set of central assumptions. The first of these is that the cluster of interacting epidemics that exists among gay men is largely socially produced, and not the result of any genetic or intrinsic set of illnesses that directly result from same gender sexual orientation. As socially produced phenomena, the conditions that gave rise to syndemics may change across generations or subpopulations of gay men. For this reason, the theory outlined here is meant to portray the situation of largely middle-class American gay men who came of age during the latter part of the 20th century. In view of the fact that much of the data on health disparities is drawn from urban gay male populations, this theory may also be most relevant to the experiences of urban gay men. The proposed theory also assumes that some proportion of men are homosexually-oriented in each generation and that some of these men, but by no means all, demonstrate nonconformity to masculine ideals at a rather early age.

The theory posits that two predominant dynamics are the cause of syndemic production among gay men: socially-produced damages associated with early adolescent male socialization among homosexual men, in combination with the added stresses associated with migration to large cities that contain "gay ghettos." The theory is thus developmental in nature, starting with socially-produced harm that begins at a very young age for gay men, continues through adolescence and early sexual awakening, and continues as men take on a gay male social identity and migrate to large urban centers. Occasionally, this urban migration is reminiscent of other urban refugee groups, particularly in the sense that men are fleeing homophobic environments to find a social setting in which they are finally free to associate with whom they please and express themselves as they see fit. In some cases—for example "throwaway" gay youth who are forced to leave their families of origin after disclosure of homosexuality, often under very dire circumstances—the use of the phrase "refugee population" is apt indeed.

Some definitions of terms central to the syndemic theory proposed here may be useful. The first of these concerns the use of the term *masculinity*. As used here, the term is not meant to convey a particular style of male gender presentation, but rather adherence to a socially-constructed male ideal that includes (among other characteristics) interest in physical sports, ready willingness to engage in physical and/or economic competition, and sexual interest in women—in short, conventional American adult male behavior and interests. The use of the phrase *gay men* in this chapter is meant to describe a man with an open social identity as homosexual; the use of the term *homosexual* is meant to convey same gender sexual attraction without social identity. "Gay ghettos" are the well-characterized neighborhoods that exist in nearly all American cities that enjoy a very high concentration of gay men.[33,53] Syndemics are the end result of epidemiological interactions found in marginalized communities in which some proportion of a population suffer from multiple health problems.

Finally, this theory draws on many different sources, not only the work of Merrill Singer and colleagues,[13,14,54] but also the seminal analyses of Ilan Meyer[55,56] and Rafael Díaz.[57] In particular, the theory of syndemic production proposed here draws on Meyer's conceptualizations of minority stressors and strengths, and Díaz's concepts of masculinity failure and sexual silence in the context of early male socialization. This theory attempts to draw upon both of these conceptualizations of the health of MSM, within a developmental framework, to explain syndemic production.

Early Masculine Socialization, Masculinity Panic, and Violence

Enormous emphasis is placed on a boy's masculine socialization, such that it is difficult to identify any organized recreational activity promoted for boys that cannot be interpreted at its core as an exercise in masculine socialization. This strong emphasis carries the implication that socialization can fail to produce sons that meet masculine ideals, an outcome that is regarded as very problematic for the boy in question as well as the boy's family. It follows that young boys who appear to be failing to reach masculine goals are punished in socially shaming ways. There are many such examples of this widespread shaming, for example, "you throw like a girl" and "sissy," which can be regarded as one of the milder of the gender policings administered by other boys and adults alike.

Research to study the health outcomes of gender policings of boys who do not conform to masculine ideals has not been a high priority for funding in the United States. Nonetheless, a substantial literature has emerged to show that boys who do not conform to these ideals meet with a surprising degree of violence. One group who appear to fail to reach masculine goals are those boys who are perceived as gender nonconforming. Some gay males exhibit gender-role nonconformity with respect to their appearance, mannerisms, and interests.[58] They are, compared to other gay youth, more likely to be physically and verbally abused.[59-62] Other youth who appear different and thus experience elevated rates of abuse are those who are perceived as less physically attractive,[63] overweight or obese,[64,65] weaker,[66] or who exhibit movement coordination problems.[67] The abuse experienced by gender nonconforming gay males, however, goes beyond the issue of difference, as these individuals are penalized for failing to achieve the masculine ideal. What is perceived as unmanly is rejected by others in an attempt to affirm their own claims of meeting ideals of masculinity.[68]

A child or adolescent need not exhibit gender-role nonconforming behavior to face the consequences of failing to meet the masculine ideal. Simply being gay or bisexual will suffice. One of the earliest studies in this area,[49] using the Youth Risk Behavior Survey, found that high-school students in

Massachusetts who reported being gay, lesbian, or bisexual (2.5% of the -sample) were about five times more likely to miss school due to fearfulness, over four times more likely to be threatened with a weapon at school, 3.5 times more likely to participate in a fight that required medical treatment, and five times more likely to carry a gun. Findings of the largest study of adolescents in the United States, the National Longitudinal Study of Adolescent Health, first implemented during the mid-1990s, found that youth who reported romantic attractions to the same sex were almost twice as likely, compared to youth who were attracted only to other-sex individuals, to be violently attacked and to require medical treatment after a fight.[69] Although none of these studies reported whether boys were gender nonconforming, it seems unlikely that the violence directed toward LGB (lesbian, gay, or bisexual) youth is experienced only by the minority of gay youth who are non-gender-conforming.

More recent studies suggest that these trends continue. Of 237,544 students surveyed in 2001–2002 in California,[70] 17,815 (7.5%) reported being harassed or bullied because they "are gay or lesbian or someone thought [they] were." An online survey conducted by Harris Interactive[71] of 3400 students from throughout the United States found that 22% of LGBT students reported not feeling safe at school and 90% of LGBT students had been harassed or assaulted during the past year (versus 7% and 62% of non-LGBT teens respectively). The problem goes beyond the direct experience of being victimized. LGBT youth who are harassed are less likely, compared to heterosexual adolescents, to report these experiences, and adults who witness such harassment are less likely to intervene.[70,71] Further, gay youth who escape being physically abused often witness the direct victimization of other gay youth,[59] itself a stressor that may contribute to psychological difficulties.

It is important to point out that in the general population, children and adolescents who are victims of bullying have been found to: (1) present a variety of physical symptoms to physicians,[72,73] (2) underachieve in school,[74,75] and (3) report higher levels of anxiety and depression[76–79] and suicide ideation and attempts.[76,80,81] The long-term consequences of being bullied may also be negative. While research on long-term outcomes is minimal, Olweus[82] found that individuals who had been bullied during adolescence reported higher levels of depression and poorer self-esteem as adults. This outcome was found even though as adults these individuals were not more likely to be bullied, otherwise harassed, or socially isolated. The consequences of victimization for gay youth also appear to be negative. Several studies have found that physical and verbal abuse of gay youth is associated with poorer mental health status.[59,83–85] One indication is that the victimization of LGBT youth by their parents may be especially damaging. For example, D'Augelli, Hershberger, and Pilkington[86] found that, compared to non-attempters, LGB youth who had attempted suicide were more likely to have experienced rejection or intolerance upon disclosing their sexual orientation to a father or mother.

The repercussions of this aggressive socialization must be far-reaching but are as yet poorly understood. Certainly a sense of being "less than," of not fitting in, of having to learn to manage identity by hiding certain behaviors for boys who do not fit the masculine ideal would be lessons learned at a very early age. In addition, even boys who are successful at meeting masculine ideals can be affected by these very aggressive socialization efforts, as they may be witnesses and perhaps even participants in meting out punishments to other boys who do not fit in. Boys who witness such events cannot escape noticing the very expensive costs of not meeting the demands of the masculine ideal, even when they themselves are successful in meeting them. Note, as well, that these very aggressive socialization efforts are imposed on boys during precisely those years when they are likely to have the weakest coping skills to deal with these stressors and so are quite impressionable. In some cases, the wounds that result from being the object of masculinity panic must be profound, indeed.

Adolescent Masculine Socialization

By adolescence, the patterns of learned careful impression management to meet masculine ideals have been well established, as well as the need to internally police actions that may not meet these norms. Since an admission of homosexual attraction ranks very high on the list of attributes that are understood to cause masculinity failure, young men are unable to talk about their urges or their actual behaviors—their sexuality is ruled by a regime of silence. Many homosexual adolescent boys may have the sense that they are alone in having strong sexual feelings for other males. The inability to discuss homosexual attraction or acts could well predispose them to strong self-censorship, disassociation during sex play with other males, sexual shaming, and a strong devaluing of other boys who are understood to be gay. Each of these processes can be thought of as definitional attributes of internalized homophobia, and each could be hypothesized in turn to predict later development of psychosocial health problems such as depression or substance abuse.

Sexual Initiation and Sexual Violence

Along with sports prowess and the physical changes that accompany male adolescence, sexual attraction to and sexual initiation with girls/women are important benchmarks of successful adolescent heterosexuality and mainstream understandings of meeting masculine ideals. Boys who do not meet these developmental benchmarks in a timely way are identified as less successful in meeting masculine ideals and so, less socially valued. Again, issues of sexual shaming emerge, so that boys who are not sexually successful with females are identified as over-intellectualized "nerds" or as physically unappealing, gay, or belonging to some other devalued male subgroup. And, again, boys who meet these socially defined sexual benchmarks but who suspect that they are homosexual learn firsthand the costs of failing to meet socially approved masculine ideals. Boys who suspect that they are vulnerable to accusations of masculinity failure are likely to withdraw from active social life to the extent that they are able and so lose the opportunity to gain important social skills such as the ability to effectively bond with a social group that confers a valued social identity. Some boys may assume social identities based on membership with groups that are regarded as marginal within adolescent social life, and so begin a career of finding refuge within marginalized and/or stigmatized social groups. Another response to vulnerability to social shaming might be that of developing only minimal connections with social groups, so that withdrawal from mainstream adolescent culture is facilitated, again at the cost of developing crucial social skills.

Some boys experience sexual initiation, but not with girls, and some of this male-to-male sexual initiation is not expressive of emotional attachment or even sexual pleasure. Although estimates of the proportion of gay men who report having been sexually abused by other men during adolescence vary considerably, even conservative estimates of this experience indicate that something on the order of one out of six gay men had early sexual socialization experiences that could be characterized as violent or abusive.[26,34] A substantial literature has now emerged to show that abusive sexual initiation is associated with numerous psychosocial health problems in later life, as well as HIV infection.[25,27,87–90] Childhood sexual abuse is discussed in greater detail in Chapter 3.

Men at the Crossroads: Initiation into Gay Male Life

By mid- to late adolescence, many homosexual youth are likely to be aware of their attractions to other males, others will have initiated sex with other males, and some may even have reached the developmental benchmark of telling others that they are homosexual or gay. However, one must consider that the achievement of these developmental benchmarks occurs within a sociocultural context in which homosexual identity is understood to be a cause of masculinity failure, of social shaming for having homosexual desire, and even of becoming a target for violence. This pervasive negative sociocultural context could make formation of strong ties with other young gay men more difficult, predisposes young men to devalue other gay men, and likely stimulates the development of internalized homophobia. Thus, many young homosexual men are reaching adulthood with strong socially mediated vulnerabilities for depression, relationship difficulties, social shaming, physical violence, and sexual violence. Each of these experiences, in turn, may make men especially vulnerable to substance abuse careers as they begin participation in gay male culture. That said, in terms of strengths, many of these young men have learned to positively manage their identities and function well within a very adverse social situation, and some even to find ways to thrive. Thus, these men enter early adulthood with a mixture of important socially shaped strengths and weaknesses.

By late adolescence, an increasing awareness of homosexual attraction as well as of the existence of gay culture itself will have manifested among many young homosexual men. Gay culture is likely to be experienced by many young men as both consistent with and divergent from the notions of masculinity with which they were raised. Where the existence of gay culture is likely to provide the greatest support of young gay men's emerging social identities, however, would be with the notions that homosexuality is natural, that it is possible to find other men who are also homosexual, that many gay men meet and even exceed conventional standards of successful masculinity, that homosexual relationships can be long-lasting and based on feelings that go beyond sexual attraction alone, and that homosexual life can be fulfilling and fun. Thus, the very existence of gay culture is likely to be experienced as a font for cultural resistance that gives young gay men permission to consider the creation of a social identity for which they had not been previously socialized by mainstream society.

Initiation into Gay Culture

Once gay men pass through the developmental hurdles of finding sexual initiation with other males, self-identification as gay/homosexual, and identifying to others that they are gay, most men will also decide to initiate contact with gay male culture. Varying routes of connection to gay life are possible, some of which will have very different repercussions in later life. The wide variety of different avenues to achieve contact with gay male life include at least: social organizations, sex venues, friendship networks, faith-based organizations, and gay bars, among other possibilities. The route of initial connection to gay culture is likely to produce different social networks, different understandings of gay social norms, different sexual outcomes, and different experiences of forming strong social bonds with other men. Thus, men who begin their connection with gay culture in public sex venues are likely to have different connections with gay culture than are men who connect to gay culture through a dense friendship network of openly gay men. Some of these modes of connection—say those that are predicated on the combination of sex and substance use—may have longer-term repercussions in terms of the emergence of later psychosocial health problems and/or exposure to STDs and HIV.

That said, one problem faced by gay men in earlier years may be resolved with open connection to gay culture: the problem of finding a social group to which men can belong and in which social shaming based on fear of failing to meet masculinity standards is nearly nonexistent. Men may find a great sense of connection to a group, for the first time in their lives, in which secrets about sexual orientation or practice are not only unnecessary but even counterproductive. For men who have been denied this sort of connection during earlier adolescence, this sense of belonging can be very powerful. Some men will want to move to large cities where they can access urban communities of openly gay men to extend this connection even further.

Stresses Associated with Moving to Gay Ghettos

When gay men discover that they have access to large communities in which being homosexual is not only normative but celebrated, they may decide to move to larger cities to be part of these communities, or, if reared in large cities, to relocate to neighborhoods that are at least gay friendly. The bulk of the literature on gay men's health has been generated through the study of urban gay neighborhoods, or "gay ghettos," and it is from these studies that the most persuasive evidence for the existence of health disparities among gay men has been generated. These data often support the conclusion that gay ghettos are characterized by substantial health disparities when compared to standard measures of health indices drawn from the general male population. Does this finding then indicate that gay men are making poor health decisions when they decide to migrate to gay ghettos to access gay community?

It is notable that the previous question contains the assumption that gay men who remain in rural or suburban settings enjoy comparable levels of health to those in the heterosexual male population; it may be that, in fact, these men suffer from even greater health disparities than do gay men who migrate to large cities. In addition, gay men who relocate to large cities may have very accurate assessments regarding their relative safety in gay ghettos as a result of their ability to find gay community, long-term relationships, refuge from homophobic attacks, economic opportunities, and so on, compared to their communities of origin. Thus, although we have relatively clear data on the health disparities suffered by gay men who reside in gay ghettos, this is not to say that the decision to migrate to these centers can be assumed to be a poor one. In summary, the ability of gay men to maintain good health in large gay ghettos relies on their ability to balance the stresses and advantages of connecting to gay community and the larger community in these settings, just as it does in small urban or rural settings.

Balancing Stressors and Resources within Gay Male Community Settings

Once men arrive in large urban settings with large gay ghettos, they can access many significant strengths. Among these are: the ability to join a community that confers a positive social identity; the ability to find membership in a social group that encourages honesty and direct conversation about sex and sex between men; and the ability to find some protection from homophobic assaults and an enhanced ability to find potential romantic/sex partners. In counterbalance to these advantages, men who move to large gay ghettos may also find that they encounter difficulties in creating new social networks in a big city: high background prevalence rates of substance abuse, violence, depression, STDs and HIV infection; and multiple stresses associated with taking on a minority identity with greater public acknowledgement of gay men.

Of the above list, the final stressor may seem the most paradoxical. With greater acknowledgment of the gay liberation movement, greater awareness of that movement is created, and greater resistance to the movement can emerge. While the emergence of open gay communities conveys enormous advantages to gay men, it also makes it more difficult for individual gay men to pass as heterosexual and to avoid homophobic attacks when they emerge. Examples of this phenomenon are common; perhaps one of the more dramatic occurred after the White Night riot at San Francisco City Hall, a riot of predominantly gay men in response to the light prison sentence given Dan White after his murder of the openly gay supervisor Harvey Milk and Mayor George Moscone in 1978. After that riot, a subset of the San Francisco police force did not need to ask for directions to the Castro when they themselves rioted and openly attacked and brutalized the patrons of a well-known gay bar at the corner of Castro and 18th Street.[91]

Some gay men may experience a "socialization disconnect" between the roles for which they were socialized as males and the possible roles that they can assume as "out" gay men in large cities. Gay men do not enter urban gay culture without socialization: rather, they have been well socialized to enter a number of important roles that become difficult to achieve within urban culture and within urban gay culture. Most of these difficulties are the result of active homophobic policies that restrict gay men from participating in roles that many adult males are socialized to perform. Among these roles are those of married spouse, membership in certain religious organizations, ability to serve in the armed forces, ability to rise to desired positions within some business or governmental organizations. Other difficulties have to do with the challenges of urban life, such as higher costs of living, in particular those associated with owning a home, making home ownership an unlikely dream for many men. Not all difficulties faced by urban gay men are restricted to gay men who live in cities; some difficulties are intrinsic to homosexual relationships, such as greater difficulties in achieving parenthood. Nonetheless, although many or even most gay men find ways to cope with these institutionalized disadvantages, other men may find the inability to meet important life goals that they assumed would come with adulthood—but which are difficult or impossible in the face of socially-constructed barriers—to be deeply frustrating. This may predispose some men to experience psychosocial problems.

For many men, then, migration to gay ghettos requires a balancing between the strengths of greater connection to gay culture, the greater stresses of life within an urban setting and the stresses of urban gay life. It is in the need to balance resources and stressors that men's earlier life histories become very important. If gay men have responded to homophobic environments by not learning important skills to find and bond with emotionally-satisfying social groups, by repeating relationships in which violence and abuse are assumed, by finding connections to other gay men only through sex or drug use, or by being afraid to access mental health or other social services based on gay identity, they will be more vulnerable to multiple psychosocial health problems.

Interconnecting Epidemics and the Rise of Syndemics

Gay men migrate to urban centers to gain freedom from oppressive cultural environments, yet then find themselves within settings that combine the pressures of urban life with the pressures of many other minority groups. The move to urban centers sometimes strips men of important social capital that they developed during early years of life, but it also gives men the opportunity to experience important connections and to build social connections within a new social milieu. However, it should also be noted that this new social milieu contains a substantial proportion of men who survived very difficult early socialization experiences; it is a social group characterized by high background prevalence rates of substance abuse, depression and other psychosocial health problems. Thus, some men within this social milieu may have attenuated abilities to form strong social connections and develop the social supports that might otherwise provide a buffering effect to the stressors with which these men are coping. Most men are able to navigate these threats to well-being, but other men apparently do not have the resources to avoid these difficulties.

Thus, many gay men bring to their adult lives a long history of experience with homophobic attacks, as well as notable skills in handling these attacks. Based on the balance of resilience and vulnerability that they bring to their adult lives, as well as the skills that gay men may possess to find social support during difficult times, they are more or less vulnerable to different psychosocial health problems. Within the urban situation, psychosocial health problems can interconnect and cascade, due to the pervasiveness of depression and/or the effects of social norms within a community that suffers relatively high rates of substance abuse. When these interconnections occur, a syndemic situation is produced.

The causal links in the theory of syndemic production that we propose are outlined in Figure 9-1.

To summarize the main themes of this chapter as illustrated in Figure 9-1, the early social and emotional development of gay men occurs within two predominant contextual influences: that of background social (demographic and class and familial) variables in combination with the influence of masculine socialization stress (i.e., the dynamics of reward and punishment for

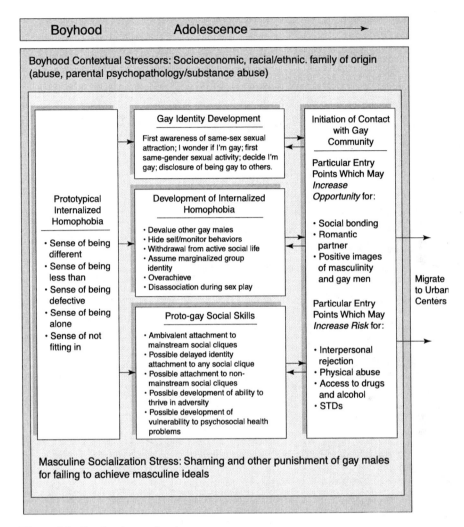

Figure 9-1. Syndemic production.

boys to encourage them to meet masculinity ideals). Within this overall so-ciocultural context, homosexually-oriented boys form their initial sense of whether they are somehow different from other boys and eventually whether they may be homosexual. This realization, within the ongoing influence of the predominant forces of sociodemographic variables and masculine socializa-tion stress, shapes how the identities of young gay men are formed, from an ini-tial sense of whether they fit into the larger sociocultural expectations placed on them (prototypical internalized homophobia), to how boys pass through a set of developmental markers for being gay (gay identity development), to possible development of internalized homophobia and specific social skills

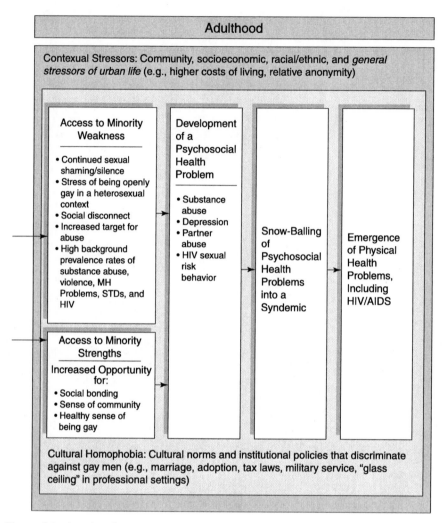

Figure 9-1. (*continued*)

that may shield boys from accusations of homosexuality. Each of these dynamics shapes in important ways the methods by which boys first make contact with the larger gay culture and probably the timing of this contact, and the eventual decision of whether to attempt migration to larger urban gay ghettos, which often occurs in early adulthood.

Analogous to the situation in early life, in adulthood two overarching forces shape how gay men navigate their connections to gay culture: that of the sociodemographic contexts of class and race and that of the remaining effects of homophobia as experienced within large American cities. Men who are attempting to access contact with gay ghettos have the opportunity of balancing important minority strengths and weaknesses, and how men balance these strengths and stressors (in combination with the vulnerabilities to biopsychosocial health problems that men have brought to adulthood from their early years) will have an important influence on whether they themselves develop psychosocial health problems. Among men vulnerable to these health problems, issues can snowball or compound within a social context with high background rates of substance abuse, depression, and violence, as is the case within many large urban gay communities. With this snowballing effect, syndemics are produced, and this interplay of epidemics is a strong predictor of whether men are vulnerable to HIV infection as well as the other biological health outcomes of syndemics.

Discussion

Our primary goal in theorizing syndemics among gay men is more than academic: we hope that with a better understanding of syndemic production, the ultimate goal of finding ways to disrupt syndemics can be realized. In addition, an important quality of a theoretical approach is also found in its utility in emphasizing variables and/or substantive topics that may have been neglected under other theoretical paradigms. We believe that a syndemic approach to gay men's health suggests a set of research and program responses that have heretofore been underemphasized and, if addressed, might well contribute to the disruption of syndemic situations among gay men. These are described below:

Enhance Gay Men's Resilience

The theory of syndemics proposed here states that the production of syndemics is due in no small part to the effects of homophobic attacks that occur early and often in many gay men's lives, and that these attacks can overwhelm the aspects of resilience and social capital that these men may possess. Although we may not be able to eradicate homophobia, we can enhance resilience among gay men, and this latter approach to gay men's health may provide as many positive effects as will efforts to remove institutionalized homophobia.

First, we must understand more about the extent to which gay men exhibit resilience to health threats and the sources of support for their resilience. Resilience among gay men must be commonplace, an observation that is based first and foremost on the finding that only a minority of gay men are caught up in syndemic situations—approximately one-fifth of the gay male population.[39] Although many different studies have focused on gay men's vulnerability to different poor health outcomes, few studies have focused on the sources of gay men's strength in high-risk situations. Redressing this imbalance will produce important insights that could enhance current research and public health practice among gay men.

Structural interventions to enhance gay men's resilience should be implemented and evaluated. One such intervention might be to study the effects of a program to lower the prevalence of school bullying, which is argued above to be especially prevalent and damaging to young gay men. An intervention study that seeks to measure the effects of enforcement of anti-bullying laws within public school settings by providing resources and training to school staff to deal directly with this issue and to enforce sanctions against bullying might well demonstrate a reduction in bullying. Syndemic theory would predict that in school settings with lowered rates of bullying, students in general will report a lowering of other high-risk health behaviors. The positive health effects of such interventions for young gay males might be especially large.

Strengthen Urban Gay Community Social Interaction

Working to further build community within gay ghettos may well yield effects toward disrupting syndemics. Groups that enhance positive social connections and friendships within large urban gay ghettos could be expected to create situations that directly and indirectly disrupt syndemic situations. Thus, the creation of gay social groups, sports teams, faith-based groups, neighborhood groups, and so on, can all be expected to increase the chances for positive social interaction and friendship-building that may well function as important social supports to help men cope with health-related stressors. Some of this community-building may be a particularly important source of support for men who are struggling with social isolation and/or men who have recently migrated to large urban centers. Efforts to ensure that the groups are welcoming to racial/ethnic minority men may need to adopt ways of supporting social interactions that are not typically thought of in terms of gay male community-building. For example, strengthening the viability of faith-based groups within the gay community may be an especially valuable effort for some minority MSM groups whose history has been shaped in powerful ways by religious life, such as is the case for African American MSM.

One of the areas in which gay community-building is evolving in important ways is in the area of relationship law. Legal recognition of gay male relationships is increasing in ways unforeseen even a decade ago. Partner benefits for same-sex partners are now often part of the benefit packages of large corporate employers, academic institutions, and other organizations. Same-sex domestic partnerships are now officially recognized by Vermont, and same-sex marriage is recognized by Massachusetts. Although this progress has not occurred without substantial resistance, it is not unlikely that gay male relationships will eventually be recognized socially and legally in most large American cities. Syndemic theory predicts that this sea change in the recognition of gay men's relationships would result in numerous health benefits among gay male populations. Certainly an important public health research question would be to study how changes in health status unfold over time in relationship to changes in social and legal recognition of gay relationships.

Adopt a Life-Course Perspective on Gay Men's Health

It is clear that gay youth are especially vulnerable to many different forms of homophobia and even homophobic attacks, with relatively few advocates in a position to defend them. The question should be asked: Who is in a better position to protect gay youth from ongoing homophobic attacks than the gay community itself? To the extent that gay communities can support programmatic and adoption services to protect and house vulnerable gay youth (e.g., runaway/throwaway gay youth), adolescents and young men who might otherwise get caught up in syndemics can be rescued from very difficult futures. Such programs could invite voluntary contributions by seniors as mentors, thereby enriching the lives of both the youngest and oldest age ranges within gay communities.

Improve Public Health Practice for Gay Men

A recent analysis argued that the dismantling of public health and police services in New York City in the 1970s fueled a syndemic of HIV, homocide, and tuberculosis[92]; it follows that improvements in public health services for gay men may help to disrupt syndemics. At present, most gay ghettos have created and supported a broad range of community-based health promotion efforts (e.g., substance abuse treatment, mental health services, HIV prevention and care, violence prevention, etc.), most of which are designed to deal with one specific health problem. But if it is true that the gay community suffers from multiple interacting epidemics, each of which function to make the others worse, then the effectiveness of these programs would be enhanced if they could operate in close partnership. To be more specific, if a violence prevention agency provides services to a young man who is being victimized by his partner, that agency should have clear procedures for screening and referral for HIV infection, substance abuse, and depression, among other possible problems. It may also be that with a conjoined effort to address all of these problems, the success rates of helping people who are trying to resolve violent relationships might be increased. The effects of careful screening for biopsychosocial health problems to facilitate treatment with well-characterized and relatively successful treatment regimens (e.g., depression) should also be studied in terms of their impact on diminishing the effects of other, interacting epidemics among gay men.

Address the Health Needs of Minority and Low-SES Gay Men

The syndemic theory outlined here is primarily concerned with how cultural marginalization impacts health among gay men; classic syndemic theory as proposed by Singer[13, 14] is also concerned with how poverty and other forms of economic marginalization create syndemics. Thus, syndemic theory predicts that racial/ethnic minority or low-SES men are especially vulnerable to syndemics: certainly, class and race play an important role in vulnerability to HIV infection. Although this dynamic has been recognized in terms of HIV infection for most of the past two decades, research and programs to address these issues have not received adequate attention. It is obvious that the health of gay men cannot be raised as a group if we neglect the health issues of important subgroups of the gay male community. Research to identify the most pressing health concerns of racial/ethnic minority and low-SES men should be accorded the highest priority, as should research to raise levels of public health services available to these men.

Fight Stigma by Supporting the Growth of Gay Communities in All American Cities

During the late 20th century, the list of cities with large and open gay communities has grown substantially, so that it is a rare major American urban center, indeed, that does not now host a large and well-defined urban "gay ghetto." And, over time, the list of smaller cities and even towns with large and open gay communities has grown. This dynamic may well mean that some of the factors encouraging syndemic production (e.g., the need to migrate to distant urban centers with the attendant social costs) are waning, and that men who are able to remain near their communities of origin will enjoy greater social cohesion and thus, better overall health. To the extent that the process of supporting open gay communities in a variety of different types of cities is achieved, both gay men and their host cities will benefit in important ways.

In closing, it should be noted that the study of syndemics is characterized by numerous paradoxes. First, the study of syndemics should not be undertaken solely to explain a phenomenon but rather to disrupt or even destroy the phenomenon under study. It is also paradoxical that, while the evidence for syndemics is drawn from individual-level data, the analysis to explain syndemic production must necessarily invoke sociocultural process. Paradox is also found in the assertion that the best way to address individual health problems is to not focus solely on a given problem, but to build partnerships so that other health problems are also addressed. And there is the final paradox: if we successfully change sociocultural processes so that gay men are not brutalized as part of a marginalization process, the physical health of individuals will be enhanced. We hope that, with attention to these paradoxes, more efficient ways to address syndemic disruption will emerge, and that gay men's health will benefit as a result.

Acknowledgments

Drs. Mike Marshal, Thomas C. Mills, David Ostrow, and Scott St. Clair offered valuable criticisms of previous versions of this chapter. Any errors or misinterpretations remaining in the chapter are the responsibility of the authors. Dr. Catania was supported by UARP ID045F008 and NIMH MH54320.

References

1. Sandfort TG, de Graaf R, Bijl RV, Schnabel P. Same-sex sexual behavior and psychiatric disorders: Findings from the Netherlands Mental Health Survey and Incidence Study (NEMESIS). *Arch Gen Psychiatry.* 2001;58(1):85–91.
2. Cochran SD, Ackerman D, Mays VM, Ross MW. Prevalence of non-medical drug use and dependence among homosexually active men and women in the US population. *Addiction.* 2004;99:989–998.
3. Gilman SE, Cochran SD, Mays VM, Hughes M, Ostrow D, Kessler R. Risk of psychiatric disorders among individuals reporting same-gender sexual partners in the National Comorbidity Survey. *Am J Public Health.* 2001;91(6):933–939.
4. Cochran SD, Sullivan JG, Mays VM. Prevalence of mental disorders, psychological distress, and mental health services use among LGB adults in the United States. *J Consult Clin Psychol.* 2003;71(1):53–61.
5. Tang H, Greenwood GL, Cowling DW, Lloyd JC, Roeseler AG, Bal DG. Cigarette smoking among lesbians, gays, and bisexuals: how serious a problem? *Cancer Causes Control.* 2004;15:797–803.
6. Stall R, Paul JP, Greenwood G, Pollack LM, Bein E, Crosby GM, et al. Alcohol use, drug use and alcohol-related problems among men who have sex with men: the Urban Men's Health Study. *Addiction.* 2001a;96:1589–1601.
7. Wolitski RJ, Valdiserri RO, Denning PH, Levine WC. Are we headed for a resurgence of the HIV epidemic among men who have sex with men? *Am J Public Health.* 2001;91(6):883–888.
8. Centers for Disease Control and Prevention. HIV prevalence, unrecognized infection, and HIV testing among men who have sex with men—five U.S. cities, June 2004-April 2005. *MMWR.* 2005;54:597–601.
9. Cochran SD, Mays VM. Lifetime prevalence of suicidal symptoms and affective disorders among men reporting same-sex sexual partners: Results from the NHANES III. *Am J Public Health.* 2000a;90(4):573–578.
10. Cochran SD, Mays VM. Relation between psychiatric syndromes and behaviorally defined sexual orientation in a sample of the U.S. population. *Am J Epidemiol.* 2000b;151(5):516–523.
11. Mills TC, Paul JP, Stall R, Pollack L, Canchola J, Chang YJ, et al. Distress and depression in men who have sex with men: The Urban Men's Health Study. *Am J Psychiatry.* 2004;161(2):278–285.
12. Jorm AF, Korten AE, Rodgers B, Jacomb PA, Christensen H. Sexual orientation and mental health: results from a community survey of young and middle-aged adults. *Br J Psychiatry.* 2002;180:423–427.
13. Singer M. AIDS and the health crisis of the US urban poor: the perspective of critical medical anthropology. *Soc Sci Med.* 1994;39:931–948.
14. Singer M. A dose of drugs, a touch of violence and case of AIDS: conceptualizing the SAVA syndemic. *Free Inquir Creative Sociology.* 1996;24(2):99–110.
15. Koblin BA, Husnik MJ, Colfax G, Huang Y, Madison M, Mayer K, et al. Risk factors for HIV infection among men who have sex with men. *AIDS.* 2006;20(5):731–739.

16. Mansergh G, Shouse RL, Marks G, Guzman R, Rader M, Buchbinder S, et al. Methamphetamine and sildenafil (Viagra) use are linked to unprotected receptive and insertive anal sex, respectively, in a sample of men who have sex with men. *Sex Transm Infect.* 2006;82(2):131–134.

17. Choi KH, Operario D, Gregorich SE, McFarland W, MacKellar D, Valleroy L. Substance use, substance choice, and unprotected anal intercourse among young Asian American and Pacific Islander men who have sex with men. *AIDS Ed Prev.* 2005;17(5):418–429.

18. Hirshfield S, Remien RH, Humberstone M, Walavalkar I, Chiasson MA. Substance use and high-risk sex among men who have sex with men: a national online study in the USA. *AIDS Care.* 2004;16(8):1036–1047.

19. Centers for Disease Control and Prevention. HIV/AIDS among men who have sex with men and inject drugs—United States, 1985–1998. *MMWR.* 2000;49(21):465–470.

20. Ruiz J, Facer M, Sun RK. Risk factors for human immunodeficiency virus infection and unprotected anal intercourse among young men who have sex with men. *Sex Transm Dis.* 1998;25(2):100–107.

21. Clement U. Psychological correlates of unprotected intercourse among HIV-positive gay men. *J Psychology Hum Sex.* 1992;5:133–155.

22. Kelly JA, Murphy DA, Brasfield TL, Koob JJ, Bahr GR, Stevenson LY, et al. Predictors of severity of depression among persons with HIV infection. *Health Psychology.* 1993;12:215–219.

23. Myers HF, Javanbakht M, Martinez M, Obediah S. Psychosocial predictors of risky sexual behaviors in African American men: implications for prevention. *AIDS.* 2003;15(Supplement A): 66–79.

24. Theodore JL, Koegel HM. The impact of depression on sexual risk-taking behavior of HIV-negative gay men. *NYS Psychologist.* 2002;41(1):22–27.

25. Bartholow BN, Doll LS. Emotional, behavioral, and HIV risks associated with sexual abuse among adult homosexual and bisexual men. *Child Abuse Neglect.* 1994;18(9):747–761.

26. Doll LS, Joy D, Bartholow BN, Harrison JS, Bolan G, Douglas JM, et al. Self-reported childhood and adolescent sexual abuse among adult homosexual and bisexual men. *Child Abuse Neglect.* 1992;16:855–864.

27. Jinich S, Paul JP, Stall R, Acree M, Kegeles S, Hoff C, et al. Childhood sexual abuse and HIV risk-taking behavior among gay and bisexual men. *AIDS Behavior.* 1998;2(1):41–51.

28. Williams JK, Wyatt GE, Resell J, Peterson J, Asuan-O'Brien A. Psychosocial issues among gay and non-gay-identifying HIV-seropositive African American and Latino MSM. *Cultur Divers Ethnic Minor Psychol.* 2004;10(3):268–286.

29. Arreola SG, Neilands TB, Pollack LM, Paul JP, Catania JA. Higher prevalence of childhood sexual abuse among Latino men who have sex with men than non-Latino men who have sex with men: Data from the Urban Men's Health Study. *Child Abuse Neglect.* 2005;29(3):285–290.

30. Catania J, Osmond D, Stall R, Pollack L, Paul JP, Blower S, et al. The continuing HIV epidemic among men who have sex with men. *Am J Public Health.* 2001;91(6): 907–914.

31. Greenwood GL, Relf MV, Huang B, Pollack LM, Canchola JA, Catania JA. Battering victimization among a probability-based sample of men who have sex with men. *Am J Public Health.* 2002;92(12):1964–1969.

32. Greenwood GL, Paul JP, Pollack LM, Binson D, Catania JA, Chang J, et al. Tobacco use and cessation among a household-based sample of us urban men who have sex with men. *Am J Public Health*. 2005;95(1):145–151.

33. Mills TC, Stall R, Pollack L, Paul JP, Binson D, Canchola J, et al. Health-related characteristics of men who have sex with men: a comparison of those living in "gay ghettos" with those who live elsewhere. *Am J Public Health*. 2001;91:980–983.

34. Paul JP, Catania J, Pollack L, Stall R. Understanding childhood sexual abuse as a predictor of sexual risk-taking among men who have sex with men: The Urban Men's Health Study. *Child Abuse Neglect*. 2001;25:557–584.

35. Paul JP, Catania J, Pollack L, Moskowitz JT, Canchola J, Mills TC, et al. Suicide attempts among gay and bisexual men: lifetime prevalence and antecedents. *Am J Public Health*. 2002;92(8):1338–1345.

36. Relf MV, Huang B, Campbell J, Catania J. Gay identity, interpersonal violence, and HIV risk behaviors: an empirical test of theoretical relationships among a probability-based sample of urban men who have sex with men. *J Assoc Nurses AIDS Care*. 2004;15(2):14–26.

37. Stall R, Greenwood G, Acree M, Paul JP, Coates TJ. Cigarette smoking among gay and bisexual men. *Am J Public Health*. 1999;89(12):1875–1878.

38. Stall R, Pollack L, Mills TC, Martin JN, Osmond D, Paul J, et al. Use of antiretroviral therapies among HIV-infected men who have sex with men: a household-based sample of 4 major American cities. *Am J Public Health*. 2001b;91(5):767–773.

39. Stall R, Mills TC, Williamson J, Hart T, Greendwood G, Paul JP, et al. Association of co-occuring psychosocial health problems and increased vulnerability to HIV/AIDS among urban men who have sex with men. *Am J Public Health*. 2003;93(6):939–942.

40. Herrell R, Goldberg J, True WR, Ramakrishnan V, Lyons M, Eisen S, et al. Sexual orientation and suicidality: a co-twin control study in adult men. *Arch Gen Psychiatry*. 1999;56:867–874.

41. Woody GE, VanEtten-Lee M, McKirnan D, Donnell D, Metzger D, Seage G, et al. Substance use among men who have sex with men: Comparison with a national household survey. *J Acquir Immune Defic Syndr*. 2001;27(1):86–90.

42. Brewer DD, Golden MR, Handsfield HH. Unsafe sexual behavior and correlates of risk in a probability sample of men who have sex with men in the era of highly active antiretroviral therapy. *Sex Transm Dis*. 2006;33(4):250–255.

43. Xia Q, Osmond DH, Tholandi M, Pollack L, Zhou W, Ruiz JD, et al. HIV prevalence and sexual risk behaviors among men who have sex with men. *J Acquir Immune Defic Syndr*. 2006;41(2):238–245.

44. Remafedi G, French S, Story M, Resnick MD, Blum R. The relationship between suicide risk and sexual orientation: results of a population-based study. *Am J Public Health*. 1998;88(1):57–60.

45. Fergusson DM, Horwood LJ, Beautrais AL. Is sexual orientation related to mental health problems and suicidality in young people? *Arch Gen Psychiatry*. 1999;5(10):876–880.

46. Garofalo R, Wolf RC, Wissow L, Woods ER, Goodman E. Sexual orientation and risk of suicide attempts among a representative sample of youth. *Arch Pediatr Adolesc Med*. 1999;153(5):487–493.

47. Mackellar DA, Valleroy LA, Anderson JE, Behel S, Secura GM, Bingham T, et al. Recent HIV testing among young men who have sex with men: correlates, contexts, and HIV seroconversion. *Sex Transm Dis*. 2006;33(3):183–192.

48. Valleroy LA, MacKellar DA, Karon JM. HIV prevalence and associated risks in young men who have sex with men: Young Men's Survey Study Group. *JAMA.* 2000;284:198–204.

49. Garofalo R, Wolf RC, Kessel S, Palfrey J, DuRant RH. The association between health risk behaviors and sexual orientation among a school-based sample of adolescents. *Pediatrics.* 1998;101(5):895–902.

50. Faulkner AH, Cranston K. Correlates of same-sex sexual behavior in a random sample of Massachusetts high school students. *Am J Public Health.* 1998;88(2):262–266.

51. Lampinen TM, McGhee D, Martin I. Use of crystal methamphetamine and other club drugs among high school students in Vancouver and Victoria. *BC Medical Journal.* 2006;48(1):22–27.

52. Safren SA, Heimberg RG. Depression, hopelessness, suicidality, and related factors in sexual minority and heterosexual adolescents. *J Cons Clin Psychol.* 1999; 67(6):859–866.

53. Levine M. Gay ghetto. *J Homosex.* 1979;4:363–367.

54. Singer M, St. Clair S. Syndemics and public health: reconceptualizing disease in bio-social context. *Med Anthropol Q.* 2003;17(4):423–441.

55. Meyer I. Minority stress and mental health in gay men. *J Health Soc Behav.* 1995; 36:38–56.

56. Meyer I. Prejudice, social stress and mental health in lesbian, gay and bisexual populations: conceptual issues and research evidence. *Psychol Bull.* 2003;129(5): 674–697.

57. Díaz R. *Latino Gay Men and HIV: Culture, Sexuality and Risk Behavior.* New York and London: Routledge; 1998.

58. Bailey JM, Zucker KJ. Childhood sex-typed behavior and sexual orientation: a conceptual analysis and quantitative review. *Dev Psychol.* 1995;31(1):43–55.

59. D'Augelli AR, Pilkington NW, Hershberger SL. Incidence and mental health impact of sexual orientation victimization of lesbian, gay, and bisexual youths in high school. *Sch Psychol Quarterly.* 2002b;17(2):148–167.

60. Friedman MS, Koeske GF, Silvestre AJ, Korr WS, Sites EW. The impact of gender-role nonconforming behavior, bullying, and social support on suicidality among gay male youth. *J Adolesc Health.* 2006;38(5):621–623.

61. Pilkington NW, D'Augelli AR. Victimization of lesbian, gay, and bisexual youth in community settings. *J Community Psychol.* 1995;23(1):34–56.

62. Waldo CR, Hesson-McInnis MS, D'Augelli AR. Antecedents and consequences of victimization of lesbian, gay, and bisexual young people: a structural model comparing rural university and urban samples. *Am J Community Psychol.* 1998;26(2): 307–344.

63. Sweeting H, West P. Being different: Correlates of the experience of teasing and bullying at age 11. *Research Papers in Education* 2001;16(3):225–246.

64. Griffiths LJ, Wolke D, Page AS, Horwood JP. Obesity and bullying: different effects for boys and girls. *Arch Dis Child.* 2006;91:121–125.

65. Janssen I, Craig WM, Boyce WF, Pickett W. Associations between overweight and obesity with bullying behaviors in school-aged children. *Pediatrics.* 2004;113(5): 1187–1194.

66. Hodges EVE, Perry DG. Personal and interpersonal antecedents and consequences of victimization by peers. *J Pers Soc Psychol.* 1999;76(4):677–685.

67. Piek JP, Barrett NC, Allen LSR, Jones A, Louise M. The relationship between bullying and self-worth in children with movement coordination problems. *Br J Educ Psychol.* 2005;75:453–463.

68. Kimmel MS. Masculinity as homophobia. In: Brod H, Kaufman M, eds. *Theorizing Masculinities.* Thousand Oaks, CA: SAGE; 1994:119–141.

69. Russell ST, Franz BT, Driscoll AK. Same-sex romantic attraction and experiences of violence in adolescence. *Am J Public Health.* 2001;91(6):903–906.

70. California Safe Schools Coalition, 4-H Center for Youth Development. *Consequences of Harrassment Based on Actual or Perceived Sexual Orientation and Gender Non-Conformity and Steps for Making Schools Safer.* Davis: University of California; 2004. Available at: http://www.glsen.org/binary-data/GLESENattachments/file/000/000/516-1.pdf. Accessed August 17, 2007.

71. Harris Interactive. From teasing to torment: School climate in America. New York: Gay, lesbian, and straight education network; 2005.

72. Sato K, Ito I, Akaboshi K. Neuroses and psychosomatic syndromes of the bullied children. *Japanese J Child Adol Psych.* 1987;28:110–115.

73. Williams K, Chambers M, Logan S, Robinson D. Association of common health symptoms with bullying in primary school children. *Br Med J.* 1996;313:17–19.

74. Hazler R, Hoover J, Oliver R. What children say about bullying. *Executive Educator.* 1992;14(11):20–22.

75. Juvonen J, Nishina A, Graham S. Peer harassment, psychological adjustment, and school functioning. *J Educ Psychol.* 2000;92(2):349–359.

76. Kaltiala-Heino R, Rimpela M, Marttunen M, Rimpela A, Rantanen P. Bullying, depression, and suicidal ideation in Finnish adolescents: School survey. *Br Med J.* 1999;319(7206):348–351.

77. Kaltiala-Heino R, Rimpela M, Rantanen P, Rimpela A. Bullying at school: an indicator of adolescents at risk for mental disorders. *J Adolesc.* 2000;23:661–674.

78. Salmon G, James A, Cassidy EL, Javaloyes MA. Bullying a review: presentations to an adolescent psychiatric service and within a school for emotionally and behaviourally disturbed childlren. *J Clin Child Psychol Psych.* 2000;5(4):563–579.

79. Salmon G, James A, Smith DM. Bullying in schools: self reported anxiety, depression and self esteem in secondary school children. *Br Med J.* 1998;317:924–925.

80. Davies M, Cunningham G. Adolescent parasuicide in the Foyle area. *Ir J Psych Medicine.* 1998;16(1):9–12.

81. Rigby K, Slee P. Suicidal ideation among adolescent school children, involvement in bully-victim problems, and perceived social support. *Suicide Life Threat Behav.* 1999;29(2):119–130.

82. Olweus D. Bully/victim problems among schoolchildren: long-term consequences and an effective intervention program. In: Hodgins S, ed. *Mental Disorder and Crime.* Newbury Park, CA: Sage Publications; 1993, 317–349.

83. Bontempo DE, D'Augelli AR. Effects of at-school victimization and sexual orientation on lesbian, gay, or bisexual youths' health risk behaviors. *J Adolesc Health.* 2002;30:364–374.

84. Hershberger S, D'Augelli AR. The impact of victimization on the mental health and suicidality of lesbian, gay, and bisexual youths. *Dev Psychol.* 1995;31(1):65–74.

85. Rosario M, Rotheram-Borus MJ, Reid H. Gay-related stress and its correlates among gay and bisexual male adolescents of predominantly black and Hispanic background. *J Community Psychol.* 1996;24:136–159.

86. D'Augelli AR, Hershberger SL, Pilkington NW. Suicidality patterns and sexual orientation-related factors among lesbian, gay, and bisexual youths. *Suicide Life Threat Behav.* 2001;31(3):250–264.
87. Boles SM, Joshi V, Grella C, Wellisch J. Childhood sexual abuse patterns, psychosocial correlates, and treatment outcomes among adults in drug abuse treatment. *J Child Sex Abuse.* 2005;14(1):39–45.
88. Liang B, M WL, Siegel JA. Relational outcomes of childhood sexual trauma in female survivors: a longitudinal study. *J Inter Violence.* 2006;21(1):42–57.
89. Murthi M, Espelage DL. Childhood sexual abuse, social support, and psychological outcomes: a loss framework. *Child Abuse Negl.* 2005;29(11):1215–1231.
90. Schuetze P, Eiden RD. The relationship between sexual abuse during childhood and parenting outcomes: Modeling direct and indirect pathways. *Child Abuse Negl.* 2005;29(6):645–659.
91. Shilts R. *The Mayor of Castro Street.* Chap. 18, The Final Act. New York: St. Martin's Press; 1982.
92. Freudenberg N, Fahs M, Galea S, Greenberg A. The impact of New York City's 1975 fiscal crisis on the Tuberculosis, HIV and Homicide syndemic. *Am J Public Health.* 2006;96(3):424–434.

10

Health Disparities for Homosexual Youth: The Children Left Behind

Gary Remafedi

It has been said that the character of a society is reflected in the condition of its children. If that were indeed the case, then history will judge us harshly by the current circumstances of gay, lesbian, bisexual, and transgender (GLBT) youth. Contemporary public heath systems have been a party to the systemic neglect of GLBT young people, threatening their health and well-being. Serious health disparities exist for GLBT youth, and existing data indicate that these problems have not remitted over time. Underlying these disparities is the stigmatization of individuals by sexual identity, race, and gender; societal problems are exacerbated by individuals' substance abuse and lack of education. Fledgling attempts have been made to alter the health outcomes of GLBT youth, but few interventions have been tested and proven effective. Still, they provide a vision for a brighter future than today.

This chapter will consider the reasons that the health of GLBT youth should concern their immediate communities and broader society, the prevalence of special health problems, contributing factors, indicators of health disparities, ways to bridge the gaps, and visions for the future. Although the focus of this book is on men who have sex with men (MSM), including young men who identify themselves as gay and bisexual, the following text refers generically to GLBT youth because they are frequently combined in research and service programs. Whenever possible, the unique experiences of young men who have sex with men (YMSM; 13–24 years of age) will be highlighted.

Several broad groups of indicators have been proposed to help evaluate the health of children and youth, including GLBT youth.[1] These include: health status (e.g., mortality rates and morbidity from illness, disability, mental health, healthy weight, accidental and unintentional injuries), risk and protective factors (e.g., family functioning, parental physical and mental health, neighborhood safety, general tobacco and alcohol use, exposure to second-hand smoke, abuse and neglect, homelessness, and victimization by violence), and the delivery of health care service and interventions (e.g., immunization rates, early learning and school readiness, educational benchmarks, social and emotional development, involvement with the juvenile justice system, children in nonparental care, economic security, and social support networks).

Although no systematic effort has been made to evaluate the condition of US GLBT youth by such health barometers, existing data indicate that they might be among the most neglected children in the United States. As will be discussed in this chapter, GLBT youth are disproportionately affected by the problems of violence, suicide, HIV/AIDS, and tobacco use; and they probably contribute substantially to mortality in US adolescents. As of 2003, unintentional injuries, homicide, and suicide were the three major killers of adolescents and young adults in the United States; and HIV/AIDS was the tenth leading cause of death among 15–24 year-old persons.[2] Despite overall declines in mortality in the general population of the United States from 1979 to 1991, adolescent and young adult mortality from violence rose 54.5%; and violent victimization rose more than 30% in the same time period.[3] Other problems such as tobacco, alcohol, and illicit drug use are major causes of adult morbidity and mortality with antecedents in the adolescent period.[4] As I discuss later in later this chapter, all of these problems appear to be over-represented in GLBT youth.

While contributing substantially to important public health problems, populations of GLBT youth were practically invisible to scientists and care providers until the 1980s.[5] Before that time, homosexuality was widely perceived to be a "lifestyle choice" made by adults. Adolescents who identified themselves as GLBT were considered to be seriously emotionally disturbed or, at best, misguided. Many considered adolescent homosexual experiences to be a passing phase on the road to adult heterosexuality, and the scientific literature was devoid of studies of adolescent homosexuality—outside of isolated case reports.

"Invisibility" of same-sex behavior had a grave impact on the spread of HIV disease. Early in the epidemic, disparities in health care and health care utilization by YMSM may have helped to fuel the spread of HIV and STDs. Although the first AIDS cases in the United States were reported in homosexual adults in 1981, the first series of AIDS cases in adolescents was described in a scientific presentation and abstract in 1987.[6] For most of the 1980s, the potential spread of HIV/AIDS among US adolescents and young adults was overlooked in many communities, in part, for lack of awareness that homosexual adolescents existed and that adolescents could be infected during unprotected sex.[7] Now, there are an estimated 40,000 new HIV infections in United States annually, with as many as half expected to occur in persons less than 25 years of age—and one-quarter in persons less than 21 years.[8]

As will be discussed further below, another example of widespread neglect involves GLBT youth suicide. Despite ample evidence of disproportionate risk that has been collected over two decades,[9] governmental and mainstream health agencies largely have failed to support research and service programs to prevent suicide among GLBT youth. Only a small percentage of all adolescent suicide attempts receive medical attention,[3] and access to care might be even worse for gay and bisexual youth whose attempts may precede disclosure of sexual orientation to others.[10,11]

Beyond saving lives during adolescence and young adulthood, early preventive interventions for at-risk youth are a cost-effective investment in reducing adult morbidity and mortality. For example, scientists report that GLBT youth are more likely to use tobacco, alcohol, and illicit drugs than their peers[12;] and early initiation of tobacco and other substances has lifelong consequences for health. First-time tobacco use almost invariably occurs before high school graduation, and individuals who avoid tobacco use in adolescence are less likely than others to initiate it in adulthood.[3] Some experts believe that the early use of tobacco, alcohol, and cannabis are gateways to more serious illicit drug use in adulthood, perhaps, by lowering barriers to the use of other illegal drugs and providing access to them.[4]

Also important—but less well understood—are the ways that adolescent sexual behavior and relationships influence adult health outcomes. Adolescence is a formative period in life, critical for the development of health-related behaviors and sexual, cognitive, moral, and personality development.[13] Some of the major psychosocial issues that teens face include: the establishment of identity, autonomy, and intimacy; academic and vocational achievement; and becoming comfortable with one's sexuality.

The real and perceived stigma and isolation associated with homosexuality can derail these normal development processes among GLBT youth. Lack of support from parents, peers, and communities can result in identity confusion, loss of self-esteem, difficulty developing intimate relationships with others, and academic and professional underachievement. Given the challenges faced by GLBT youth, it is surprising that so many people who assume a homosexual identity at young ages survive and flourish in adulthood.

Methodological Issues in Research

Thus far, little has been done to monitor the scope and evolution of health problems among GLBT youth. To date, the main sources of information about the health problems in GLBT youth have been:

- *Qualitative and quantitative research involving convenience samples.* Although such studies are limited by sample biases, they provide detailed information that is difficult to glean from population-based surveys. Qualitative studies have used techniques such as purposive and maximum variation sampling to attain a wide range of responses to research questions of interest.
- *Surveys of representative samples* selected from schools and community settings. Existing population-based studies have used censuses (e.g.,

military cohorts, or twin sibling databases), cluster sampling (e.g., school and household surveys), and time/place sampling techniques (e.g., randomly selecting participants from venues frequented by the GLBT youth) to select participants. The different approaches have corresponding strengths and weaknesses. In general, they offer promising ways to sample difficult-to-reach populations, but results cannot be generalized beyond the studies' settings. Another limitation is the lack of standardized definitions and measures of homosexuality used in research.

- A third source of information is surveillance data—available for AIDS cases in all states, non-AIDS HIV cases in most states, and certain STDs and sexually-based hate crimes in some localities. Unfortunately, the actual size of GLBT and YMSM populations is unknown, and accurate per capita prevalence estimates of health problems are unavailable. Also, information about sexual identity generally is missing from death certificate data and most disease surveillance databases. Such data could shed light on the relationship between sexual orientation and morbidity and mortality due to suicide, homicide, or other chronic health issues, such as those related to the use of tobacco, alcohol, and illicit drugs.

Etiology and Epidemiology of Common Problems

Externalized and internalized homophobia likely contribute to health disparities among GLBT youth. *Homophobia* is an irrational fear or hatred of homosexuality or otherwise distorted perception of homosexuality that can be manifested by stigmatization, stereotyping, prejudice, or general discomfort. *Externalized homophobia* refers to the overt expression of negative attitudes, ranging from lack of support to verbal and physical abuse. *Internalized homophobia* refers to homophobic prejudices directed against oneself.

At a time in life when peers play a critical role in healthy personal and social development, isolation and stigma can be highly traumatic. Gay and bisexual youth have reported that the greatest stressors in their lives are related to parental disapproval, loss of friendships, and victimization by violence. In a national study of adolescent health,[14] youth who were attracted to the same sex and to both sexes were more likely than youth attracted to the other sex to have been "jumped" or attacked and to have been in a fight that resulted in the need for medical treatment. Peers, other students, and roommates usually were responsible for such incidents.

More than half of gay and lesbian students have expressed worries about their future personal safety.[15] According to Pilkington and D'Augelli, "research has consistently demonstrated that victimization based on known or presumed lesbian or gay sexual orientation is the most common form of bias-related violence."[15] In their own study of lesbian, gay, and bisexual youth volunteers recruited from US lesbian and gay community centers,[15] more than 80% encountered some form of victimization due to their sexual orientation. Victimization was not confined to a particular setting, but pervaded family, school, work, and community settings.

Through repeated exposure, many homosexual youth incorporate negative societal attitudes into self-image, resulting in internalized homophobia. Overt manifestations include self-doubt and self-destructive behaviors. Subtler forms include resignation to mistreatment by others, abandonment of educational goals, and self-compromising behaviors. Accordingly, most of the difficulties experienced by GLBT youth are thought to be directly or indirectly related to isolation and stigma.[16]

The following is a brief overview of the most common medical and psychosocial problems that confront GLBT youth—typically at rates higher than heterosexual peers.

School Problems

Academic underachievement, truancy, and drop-out have been described as the common consequences of violence and verbal and physical abuse at school; and dropout rates are thought to be higher among GLBT youth than in the general population.[17]

Running Away, Homelessness, Prostitution, and Illegal Conduct

Although precise figures are unavailable, homosexual youth are overrepresented among homeless and runaway youth in the US.[18] Some parents do not adopt a supportive attitude, and a substantial number of homosexual adolescents run away or are evicted because of parental disapproval. Life on the streets exposes youth to drugs and sexual abuse and promotes illegal conduct for survival.

Substance Abuse

Levels of substance abuse in homosexual communities exceed those of the general population.[16] As compared to heterosexual peers, homosexual youth initiate tobacco use at younger ages and are more likely to smoke regularly.[12] In a study of 13–21-year-old gay and bisexual male adolescents, frequent (i.e.. more than 40 times per year) use of alcohol was reported by 24.5% of participants; frequent marijuana use, by 8.4%; and frequent cocaine/crack use, by 2.4%. More than 4% had used intravenous drugs in the previous year. When compared with normative samples, overall drug use was higher in the gay and bisexual group, 19.1% of whom met criteria for further substance abuse evaluation, as compared to 9% of a high school sample.[19]

Suicidality

Rates of attempted suicide among YMSM have been found to be consistently higher than expected in the general population of adolescents.[9] The severity of attempts is comparable to other adolescents.[10] A recent study of YMSM randomly sampled from venues frequented by GLBT youth is one of the latest generations of studies involving representative samples of participants selected from community settings (e.g., bars, cafes, retail outlets, drop-in centers) outside of schools.[20] One-third of respondents in the study reported at least one suicide attempt in their lives. Nearly 5% of participants had attempted suicide in the past year. In the past month alone, nearly one in five individuals contemplated suicide, and 6.3% of them said they "would like to kill (themselves)." Ingestion of drugs, cutting, or stabbing were the most common methods used by attempters, accounting for 82.1% of all attempts. Attempted drowning, asphyxiation, or strangulation contributed an additional 7.1%; and two individuals attempted suicide by jumping or by shooting themselves. The remaining attempters reported a combination of the previous methods, automobile injury, and "unsafe sex"; or they refused further description. One-third of all attempts resulted in hospital admission for routine or intensive care. An additional 22.6% of cases reportedly received first aid or emergency room care.

Only two "psychological autopsy" studies have examined the sexual orientation of youth who actually completed suicide. One found that 11% of young men who committed suicide in San Diego were known to be gay.[21] A second study in New York found that 3.2% of adolescent male suicides and none of the living comparison group were known to have had homosexual experiences.[22]

Eating Disorders

Theoretically, gay men and heterosexual women are predisposed to weight dissatisfaction and eating disorders by a common desire to appear physically attractive to men.[23] However, empirical epidemiological data regarding different types of disordered eating behaviors and cognitions are sparse and somewhat conflicting. In a population-based study of adolescents, one-quarter of gay youth reported a poor body image, and about one in ten dieted frequently or purged. As compared to heterosexual males, all indicators of eating problems were more prevalent in gay youth.[24]

Medical Threats to Health

Homosexual adolescents generally have the same medical concerns as heterosexual youth. Specific sexual behaviors, not sexual orientation, pose medical risks.[16] Unprotected oral sex can lead to oropharyngeal disease and gonococcal and nongonococcal urethritis for the insertive partner.[25] Among men with urethritis attending a San Francisco STD clinic, heterosexual and homosexual men had similar rates of infection with *Chlamydia trachomatis*, but young age was associated with infection in the MSM.[26]

The most common and dangerous sexually-related conditions arise from unprotected anal intercourse (UAI). The epithelial surface of the fragile rectal mucosa is easily damaged during anal penetration, facilitating the transmission of pathogens. Anal intercourse has been shown to be the most efficient route of sexual infection by hepatitis B, cytomegalovirus, and HIV.[27] Oral-anal or digital-anal contact can transmit enteric pathogens such as the hepatitis A virus. There are a paucity of comparative data on STDs, but a screening program for youth at risk of hepatitis A found higher rates of infection among YMSM than among heterosexual males.[28] Sexually transmitted diseases (STDs), particularly ulcerative diseases like syphilis and herpes simplex virus infection, can facilitate the spread of human immunodeficiency virus (HIV) infection.[29]

The Extent of Heath Disparities

Because of incomplete information regarding many of the previous problems, the remainder of this chapter will focus on three important public health issues for which the greatest amount of information is available: suicidality, tobacco use, and HIV/AIDS.

Suicidality

Over the past 25 years, researchers have reported consistently high rates of suicidality (including suicidal thoughts, intentions, and attempts) among homosexual persons, particularly among adolescents and young adults.[9] Based on the data available at the time of its release, the 1989 Report of the Secretary's Task Force on Youth Suicide concluded that "gay youth are 2 to 3 times more likely to attempt suicide than other young people. They may comprise up to 30% of completed youth suicides annually."[30]

The report ignited a controversy that has persisted to the present day. In response to public and Congressional inquiries, the American Association of Suicidology, the Centers for Disease Control and Prevention (CDC), and the National Institute of Mental Health (NIMH) convened a workshop in 1994 regarding rates of suicide among gay and lesbian people.[31] Some of the meeting attendees concluded that "there is no population-based evidence that sexual orientation and suicidality are linked in some direct or indirect manner."[32] In light of the research that appeared soon thereafter, that conclusion was premature and overstated.

To date, multiple peer-reviewed studies have found unusually high rates of attempted suicide, in the range of 20% to 42%, among young bisexual and homosexual research volunteers.[9] Initial studies of sexual orientation and suicidality used convenience samples that were limited by participant biases or school-based samples that could not capture out-of-school youth. Since 1997, however, more than half a dozen population-based and controlled studies have corroborated the findings of earlier studies. All have found a clinically and statistically significant association between suicide attempts and homosexuality, strongest among males.[9] Some of the school-based surveys have been unable to ascertain the sexual orientation of subjects *per se* and rely on sexual behavior or sexual attraction as a proxy measure of sexual identity. Only two of the largest studies of students in Minnesota[33] and Massachusetts[34] have had sufficient statistical power to examine gender differences, finding an association between homosexuality and suicidality among males. In the two states, the relative risks of attempted suicide for bisexual and homosexual male students were respectively 7.10 and 3.40 times higher than heterosexual male peers.

Tobacco Use

Tobacco use is a common and life-threatening problem in the lives of GLBT people. A rapidly expanding body of scientific knowledge, based on the experiences of GLBT youth and adults, chronicles the magnitude of tobacco-related harm and health risk across their lifespan. Since the 1980s, four different studies have examined tobacco use by GLBT teens and young adults (13–21 years of age), finding consistently higher rates of smoking among GLBT youth than heterosexual comparison groups or the general population. Two of these studies[17,35] involved convenience samples of youth. The first study reported current daily smoking among gay and bisexual male Minnesotans less than 18 years of age.[17] Daily smoking was found to be more prevalent than in the general population during the same time frame. The second[35] described lifetime cigarette use by young men and women in a New York City alternative school for GLBT youth, finding the lifetime prevalence of tobacco use among lesbians—but not gay and bisexual males—higher than national norms for same-gender students.[36]

Subsequent school-based surveys in Massachusetts[12] and Vermont[37] also have found that GLBT students were more likely than their heterosexual peers to use tobacco. Approximately 4% of students identified as gay, lesbian, or bisexual (GLB) or "unsure" in the 1995 Massachusetts Youth Risk Behavior Survey; 70% of them had smoked cigarettes, and 33% had used smokeless tobacco.[34] GLB students were significantly more likely than non-GLB peers to: smoke at school (37% vs. 18%), initiate cigarette use before 13 years of age (48% vs. 23%), and smoke cigarettes in the past month (59% vs. 35%).[12]

Further analysis of the Massachusetts data revealed that tobacco use by GLB students also was associated with recent suicide attempts.[12] By way of explanation, the authors concluded, "Homosexual, bisexual, and other adolescents confronting issues of sexual expression or orientation have been identified as facing stresses including emotional isolation, social rejection, and lowered self-esteem. These issues challenge many adolescents' emotional and psychological development and most likely contribute to the risk of developing the syndrome of risk behavior" (p. 899).[12]

HIV/AIDS

Although fewer than 3% of US high school-aged males report same sex experiences,[12,38] YMSM accounted for 57% of all reported AIDS cases in adolescents and young adults in 2001, the last year for which age-specific transmission category data are available.[39] In a study of HIV risk among 15- to 22-year-old YMSM in seven US cities from 1994 to 1998, Valleroy and colleagues[40] interviewed and tested approximately 3500 young men who were recruited in public venues. Four out of ten participants (41%) reported unprotected anal intercourse (UAI) in the past six months (range: 33% to 49% across cities), and the prevalence of HIV infection was 7.2% (range: 2.2% to 12.1%). In a subsequent study of 23- to 29-year-old MSM in six US cities from 1998 to 2000,[41] Valleroy and colleagues found 46% of 2401 men reported UAI in the past six months (range: 41% to 53%) and HIV prevalence was 12.3% (range: 4.7% to 18%).

In the combined sample of 13- to 29-year-old men participating in the two studies, 10% tested positive for HIV, and 77% of them had been unaware of their infection.[42] HIV prevalence was found to be higher in YMSM of color than among Caucasian YMSM.[40,41] Among 23- to 29-year-old persons, HIV prevalence was higher for African American men—with nearly one in three (30%) found to be infected with HIV—and Hispanic/Latino men (15%) than for white (7%) or Asian men (3%).[41]

Risk and Protective Factors Associated with Common Medical and Psychosocial Problems

GLBT youth are not a single monolithic population with uniform risk for health problems. Some individuals identify their homosexuality during adolescence without any adverse consequences, while others encounter obstacles. A sound understanding of risk and resiliency factors is necessary to assure the best health outcomes for all.

Within the broader populations of GLBT youth, there is evidence that medical and psychosocial problems might be more prevalent in males, African Americans, homeless young people, and substance abusers. Problems also appear to be exacerbated by the stress of the "coming out" process, especially when "coming out" occurs at a young age.[16] Adolescence is a period of dramatic physical, psychological, and social change. Because healthy development hinges on the support of families, schools, peers, and communities, the experience of isolation and stigma associated with a homosexual identity can be especially traumatic. Enrollment in school may, to a greater or lesser degree, be protective by providing constructive connections to others, supervision, and opportunities for learning and personal advancement. Beyond these commonalities, each of the aforementioned problems also has a unique set of risk factors that defy simplistic or one-dimensional solutions.

Suicidality

Studies comparing homosexually-oriented attempters to nonattempters have highlighted social risk factors such as gender nonconformity, early awareness of homosexuality, gay-related stress, victimization by violence, lack of social support, school dropout, family problems, suicide attempts by friends or relatives, and homelessness.[9] Several works[43–45] have found a significant association between reported suicide attempts and substance abuse or mental health symptoms in GLB youth. Although some investigators have attributed suicidality to psychological disorders, others have found that the association between suicidality and same-gender orientation in adolescent and adult men is independent of the confounding effects of substance use and mental health diagnoses.[12,46,47]

In the aforementioned study of YMSM sampled from community settings,[20] African Americans had the highest prevalence of suicide attempts (54.5%). As compared to nonattempters in bivariate analyses, attempters also were significantly more likely to be urban residents and not enrolled in school and to have completed fewer years of education. There were no statistically significant associations between suicide attempts and age, self-identified sexual orientation, employment, and US citizenship.

When the significant independent variables were entered into a multiple logistic regression analysis, only school enrollment was associated with a prior suicide attempt. There were significantly lower odds of an attempt among those in school (Adjusted OR = .55; 95% CI = .31, .97). Leaving school may be a symptom of the underlying emotional and social difficulties that may predispose youth to suicide. As previously noted, GLBT students often experience school problems related to maltreatment. Conversely, "school connectedness" may operate as a protective factor, accounting for the observed lower attempt rates among students (regardless of sexual orientation).[48]

Tobacco Use

GLBT people typically start smoking during early and middle adolescence; and tobacco use may be the gateway to other drugs.[4] A study of 455 homosexual men and women who were 18 years of age or older and living in a southern state found that lifetime, annual, and monthly use of cigarettes, alcohol, and illicit drugs was greatest in the youngest (18–25 years) age group.[49] For both men and women, cigarette and marijuana use was significantly associated with lower levels of education.

Investigators[36,50,51] have postulated that various factors predispose GLBT people to tobacco use: (1) GLBT people may face an inordinate amount of stress that predisposes them to tobacco use; (2) historically, GLBT people have socialized in venues, such as bars, where smoking is prevalent; (3) other behaviors that are associated with smoking (e.g., illicit substance abuse) may be more common among GLBT than their heterosexual counterparts; and (4) the tobacco industry has targeted the gay market through advertisements, sponsorships, and promotional events.

In recent qualitative research with GLBT youth and people with whom they interact,[52] almost a third of participants said that *all* GLBT youth are at risk for smoking; and the other respondents named a wide range of subpopulations that, combined, represent most GLBT youth. Many contributing factors were cited, including personal characteristics (e.g., stress, rebelliousness, and predisposition to addiction), interpersonal issues (e.g., peer pressure, desire to "fit in," and lack of positive role models); environmental conditions (e.g., homophobia, homelessness, and exposure to secondhand smoke); and structural issues (i.e., tobacco marketing and poor access to heath care and information).

More than a third of youth who were interviewed were not acquainted with GLBT nonsmokers and could not imagine how they avoid using tobacco. Others emphasized the importance of refusal skills, avoidance strategies, and concern for personal health, appearance, and well-being. Some risk factors (e.g., limited opportunities to socialize with GLBT peers outside of smoking venues, a desire among both young men and women to appear more masculine, and sexuality-related stress) may be unique to GLBT populations, reinforcing the need for culturally specific interventions. Highlighting the positive attributes of nonsmokers and encouraging healthy self-esteem might prove useful in prevention campaigns.

Unprotected Intercourse and HIV/AIDS/STDs

Why are YMSM having unprotected sex? Multiple themes emerge from diverse populations of adolescent and young adult MSM in different parts of the United States Risk factors for unprotected anal intercourse (UAI) include self-identification as gay,[53] less acceptance of sexual identity,[54] less involvement in gay communities,[55] having a steady male partner,[55-57] frequent intercourse,[56] multiple sexual partners,[58] noncommunication with partners about risk reduction,[55-58] less perceived peer support for risk reduction,[53,54] perceived personal likelihood of acquiring HIV infection,[56] having been tested for HIV,[53] impulsivity,[57] and substance use.[54,59]

From studies such as these, we can conclude that UAI in YMSM is associated with higher levels of sexual activity (as reflected in numbers of partners and frequency of intercourse)—perhaps because of greater opportunities for unsafe sex. Substance use, impulsivity, and other factors that impair deliberation and communication with partners about condom use adversely affect risk reduction. Also, highlighting the importance of healthy psychosocial development, engaging in UAI is related to the adolescents' perceptions of self (i.e., self-efficacy, identity, self-acceptance), perceived peer norms of behavior, and relationship status.

Temporal Trends

Suicidality

Herrell and colleagues[46] analyzed data on suicidality and same-sex-sexual behavior from a unique database of male, military-veteran twin pairs. The study involved 48 monozygotic and 55 dizygotic twin pairs born between 1939 and 1957, who were discordant for sex with same-sex partners during adulthood. An elegant co-twin control methodology was used to examine the relationship between same sex sexual behavior and suicidality. Conditional logistic regression analysis for matched pairs was used to examine how demographic, military service, and psychiatric comorbidity variables affected the association between sexual orientation and suicidality. The investigators found that men with same-gender sexual partners were 6.5 (95% CI = 1.5–28.8) times as likely as their co-twins to have attempted suicide, and the relatively high risk was not explained by mental health or substance abuse disorders.

Another study by Fergusson and colleagues[60] examined the extent to which 28 GLB youth in a New Zealand birth cohort were at risk of suicidal behaviors and psychiatric disorders. Different from the work of Herrell and colleagues,[46] this study treated mental health diagnoses as main outcomes, rather than covariates of suicidality. The subjects were persons in the birth cohort who either self-identified as GLB (9 male, 11 female) or otherwise reported sex with same sex partners (2 male, 6 female). GLB youth were found to be at increased risk of a variety of psychiatric disorders, nicotine dependence, suicidal ideation and attempts (OR 6.2, 95% CI, 2.7–14.3). The odds of a suicide attempt among homosexual persons from the two studies were quite similar, and closely resemble figures from a population-based study of Minnesota students.[33]

Based on the results of these studies, there appears to have been no decline in the risk of suicide for GLB individuals born from 1949 (the mean birth year of the veteran's sample) to 1977 (the birth year of the New Zealand sample) and to present-day school and community-based samples. As the authors of the twin study allude, whatever societal progress has been made in the interim might not have benefited adolescents struggling with the issue of sexual orientation.

Unprotected Intercourse and HIV/AIDS/STDs

Since the mid-1990s, there has been growing concern about a resurgence of risky sexual behavior in MSM, possibly leading to an increase in HIV transmission.[61,62] Reviews of sexual behavior data suggest that rates of UAI have been increasing among MSM.[61,62] There have been outbreaks of syphilis and gonorrhea among MSM in various US cities[63] and a statistically significant increase in newly diagnosed HIV infections among MSM between 2003 and 2004 in 33 states reporting HIV by name.[64]

However, few studies have examined temporal trends in sexual risk-taking. Such data are needed to understand behavioral trends within subpopulations and to direct HIV prevention resources to areas of greatest need. As part of the Community Intervention Trial for Youth, an HIV prevention study, YMSM of different races and ethnicities were surveyed annually in six communities in the United States during the summers of 1999 to 2002.[65] Data from these sites provided an opportunity to examine trends in the prevalence of UAI in different ethnic groups and geographic areas.

These data presented a complex picture of trends in UAI among YMSM, highlighting the importance of population-specific behavioral surveillance. The prevalence of UAI reported by these six subsets of YMSM was similar in 1999 (between 27% and 35%) but varied widely by 2002 (from 14% to 39%). The most consistent trend was the significant reduction in UAI in the two metropolitan areas where Latino/Hispanic YMSM were sampled. No statistically significant trends in UAI were observed among Asian/Pacific Islanders in San Diego and African Americans in Atlanta. Among predominately Caucasian samples of YMSM, there was an initial increase in UAI in Detroit and a steady, but nonsignificant, increase in the Twin Cities (i.e., the seven-county metropolitan area of Minneapolis and St. Paul, Minnesota). Between 2000 and 2002, UAI declined significantly in Detroit, but not in the Twin Cities. These data indicate that behavioral trends, even within similar subpopulations, may vary considerably by geographic region; and they underscore the potential dangers of generalizing findings beyond a study sample. Although UAI declined in two localities where Latino/Hispanic men were sampled, newly diagnosed HIV infections among MSM increased in 29 states during the same period of time;[66] and HIV prevalence[40] and incidence[67] in YMSM were highest among African American and Latino/Hispanic men. By way of explanation for discrepancies between rates of UAI and HIV infection, other factors besides UAI—such as size and density of sexual networks and background seroprevalence—would influence rates of HIV transmission.[68] Injection drug use, concomitant sexually transmitted disease, and use of highly active antiretroviral treatment (HAART) also might affect HIV transmission among YMSM.[63]

Promising Responses to Resolving the Disparities

The serious and complex problems previously described can only be addressed by multifaceted and comprehensive approaches aimed at influencing and changing public policy, fostering equal representation in research, building community awareness, protecting children and youth against maltreatment, implementing programs known to be effective, and fostering inclusive clinical service systems.

Health Care Policies

Organizational statements and policies can serve important functions: providing appropriate clinical guidelines, encouraging provider training, eliminating harmful practices such as reparative therapy, and protecting providers and patients alike. Although many organizations have issued policies or guidelines on the general treatment of homosexual persons, few have taken specific stands on youth issues. The following are notable exceptions:

- The American Academy of Pediatrics (AAP)[69] issued its first statement of policy on Adolescent Homosexuality in 1983, recognizing the pediatricians' responsibility to care for "homosexual youth and other young people struggling with the problem of sexual expression."
- The American Counseling Association and the American Psychological Association have adopted resolutions that oppose the portrayal of GLBT youth and adults as mentally ill and promote the provision of accurate information and appropriate interventions to counteract bias.[70]
- The Society for Adolescent Medicine (SAM) has decried abstinence-only sexual education policies and programs as "flawed from scientific and medical ethics viewpoints." Citing US laws that limit marriage to heterosexual couples, SAM takes the stand that federally-funded abstinence-until-marriage programs discriminate against GLBT youth and "stigmatize homosexuality as deviant and unnatural behavior."[71]

Social Support for GLBT Youth

Many experts consider social support to be an essential component of primary prevention interventions.[71–74] Normalizing the adolescent experiences of GLBT youth—that is, creating opportunities for friendship, support, and socializing in safe environments—could reduce or avert many of the problems discussed in this chapter. Although the effect has not been formally evaluated, it is widely believed that referral to special social support groups, known as gay-straight alliances (GSAs), can relieve many of the minor psychosocial problems that GLBT youth might experience.

GSAs are student-organized and student-led clubs in U.S. public high schools that support gay, lesbian, bisexual, and transsexual students in their struggle for equal rights and treatment.[75] Advocates have argued successfully that the Federal Equal Access Act (20 U.S.C. §§ 4071–74) requires public secondary schools with any noncurriculum clubs to also allow the creation of GSAs, under penalty of losing federal funding.[76]

According to the executive director of the Gay Lesbian Straight Educational Network (GLSEN), "Nearly 3,000 schools have Gay-Straight Alliances (GSAs) or other student clubs that deal with GLBT issues. Over fifty national education and social justice organizations, including the National Education Association (NEA), have joined GLSEN in its work to create safe schools for our nation's children through projects like "No Name-Calling Week."[75] In many localities, specialized social service agencies located outside the school setting also can help GLBT youth with social, educational, and other unmet needs.

Implementation of Successful Programs

HIV/AIDS Prevention

The CDC's Diffusion of Effective Behavioral Interventions (DEBI) project is a national-level strategy to provide training and ongoing technical assistance on selected evidence-based HIV/STD interventions to state and community grantees.[77] The DEBI project has featured several interventions that have proven to be effective in preventing HIV infection among YMSM.

Mpowerment, an intervention for young gay men, has five key elements: (1) a core group of young gay men who help direct the project, (2) informal outreach to spread safer sex norms, (3) formal outreach to distribute safer sex materials into venues where young gay men can be accessed, (4) M-groups that build social and safer sex skills for young gay men, and (5) social marketing of norms and social events that reach young gay men who may not be reached by other components of the intervention.[78]

Another intervention, Street Smart,[79] is an eight-session, skills-building program to help runaway and homeless youth practice safer sexual behaviors and reduce substance use. Sessions help improve social skills, assertiveness, and coping through problem-solving exercises, identifying triggers of risky behavior, and reducing harmful behaviors. Program personnel offer individual counseling and accompaniment to community health providers. Street Smart was able to increase condom use with homeless and runaway adolescents.[79]

Though not part of the DEBI project, EXPLORE is another program worthy of mention, although youth (16–25 years of age) constituted only 19% of the study population. The intervention consisted of ten one-on-one counseling sessions followed by quarterly maintenance sessions and biannual follow-up visits, including HIV testing and assessment of behavioral outcomes. The intervention was designed to address individual, interpersonal, and situational factors associated with risk-taking. In the trial of the intervention, there were significant reductions in the occurrence of UAI; and the rate of HIV infection was 18.2% lower in the intervention group than in the standard group (though not statistically significant).[80]

Tobacco Prevention Programs

Programs to prevent youth tobacco use among GLBT youth still are in formative stages. A recently completed study used qualitative methods to identify subpopulations at risk of tobacco use, protective factors, patterns of use, and approaches to prevention. The published report[52] focused on participants' recommendations for the development of preventive interventions and concluded that prevention programs should: involve young people in enjoyable and engaging activities, address the psychosocial and cultural underpinnings of tobacco use, support healthy psychosocial development, and consider offering pharmacological smoking cessation aids.

Collaborating community agencies in San Francisco have conducted a smoking cessation needs assessment survey at four GLBT youth events and one educational/social event for transgender individuals.[81] Approximately two-thirds of smokers said they were interested in quitting at some time. Subjects responded that they would like GLBT specific services (90%) and recommended that GLBT ex-smokers (56%) and physicians (55%) teach classes. Based on their responses and best practice models, the collaborators developed a smoking cessation manual tailored for GLBT persons and pilot tested the curriculum in class with 18 persons. Satisfaction reportedly was high, but mostly older (35+ years) white GLB persons attended the class.

Suicide Prevention Programs

As previously discussed, some authorities have disregarded research finding pertaining to suicide and sexual orientation. Writing in 1993, Dr. David Shaffer, expert psychiatrist and former president of the American Foundation of Suicide Prevention (AFSP), dismissed existing data on the risk of suicide for homosexual youth based on his perception that participants have been "unusual groups of gays" and criticized advocates for using the data to justify social tolerance. He concluded: "Suicide is usually the story of misperceptions and misunderstandings, of feelings of despair and lack of control; it cannot be attributed simply to having a difficult life. And it has no place in anyone's political agenda, no matter how worthy."[82] As of August 2006, Web sites for AFSP and American Association of Suicidology currently did not list homosexuality among the named risk factors for suicidality.

Also reflecting skepticism about the data and the prospects of school-based suicide prevention interventions for GLBT youth, the NIMH Web site notes in "Frequently Asked Questions about Suicide":

> Experts have not been in complete agreement about the best way to measure reports of adolescent suicide attempts, or sexual orientation, so the data are subject to question. . . . Because school based suicide awareness programs have not proven effective for youth in general, and in some cases have caused increased distress in vulnerable youth, they are not likely to be helpful for GLB youth either. Because young people should not be exposed to programs that do not work, and certainly not to programs that increase risk, more research is needed to develop safe and effective programs.[83]

To the contrary, other scholars have proposed a model of preventing GLBT youth suicide that entails "treating the environments that interface with GLBQ youth in addition to treating the adolescents themselves."[84] They argue that multi-level assessment and intervention that considers social, as well as individual, risk factors might help clients "reframe" their environments, instead of seeing suicide as the only alternative to their pain.

Visions for the Future

Appropriate Representation in Research

Lack of adequate scientific information poses a threat to the health of young GLBT Americans. The difficulty of raising awareness and acquiring adequate resources to address health concerns without scientifically obtained data and published reports has long been recognized.[85] With the exception of HIV-related research, few studies regarding the medical and psychosocial implications of sexual orientation have been publicly funded. Considerable advances in knowledge could be made with the simple inclusion of questions about the sexual identity of respondents in population-based surveys, allowing scientists to study the prevalence of health-related parameters and the extent of health disparities in relation to dimensions of sexual orientation.

Questions about one or more dimension of sexual identity already have appeared in the National Survey of Adolescent Males, the National Longitudinal Study of Adolescent Health, and miscellaneous state-wide school based surveys.[86] Including questions about sexual identity in research that involves youth should continue to be promulgated as a matter of parity, in the same manner that researchers are asked to assure that persons of any gender and special racial and ethnic subpopulations are represented in their work. In addition, such information should be routinely collected in public disease-surveillance systems and death certificates.

According to Sell and Bradford, the US Department of Health and Human Services (DHHS) identified 29 areas in which disparities exist between homosexual or bisexual persons and heterosexual persons. They include access to care, educational and community-based programs, family planning, immunization and infectious disease, STDs including HIV infection, injury and violence prevention, mental health and mental disorders, substance abuse, and tobacco use.[87] However, only half of the 12 systems used to monitor the Healthy People 2010 objectives measure some aspect of sexual orientation: the National Household Survey on Drug Abuse (NHSDA), the National Crime Victimization Survey (NCVS), the HIV/AIDS Surveillance System, the National Health and Nutrition Examination Survey (NHANES), the National Survey of Family Growth (NSFG), and the Youth Risk Behavior Surveillance System (YRBSS).[87]

A paper supported by funding from the Office of the Assistant Secretary for Planning and Evaluation explored these concerns and suggested that the DHHS: (1) create work groups to examine the collection of sexual orientation data in DHHS data collection and reporting activities; (2) create a set of guiding principles to govern the process of selecting standard definitions and measures; (3) recognize that racial/ethnic, immigrant-status, age, socioeconomic, and geographic differences must be taken into account when standard measures of sexual orientation are selected; (4) select a minimum set of standard sexual orientation measures; and (5) develop a long-range strategic plan for the collection of sexual orientation data.[85]

Core Research Needs

Despite significant advances in research methodology, many difficulties challenge research with populations of GLBT youth:

- Researchers face the hurdle of selecting representative samples from a "hidden" population. Consideration of youth populations who have same-sex desires but who do not identify as gay, lesbian, or bisexual might lead to a broader understanding of sexual minority youth.[88]
- Questions remain about the ways adolescents conceptualize their sexual orientation, which dimensions of orientation are most salient to particular health problems, and how to administer such questions in a uniform way across surveys.
- Collecting reliable and valid data—especially from young people who might not have previously disclosed their sexual behavior or foreclosed their sexual identity—is challenging.
- In other than the largest national and state surveys, it is difficult to achieve sample sizes that are sufficient to compare subgroups within GLBT populations—without some way of boosting samples of the relevant groups, such as the established practice of oversampling minority ethnic populations.[89]

Regarding general research topics of importance at this time, there is a fundamental need for cross-cultural research to understand the development of sexual identity in childhood and adolescence and how it influences health and psychosocial well-being throughout the lifespan. This type of basic research would advance understanding of the health problems identified in this chapter and help identify ways to improve health outcomes. Also, there also is a pressing need to develop and evaluate interventions to prevent morbidity and mortality among GLBT youth. Few studies outside of the arena of HIV prevention have evaluated interventions to moderate health and psychosocial outcomes. There is a particular need to understand the impact of social support groups and GSAs on the primary prevention of problems.

Research Pertaining to Tobacco Use, HIV/AIDS/STDs, and Suicidality

There are limitless numbers of research questions regarding these important public health issues, but the following are especially pressing issues:

- As previously discussed, UAI is prevalent among YMSM in all US localities, underscoring the need to assess the appropriateness, availability and use of local prevention services and to provide innovative interventions that motivate diverse subpopulations of YMSM to adopt safer sex practices.
- Beyond the epidemiological evidence of disparities in smoking rates related to sexual orientation, program developers need more information about the smoking prevention and cessation needs of GLBT youth and clinical trials of culturally appropriate prevention and cessation strategies.
- While acknowledging the absence of empirical data on completed suicides, the Surgeon General's Call to Action to Prevent Suicide recognized the growing concern about an association between suicide risk and bisexuality or homosexuality for youth, particularly males.[90] In reply to the call for action, the Division of Violence Prevention at the Centers for Disease Control (CDC) commissioned papers for a National Suicide Prevention Conference, including a report on suicide and sexual orientation.[91] The recommendations for future research included additional study of risk factors for suicide attempts and completions across the lifespan, ethnic differences, and measures of resiliency in representative populations of GLBT persons.

Assuring the Safety of GLBT Youth

There is a need to address institutions that interact with GLBT youth. It is imperative that schools become safe places for GLBT students, especially since dropout rates for GLBT youth are high and school attendance seems to be associated with better health outcomes. As indicated by the CDC:[92]

> Regardless of a child's ethnic, socioeconomic, religious, sexual orientation, or physical status, all children have a right to safety. When victimization through bullying, verbal abuse, and physical violence is prevalent in a school, the entire school community experiences the consequences. . . . Students who are different from the majority of their classmates because of their race, ethnicity, sexual orientation, religion, or other personal characteristics are at increased risk for being bullied. Gay, lesbian, or bisexual students, and students perceived to be gay by their peers are often victims of repeated verbal abuse and physical assault. (p. 18)

As of April 2005, 17 states and Guam have enacted some form of anti-bullying legislation.[93] Comprehensive policies include the following components:

- Defines bullying
- Prohibits bullying by students

- Informs students and others of anti-bullying policy
- Enables students and parents to report bullying incidents
- Provides immunity to those reporting incidents
- Requires administrators to investigate reports
- Encourages preventive education.

In lieu of empirical data, one can only surmise that exclusion from mainstream social institutions harms GLBT youth by restricting equal opportunity. Such bias can damage self-esteem during adolescence and have a longer-term impact on personal, academic, professional, and financial advancement and achievement. Besides schools, there is a need to address other institutions and policies that exclude GLBT youth from activities, clubs, occupations, and social institutions (such as Boys Scouts of America, military service, domestic partnership, and marriage).

Building Community Awareness and Capacity

There is a need to build communities' awareness and capacity to address the previously mentioned problems of HIV/AIDS, tobacco use, and suicide. Although some members of GLBT communities are aware of published research regarding suicide and sexual identity, the actual suicides of GLBT youth and adults are not publicized and easily escape the attention of the general public. States do not systematically collect and report information about the sexual orientation of suicide cases.

Similarly, older gay adults may be familiar with the scourge of AIDS; but most young people today have no firsthand experience of facing the illness and deaths of friends and loved ones. They have not had the benefit of the aggressive mass education and prevention campaigns that older generations experienced.

Awareness of tobacco-related problems and resources for smoking prevention and cessation also are inadequate within GLBT communities. A recent online survey of US adults found that GLBT respondents were more likely than heterosexuals to smoke cigarettes (34% vs. 24%) and to smoke more than one pack per day (47% vs. 36%). However, fewer GLBT persons (4% vs. 7%) considered smoking to be a personal health risk[94]; and 89% said they had not seen an anti-smoking education or awareness campaign targeted toward them.[95]

Eliminating the Diagnosis of Childhood
Gender Identity Disorder

Circumventing professional condemnation of reparative therapy for homosexuality in adulthood, some groups have redirected their attention to the treatment of "gender identity disorder" in childhood and adolescents as a way to prevent homosexuality.[96] Gender identity disorder refers to strong and persistent cross-gender identification and by continuous discomfort about one's assigned sex or by a sense of inappropriateness in the gender role of that sex. The American Psychiatric Association introduced it to the third edition of the *Diagnostic and Statistical Manual of Mental Disorders* (DSM-III) in 1980.[97] However, as recognized in DSM-IV,[98] longitudinal studies have found that about three-quarters of boys with a childhood history of gender identity disorder report a homosexual or bisexual orientation by adolescence, without lingering evidence of the gender disorder.

Assigning pathology to childhood precursors of homosexuality is objectionable because it perpetuates the stigmatization and maltreatment of homosexual people and potentially widens the chasm of health disparities. Experts "disagree with the DSM-IV labeling of gender variance as a mental disorder, since neither homosexuality nor transexuality is classified as a mental disorder, and significant distress or functional impairment are not necessarily intrinsic to this condition."[99] While some transgender advocates argue on behalf of maintaining the diagnosis just to permit reimbursement of therapy and hormonal replacement, others recommend finding alternative strategies to legitimize care that do not the risk harming children who do not fit dominant norms of gender.[100]

Access to Appropriate Health Care Services

Health care services should be inclusive of all young people, regardless of sexual orientation. A trusting, mutual relationship between the patient and provider is the basis of effective communication. Waiting room materials addressing sexual orientation, information about support groups, and other community resources indicate that the staff is open to discussing homosexuality. Interviewing the teen with and without parents present and assuring confidentiality set the stage for honest communication. For some teens, multiple visits might be necessary to complete an evaluation sensitively. Caution should be exercised when recording sensitive information in accessible parts of the medical chart.

Providers should be aware of the various threats to the medical and psychosocial health of homosexual teenagers and screen for them appropriately. The basic physical examination and laboratory evaluation are the same for all sexually active teenagers, with additional work-up guided by the sexual risk assessment. Voluntary HIV antibody counseling and testing should be routinely offered to adolescents who have engaged in unprotected sex.[16,73] The CDC has recommended that MSM who are sexually active be tested annually for HIV, chlamydia, syphilis, and gonorrhea and that they should be vaccinated against hepatitis A and B.[101]

Special emphasis should be placed on education and counseling to prevent the spread of HIV and STDs through safer sexual behavior, including limiting numbers of sexual partners, avoiding anal intercourse, staying sober in sexual situations, and consistently using condoms. Testing for HIV and the treatment of STDs should follow the latest recommendations of the CDC. Complicated STDs and HIV infection warrant referral to medical subspecialists.

Well-informed professionals can help adolescents and their parents to explore their feelings and learn about topics related to homosexuality and its etiology, psychological normalcy, spiritual and cultural implications, disclosure to significant others, preventive care, and community resources. Health care providers should inquire about the health problems discussed in this chapter, including mental health concerns, and refer clients to culturally and developmentally appropriate prevention and intervention services when problems are detected. The AAP Committee on Adolescence recommends that professionals help raise awareness of school and community leaders of issues relevant to homosexual youth and support the development and maintenance of social support groups for affected youth, friends, and parents.[73]

In the last two decades, the visibility of GLBT youth in clinics, schools, and other community settings has increased dramatically. Within a short amount of time, considerable information has been amassed about their social experiences and health concerns. Existing research focuses on several major public health issues that carry with them serious risk of morbidity and mortality, such as violence, suicide, HIV/AIDS, and tobacco use. The data from these areas paints a bleak picture of the children left behind in a cultural battle between pro- and anti-gay social factions.

The problems of GLBT youth are the direct and indirect consequence of neglect and maltreatment within families, peers groups, and larger communities. Much remains to be learned about the full gamut of health and psychosocial concerns, protective factors, and intervention strategies. Uniformly introducing questions about respondents' sexual identity to population-based surveys is a practical, efficient, and cost-effective way to collect additional information quickly.

Because the health problems of GLBT youth stem from externalized and internalized homophobia, intervening at multiple levels with individuals, social networks, and larger communities is needed to close the gap in disparities. Successful HIV prevention programs demonstrate the possibility of intervening effectively. There is every reason to believe that, with appropriate support from families, school, and communities, GLBT youth have the same potential as others to lead happy, healthy, and productive lives.

References

1. Australian Institute of Health and Welfare. Key national indicators of children's health, development, and wellbeing. http://www.aihw.gov.au/publications/aus/bulletin20/bulletin20.pdf. 2004. Accessed August 22, 2005.
2. Hoyert DL, Kung HC, Smith BL. *Deaths: Preliminary Data for 2003*. 53rd ed. Hyattsville, MD: National Center for Health Statistics; 2005.
3. Sells CW, Blum RW. Morbidity and mortality among US adolescents: An overview of data and trends. *Am J Public Health*. 1996;86:513–519.

4. Lynskey MT, Heath AC, Bucholz KK et al. Escalation of drug use in early-onset cannabis users vs co-twin controls. *JAMA.* 2003;289:427–433.

5. Remafedi G. Homosexual youth: a challenge to contemporary society. *JAMA.* 1987;258:222–225.

6. Manoff SB, Rogers MF, D'Angelo LJ, et al. The epidemiology of AIDS in adolescents and young adults. *J Adolesc Health Care.* 1987;8:307.

7. Remafedi GJ. Preventing the sexual transmission of AIDS during adolescence. *J Adolesc Health Care.* 1988;9:139–143.

8. Rosenberg PS, Biggar RJ, Goedert JJ. Declining age at HIV infection in the United States. *N Engl J Med.* 1994;330:789–790.

9. Remafedi G. Sexual orientation and youth suicide. *JAMA.* 1999;282:1291–1292.

10. Remafedi G, Farrow JA, Deisher RW. Risk factors for attempted suicide in gay and bisexual youth. *Pediatrics.* 1991;87:869–875.

11. D'Augelli AR, Hershberger SL, Pilkington NW. Suicidality patterns and sexual orientation-related factors among lesbian, gay, and bisexual youths. *Suicide Life Threat Behav.* 2001;31:250–264.

12. Garofalo R, Wolf RC, Kessel S, Palfrey SJ, DuRant RH. The association between health risk behaviors and sexual orientation among a school-based sample of adolescents. *Pediatrics.* 1998;101:895–902.

13. Steinberg L. *Adolescence.* 5th ed. McGraw-Hill; 1999.

14. Russell ST, Franz BT, Driscoll AK. Same-sex romantic attraction and experiences of violence in adolescence. *Am J Public Health.* 2001;91:903–906.

15. Pilkington N, D'Augelli A. Victimization of lesbian, gay, and bisexual youth in community settings. *J Community Psychol.* 1995;23:33–55.

16. Stronski Huwiler SM, Remafedi G. Adolescent homosexuality. *Adv Pediatr.* 1998;45:107–144.

17. Remafedi G. Adolescent homosexuality: psychosocial and medical implications. *Pediatrics.* 1987;79:331–337.

18. Kruks G. Gay and lesbian homeless/street youth: special issues and concerns. *J Adolesc Health.* 1991;12:515–518.

19. Winters KC, Remafedi G, Chan BY. Assessing drug abuse among gay-bisexual young men. *Psychology of Addictive Behaviors.* 1996;10:228–236.

20. Remafedi G. Suicidality in a venue-based sample of young men who have sex with men. *J Adolesc Health.* 2002;31:305–310.

21. Rich CL, Fowler RC, Young D, Blenkush M. San Diego suicide study: comparison of gay to straight males. *Suicide Life Threat Behav.* 1986;16:448–457.

22. Shaffer D, Fisher P, Hicks RH, Parides M, Gould M. Sexual orientation in adolescents who commit suicide. *Suicide Life Threat Behav.* 1995;25 Suppl:64–71.

23. Siever MD. Sexual orientation and gender as factors in socioculturally acquired vulnerability to body dissatisfaction and eating disorders. *J Consult Clin Psychol.* 1994;62:252–260.

24. French SA, Story M, Remafedi G, Resnick MD, Blum RW. Sexual orientation and prevalence of body dissatisfaction and eating disordered behaviors: a population-based study of adolescents. *Int J Eat Disord.* 1996;19:119–126.

25. Remafedi G. Sexually transmitted diseases in homosexual youth. *Adolesc Med.* 1990;1:565–582.

26. Ciemins EL, Flood J, Kent CK et al. Reexamining the prevalence of Chlamydia trachomatis infection among gay men with urethritis: implications for STD policy and HIV prevention activities. *Sex Transm Dis.* 2000;27:249–251.

27. Collier AC, Meyers JD, Corey L, Murphy VL, Roberts PL, Handsfield HH. Cytomegalovirus infection in homosexual men: relationship to sexual practices, antibody to human immunodeficiency virus, and cell-mediated immunity. *Am J Med.* 1987;82:593–601.

28. Ochnio JJ, Patrick D, Ho M, Talling DN, Dobson SR. Past infection with hepatitis A virus among Vancouver street youth, injection drug users and men who have sex with men: implications for vaccination programs. *CMAJ.* 2001;165:293–297.

29. Stamm WE, Handsfield HH, Rompalo AM, Ashley RL, Roberts PL, Corey L. The association between genital ulcer disease and acquisition of HIV infection in homosexual men. *JAMA.* 1988;260:1429–1433.

30. Gibson P. Gay male and lesbian youth suicide. In: US Dept of Health and Human Services, ed. *Report of the Secretary's Task Force on Youth Suicide.* Rockville, MD: DHHS publication ADM 89–1623; 1987:110–42.

31. Moscicki EK, Muehrer P, Potter LB. Introduction to supplemental issue: research issues in suicide and sexual orientation. *Suicide Life Threat Behav.* 1995;25 Suppl:1–3.

32. Working Groups, Workshop on Suicide and Sexual Orientation. Recommendations for a research agenda in suicide and sexual orientation.*Suicide Life Threat Behav.* 1995;25 Suppl:82–94.

33. Remafedi G, French S, Story M, Resnick MD, Blum R. The relationship between suicide risk and sexual orientation: results of a population-based study. *Am J Public Health.* 1998;88:57–60.

34. Garofalo R, Wolf RC, Wissow LS, Woods ER, Goodman E. Sexual orientation and risk of suicide attempts among a representative sample of youth. *Arch Pediatr Adolesc Med.* 1999;153:487–493.

35. Rosario M, Hunter J, Gwadz M. Exploration of substance use among lesbian, gay, and bisexual youth: prevalence and correlates. *J Adolesc Research.* 1997;12:454–476.

36. Ryan H, Wortley PM, Easton A, Pederson L, Greenwood G. Smoking among lesbians, gays, and bisexuals: a review of the literature. *Am J Prev Med.* 2001;21:142–149.

37. DuRant RH, Krowchuk DP, Sinal SH. Victimization, use of violence, and drug use at school among male adolescents who engage in same-sex sexual behavior. *J Pediatr.* 1998;133:113–118.

38. Remafedi G, Resnick M, Blum R, Harris L. Demography of sexual orientation in adolescents. *Pediatrics.* 1992;89:714–721.

39. Centers for Disease Control and Prevention. Table 24. Estimated AIDS incidence in adolescents and adults under age 25, by sex and exposure category, diagnosed in 2001, and cumulative totals though 2001, United States. *HIV/AIDS Surveillance Report* 13(2). 9–24–2002. 6–23–2006.

40. Valleroy LA, Mackellar DA, Karon JM et al. HIV prevalence and associated risks in young men who have sex with men. Young Men's Survey Study Group. *JAMA.* 2000;284:198–204.

41. Valleroy L, MacKellar MA, Karon JM, and et al. High HIV and risk behavior prevalence among 23- to 29-year-old men who have sex with men in 6 US cities. 8th Conference on Retroviruses and Opportunistic Infections. 2001.

42. MacKellar DA, Valleroy LA, Secura GM et al. Unrecognized HIV infection, risk behaviors, and perceptions of risk among young men who have sex with men: opportunities for advancing HIV prevention in the third decade of HIV/AIDS. *J Acquir Immune Defic Syndr.* 2005;38:603–614.

43. Hershberger SL, Pilkington NW, D'Augelli AR. Predictors of suicide attempts among gay, lesbian, and bisexual youth. *J Adolesc Res*. 2005;12:477–497.

44. Nicholas J, Howard J. Better dead than gay: depression, suicide ideation, and attempt among a sample of gay and straight-identified males aged 18–24. *Youth Stud Aust*. 1998;17:28–33.

45. D'Augelli AR, Hershberger SL. Lesbian, gay, and bisexual youth in community settings: personal challenges and mental health problems. *Am J Community Psychol*. 1993;21:421–448.

46. Herrell R, Goldberg J, True WR et al. Sexual orientation and suicidality: a co-twin control study in adult men. *Arch Gen Psychiatry*. 1999;56:867–874.

47. Cochran SD, Mays VM. Lifetime prevalence of suicide symptoms and affective disorders among men reporting same-sex sexual partners: results from NHANES III. *Am J Public Health*. 2000;90:573–578.

48. Resnick MD, Blum RW, Hector J. Adolescent perceptions of the school nurse. *J Sch Health*. 1980;50:551–554.

49. Skinner WF. The prevalence and demographic predictors of illicit and licit drug use among lesbians and gay men. *Am J Public Health*. 1994;84:1307–1310.

50. Aaron DJ, Markovic N, Danielson ME, Honnold JA, Janosky JE, Schmidt NJ. Behavioral risk factors for disease and preventive health practices among lesbians. *Am J Public Health*. 2001;91:972–975.

51. Gruskin EP, Hart S, Gordon N, Ackerson L. Patterns of cigarette smoking and alcohol use among lesbians and bisexual women enrolled in a large health maintenance organization. *Am J Public Health*. 2001;91:976–979.

52. Remafedi G, Carol H. Preventing tobacco use among lesbian, gay, bisexual, and transgender youth. *Nicotine Tob Res*. 2005;7:249–256.

53. Choi KH, Han CS, Hudes ES, Kegeles S. Unprotected sex and associated risk factors among young Asian and Pacific Islander men who have sex with men. *AIDS Educ Prev*. 2002;14:472–481.

54. Waldo CR, McFarland W, Katz MH, MacKellar D, Valleroy LA. Very young gay and bisexual men are at risk for HIV infection: the San Francisco Bay Area Young Men's Survey II. *J Acquir Immune Defic Syndr*. 2000;24:168–174.

55. Hays RB, Kegeles SM, Coates TJ. Unprotected sex and HIV risk taking among young gay men within boyfriend relationships. *AIDS Educ Prev*. 1997;9:314–329.

56. Remafedi G. Predictors of unprotected intercourse among gay and bisexual youth: knowledge, beliefs, and behavior. *Pediatrics*. 1994;94:163–168.

57. Hays RB, Paul J, Ekstrand M, Kegeles SM, Stall R, Coates TJ. Actual versus perceived HIV status, sexual behaviors and predictors of unprotected sex among young gay and bisexual men who identify as HIV-negative, HIV-positive and untested. *AIDS*. 1997;11:1495–1502.

58. Molitor F, Facer M, Ruiz JD. Safer sex communication and unsafe sexual behavior among young men who have sex with men in California. *Arch Sex Behav*. 1999;28:335–343.

59. Stueve A, O'Donnell L, Duran R, San DA, Geier J. Being high and taking sexual risks: findings from a multisite survey of urban young men who have sex with men. *AIDS Educ Prev*. 2002;14:482–495.

60. Fergusson DM, Horwood LJ, Beautrais AL. Is sexual orientation related to mental health problems and suicidality in young people? *Arch Gen Psychiatry*. 1999;56:876–880.

61. Stall RD, Hays RB, Waldo CR, Ekstrand M, McFarland W. The Gay '90s: a review of research in the 1990s on sexual behavior and HIV risk among men who have sex with men. *AIDS*. 2000;14 Suppl 3:S101–S114.
62. Wolitski RJ, Valdiserri RO, Denning PH, Levine WC. Are we headed for a resurgence of the HIV epidemic among men who have sex with men? *Am J Public Health*. 2001;91:883–888.
63. Ciesielski CA. Sexually transmitted diseases in men who have sex with men: an epidemiologic review. *Curr Infect Dis Rep*. 2003;5:145–152.
64. Centers for Disease Control and Prevention. Trends in HIV/AIDS Diagnosis—33 States, 2001–2004. *MMWR*. 2005;54:1149–1153.
65. Guenther-Grey CA, Varnell S, Weiser JI et al. Trends in sexual risk-taking among urban young men who have sex with men, 1999–2002. *J Natl Med Assoc*. 2005;97:38S–43S.
66. Centers for Disease Control and Prevention. Increases in HIV diagnoses—29 states, 1999–2002. *MMWR*. 2003;52:1145–1148.
67. McFarland W, Katz MH, Stoyanoff SR, et al. HIV incidence among young men who have sex with men—seven U.S.cities, 1994–2000. *MMWR*. 2001;50:440–444.
68. Bingham TA, Harawa NT, Johnson DF, Secura GM, MacKellar DA, Valleroy LA. The effect of partner characteristics on HIV infection among African American men who have sex with men in the Young Men's Survey, Los Angeles, 1999–2000. *AIDS Educ Prev*. 2003;15:39–52.
69. American Academy of Pediatrics' Committee on Adolescence LWC. Homosexuality and adolescence. *Pediatrics*. 1983;72:249–250.
70. Just the facts about sexual orientation and youth: a primer for prinicipals, educators, and school personnel. http://www.apa.org/pi/lgbc/facts.pdf. 1999. Accessed January 17. 2006.
71. Santelli J, Ott MA, Lyon M, Rogers J, Summers D. Abstinence-only education policies and programs: a position paper of the Society for Adolescent Medicine. *J Adolesc Health*. 2006;38:83–87.
72. Remafedi G. Fundamental issues in the care of homosexual youth. *Med Clin North Am*. 1990;74:1169–1179.
73. Frankowski BL, Committee on Adolescence. Sexual orientation and adolescents. *Pediatrics*. 2004;113:1827–1832.
74. Gonsiorek JC. Mental health issues of gay and lesbian adolescents. *J Adolesc Health Care*. 1988;9:114–122.
75. Jennings K. Lesbian and Straight Education Network. http://www.glsen.org/cgi-bin/iowa/student/about/index.html. 2005. Accessed August 22, 2005.
76. Wall L. School sued for indecision on gay club. *Houston Chronicle*. 2003. Available at: http//www.jsc.nasa.gov/news/columbia/107_onboard_archive/messages/nfhJan232003.pdf. Accessed August 20, 2007.
77. Centers for Disease Control and Prevention. Diffusion of Effective Behavioral Interventions. http://www.effectiveinterventions.org/. 2005. Accessed June 15, 2006.
78. Kegeles SM, Hays RB, Coates TJ. The Mpowerment Project: a community-level HIV prevention intervention for young gay men. *Am J Public Health*. 1996;86:1129–1136.
79. Rotheram-Borus MJ, Song J, Gwadz M, Lee M, Van RR, Koopman C. Reductions in HIV risk among runaway youth. *Prev Sci*. 2003;4:173–187.

80. Koblin B, Chesney M, Coates T. Effects of a behavioural intervention to reduce acquisition of HIV infection among men who have sex with men: the EXPLORE randomised controlled study. *Lancet.* 2004;364:41–50.

81. Center for AIDS Prevention Studies. Smoking cessation interventions in San Francisco's queer communities. *Science to Community.* 2005.

82. Shaffer D. Political science. The New Yorker, 116. 5–3–1993.

83. National Institute of Mental Health. Frequently asked questions about suicide. http://www.nimh.nih.gov/suicideprevention/suicidefaq.cfm. 2005. Accessed August 22, 2005.

84. Morrison LL, L'Heureux J. Suicide and gay/lesbian/bisexual youth: implications for clinicians. *J Adolesc.* 2001;24:39–49.

85. Sell RL, Becker JB. Sexual orientation data collection and progress toward Healthy People 2010. *Am J Public Health.* 2001;91:876–882.

86. Saewyc EM, Bauer GR, Skay CL et al. Measuring sexual orientation in adolescent health surveys: evaluation of eight school-based surveys. *J Adolesc Health.* 2004;35:345–15.

87. Sell RL and Bradford J. Elimination of health disparities based upon sexual orientation: Inclusion of sexual orientation as a demographic variable in Healthy People 2010 Objectives. http://www.glma.org/policy/hp2010/hp2010final.shtml. 2000. Accessed August 22, 2005.

88. Savin-Williams RC. A critique of research on sexual-minority youth. *J Adolesc.* 2001;24:5–13.

89. McManus S. Sexual orientation research phase 1: A review of methodological approaches. http://www.scotland.gov.uk/publications/note.asp. 1–76. 2003. Scottish Executive Publications. Accessed January 17, 2006.

90. U.S. Public Health Service. The Surgeon General's call to action to prevent suicide. http://www.surgeongeneral.gov/library/calltoaction/calltoaction.pdf. 1999. Accessed August 22, 2005.

91. MacDaniel JS, Purcell D, D'Augelli AR. The relationship between sexual orientation and risk for suicide: Research findings and future directions for research and prevention. *Suicide and Life-Threatening Behavior.* 2001;31:84–105.

92. Centers for Disease Control and Prevention. School health guidelines to prevent unintentional injuries and violence. *MMWR.* 2001;50 (No. RR-22):1–46.

93. Dounay J. State Anti-bullying Statutes. In Education Commission of the States, StateNotes. http://www.ecs.org/clearinghouse/60/41/6041.pdf. 2005. Accessed August 22, 2005.

94. Harris Interactive. HIV/AIDS and heart disease should be nation's top health care priorities, according to new national survey of gays and non-gays. http://www.harrisinteractive.com/news/allnewsbydate.asp?NewsID=598. Accessed August 22, 2005.

95. Harris Interactive. Six out of ten adults surveyed prefer smoke-free bars and clubs. http://www.harrisinteractive.com/news/allnewsbydate.asp?NewsID=566. Accessed August 22, 2005.

96. Reckers GA. Gender identity disorder. http://www.leaderu.com/jhs/rekers.html. 2002. Accessed August 22, 2005.

97. American Psychiatric Association. *Diagnostic and Statistical Manual of Mental Disorders.* 3rd ed. Washington, DC: A.P.A.; 1980.

98. American Psychiatric Association. *Diagnostic and Statistical Manual of Mental Disorders.* 4th ed. Washington, DC: A.P.A.; 1994.

99. Perrin EC, Menvielle EJ, Tuerk C. To the beat of a different drummer: The gender-variant child. http://www.contemporarypediatrics.com/contpeds/article/articleDetail.jsp?id=147767. Accessed July 19, 2006.

100. Dean L, Meyer IH, Robinson K, et al. Lesbian, gay, bisexual, and transgender health: findings and concerns. *J Gay Lesbian Med Assoc.* 2000;4:101–151.

101. Centers for Disease Control and Prevention. Sexually transmitted diseases treatment guidelines 2002. *MMWR.* 2002;51(RR06):1–80.

11

The Unique Experiences of Older Gay and Bisexual Men: Associations with Health and Well-Being

Arnold H. Grossman

Many members of the "gay community" and heterosexual society think that there are no older gay and bisexual men in the United States. "The stereotype is that older gay [and bisexual] men don't exist, they burn out like a candle at both ends, they die, vanish, kaput!"[1[p213]] This stereotype has been exacerbated by: (1) the HIV/AIDS epidemic, as many people believe that so many gay men died at the beginning of the epidemic that there are few left to grow old; (2) ageism (i.e., devaluing or discriminating against people because of their age) in the gay community; and (3) heterosexism (i.e., devaluing or discriminating against people because they are not heterosexual) in mainstream society. Although not completely out of the sight of researchers, accurate numbers of older gay and bisexual men living in the United States are not available. While this lack of information may be due to acts of omission by gerontologists and designers of population studies, it also reflects choices made by many of today's older gay and bisexual men; many have chosen not to disclose their sexual identity because of their experiences with homophobia, stigmatization, and discrimination in their younger years. Having lived life in the closet for years, many have decided not to reveal their romantic attractions, sexual behaviors or sexual identities in their later lives.[2]

The Census 2000 count of same-sex partners sharing households represents the largest and most comprehensive data on gay and lesbian couples living in the United States. Findings from Census 2000 indicate that there are 601,209 unmarried partner households in the United States, of which 304,148 households are same-sex male (gay) partners.[3] However, due to the continuing prejudice and discrimination against gay people, the confusing wording of the census question, as well as not asking about sexual orientation per se, Smith and Gates have determined that these figures may represent an undercount of as much as 62%.[3] Additionally, Census 2000 did not count single gay and bisexual men, or gay and bisexual men in committed relationships not living together in the same residence.

Smith and Gates[3] also found that 11.8% of the unmarried same-sex partner households included one senior 65 years or older; and 23.4% included at least one partner 55 years or older. Using the 62% correction for undercounting of same-sex households and the figure for gay male households, there may be 44,556 gay male households with at least one senior 65 years or older, and there may be 88,357 with at least one senior 55 or older. These estimates do not include figures for gay and bisexual single adults and those older gay and bisexual male adults in same-sex committed relationships not living in the same residence. Consequently, there are likely significant numbers of older gay and bisexual men living in the United States; according to Smith and Gates they are living throughout the country, from big cities to small farming towns, and from the Deep South to the Pacific Northwest. Older gay and bisexual men are not only in major urban centers on the East and West Coasts, as another stereotype suggests.

The goal of this chapter is to look at the mental and physical health aspects of the lives of older gay and bisexual men. Its specific aims are to: (1) provide a contextual framework for examining the mental and physical health of older gay and bisexual men; (2) examine what we currently know about the mental and physical health of older gay and bisexual men; (3) enumerate the barriers to gay and bisexual men in accessing and receiving health care; and (4) discuss gaps in knowledge, needed interventions, and recommendations to reduce the disparities in the provision of health services between older gay and bisexual men and their heterosexual counterparts.

Unique Experiences

Today's older gay and bisexual men comprise a distinctive cohort that shares unique experiences. As indicated above, primary among them is their invisibility. Also, in relation to mainstream society, they are viewed as a "double minority" being gay/bisexual (facing homophobia and its sequelae) and being old (facing ageism and its consequences). They remember the police entrapments, and many experienced the police raids on gay bars, including the Stonewall Inn, which led to the Stonewall Riots (see below). Furthermore, they lived most of their early developmental years when homosexuality was listed as a mental disorder by the American Psychiatric Association and sodomy was unlawful in all 50 states of the United States. Many of today's older gay and bisexual men directly experienced the beginning of the AIDS epidemic 25 years ago, losing many partners, friends, and colleagues to a disease that initially had no name, no known routes of transmission, and was unstoppable.[2]

A Cohort Born before the Stonewall Riots

Knowing the historical and social cohort effects of older gay and bisexual men is vital to understanding their unique experiences and health needs. Different cohorts have different degrees of comfort in acknowledging and disclosing their sexual attractions and behaviors to health professionals, which is important to preventive heath education and health care. In talking about older gay and bisexual men, this chapter takes as its definition those who are 60 years and older. In the National Survey of Midlife Development in the United States (MIDUS) 1730 men, who identified themselves as attracted to men or to both men and women, estimated middle-age as beginning at 43 and ending at 58.[4] Thus, it follows that old age would begin in the early sixties. This definition coincides with one that human development psychologists tend to use, with middle adulthood including the forties and fifties and late adulthood being age 60 and over.[5] The age of 60 as the start of being an older adult was used by both Friend,[6] in his studies of older lesbian and gay people, and by Grossman, D'Augelli, and O'Connell in their recent national study: "Being Lesbian, Gay, Bisexual, and Sixty or Older in North America."[7] Some gerontologists make a distinction between two groups of older adults: the "young old" (i.e., people in their mid-sixties to mid-seventies,) and "old-old" (people in their late seventies and beyond).[8]

Of the 416 older lesbian, gay, and bisexual people in the Grossman et al. study,[7] 71% ($n = 297$) were gay and bisexual men. Data were collected in 1997–1998, and the average age of the gay and bisexual male study participants was 68.9 ($SD = 5.9$; range 60 to 91). This means that they were born about 1930, and were about 40 years of age when the Stonewall Riots of 1969 occurred in New York City's Greenwich Village (which has traditionally been used as a marker of the start of the modern US movement for gay, lesbian, bisexual, and transgender liberation).

For about the first 45 years of their lives, this cohort was told that gay and bisexual men were mentally ill, as "homosexuality" was not removed from the Diagnostic and Statistical Manual of Mental Health Disorders until 1973.[9] Additionally, most grew up hearing negative stereotypes about homosexual men, and they frequently learned that having sex with other men was not only unnatural and immoral, but also unlawful. Sodomy laws existed in all states until 1961. Therefore, these older gay and bisexual adults heard that the ways in which individuals with same-sex attractions expressed their love for one another were "criminal" for approximately the first 30 years of their lives. In fact, the sodomy laws of the last 13 states were not declared unconstitutional by the United States Supreme Court until 2003. Today's older gay and bisexual men were about age 52 in 1981, when AIDS was first diagnosed among gay men and prior to July 1982 was named Gay-Related Immune Deficiency (GRID). The older gay and bisexual men in the Grossman et al. study[7] were nearly 70 years old when relatively positive images of gay men were portrayed on television in the "Will and Grace" series.

Invisibility

The ubiquitous experience of the majority of older gay and bisexual men is their invisibility. As media images of them are not portrayed realistically and their lives and relationships are not celebrated, older gay and bisexual men are assumed not to exist by many people in heteronormative (i.e., based on heterosexual norms) communities. Younger gay and bisexual males, with their focus on youth, tend not only to ignore older gay and bisexual men, but also to distance themselves from them; therefore, the invisibility of old age in the gay community is compounded by the stress of being socially unaccept-able within the community.[10] Older gay and bisexual men may also be invis-ible to gerontologists and health professionals, as questions about sexual identity and sexual behaviors are not routinely asked in studies about older adults, and health professionals often assume that older people are asexual, not interested in dating, and not desirous of a romantic partner.[11] Most health professionals are even less likely to think of older gay male clients as being gay or bisexual. However, among the scarce research that has been conducted about aging gay men, Pope and Schulz, surveying 87 gay men between the ages of 40 and 77, reported that 91% said they were still sexually active, with the majority indicating no change in their level of interest in or enjoyment of sexual activity.[12]

Most of the current cohort of older gay and bisexual men tends to remain silent and invisible for self-preservation and survival, having come of age when hiding one's sexual orientation was a prominent coping mechanism.[13] Therefore, older gay and bisexual men tend not to be the spokespersons for the gay community. They are usually not found on the frontlines of people advocating for same-sex marriage or other rights for same-sex partners, such as inheritance or making health care decisions for a partner. This further leads to their invisibility in the gay community—in addition to their invisibility in mainstream society.

Being a Double Minority: Old and Gay or Bisexual

Although it is important to recognize the diversity among older gay and bi-sexual men, it is also critical to understand their common experience of being members of at least two minority groups characterized by their sexual orien-tation and age. Stigmatizing qualities tend to assume primacy, anchoring "master status," that is, a lens through which everything about gay and bi-sexual (and lesbian) people or aging persons is viewed. In other words, they are primarily understood in terms of the stigmatization attached to their being gay or bisexual or old, even when it is irrelevant.[14] For example, they come to be known primarily as the "gay man" on the fourth floor or the "old man" on the second floor. These two stigmas overshadow their other social identities such as being professionals, parents, grandparents, and family and community members.[2] This incongruence between their personal identities and experiences and societal structures leads to their enduring "minority stress" from a variety of perspectives. Having to employ stigma management, that is, careful management of disclosure and nondisclosure of their sexual orientation and age, leads to a pervasive series of stressors that can have a negative effect on their mental and physical health over the life-course.[15]

DiPlacido[16] and Meyer[15,17] have cited findings that link minority stress to greater mental health problems, emotional distress, and depressive mood among gay men. However, they have also indicated that some gay and bisexual individuals deal successfully with minority stress so that it does not lead to negative health outcomes. Social support and personality characteristics, such as hardiness and high self-esteem, have been found to moderate the negative effects of minority stress.[17,18]

Developmental Trajectories of Older Gay and Bisexual Men, and Differences between Them and Young Men

The older gay and bisexual men in the Grossman et al. study[7] reported becoming aware that they were attracted to people of the same sex (although they may not have labeled these feelings) at a mean age of 12.9 years ($SD = 6.9$). They had their first same-sex fantasy at a mean age of 13.0 years ($SD = 5.8$) and their first same-sex experience at a mean age of 18.6 years ($SD = 10.4$). However, they did not label themselves as homosexual/gay/bi-bisexual until a mean age of 22.6 years ($SD = 10.5$), and they first told some-one else that they were gay or bisexual at a mean age of 28.7 years ($SD = 13.6$). Consequently, there were approximately four years between their first same-sex experience and first labeling themselves as homosexual/gay/bisexual, and there were an additional six years of passing and hiding before they first told someone else about their sexual orientation. Therefore, during a 10-year period of having same-sex experiences, it is likely that they were not only se-cretive and trying to pass as heterosexual, but they were also keeping the truth about their sexual orientation and behaviors from their health care providers as well as everyone else.

To demonstrate the salience of these sexual identity milestones in the lives of today's older gay and bisexual men, some brief comparisons with the gay and bisexual youth are provided. The data were collected between 1999 and 2001 among 274 gay and bisexual male youth who had a mean age of 17.01 years ($SD = 1.27$; range 15–19).[19] These youth reported becoming aware that they were attracted to people of the same sex at a mean age of 9.8 years ($SD = 3.5$), had their first sex-sex fantasy at a mean age of 12.6 years ($SD = 7.2$), and their first same-sex experience at a mean age of 13.7 years ($SD = 3.2$). They considered themselves gay at a mean age of 13.6 years ($SD = 2.6$) and first told someone else that they were gay at a mean age of 14.5 years ($SD = 14.5$).[19] Therefore, the total number of years between the gay and bisexual male youths' first same-sex experience and first telling someone was approximately one year compared to the 10-year interval of the older gay and bisexual adults. While many of the older gay and bisexual male adults may have experienced negative mental and physical health effects associated with hiding their sexual orientation (see below), they also reported significantly fewer verbal and physical victimization experiences than those in the youth study. In both studies, those who disclosed their sexual identity at a younger age experienced more victimization based on sexual orientation.

The Consequences of Hiding or Disclosing Sexual Orientation

Friend has developed a model of identity formation to explain the diverse types of lives that older gay and lesbian people lead.[6,20] He suggested that responses to developing a gay identity within a heterosexist sociohistoric context that devalues and abhors homosexuality occurred along a set of two continuums. The first continuum represents cognitive/behavioral responses. One end point of this continuum results from internalizing the pervasive heterosexist and negative ideologies about homosexuality, such as the belief that gay people are sick or otherwise inferior. According to Friend's model, these older gay and lesbian people conform to the stereotype of loneliness, depression, and alienation. They respond to heterosexism by internalizing the negative beliefs, and as a result they experience extreme internalized homophobia. Friend labeled this group "Stereotypic Older Lesbian and Gay People"; he described the process that they experience as leading to feelings of guilt, anxiety, self-hatred, and low self esteem, which can interfere with their ability to form close relationships and lead to despair, depression, and suicide.

The other end point of Friend's continuum results from responses to heterosexism that challenge or question the validity of negative messages; reconstructing what it means to be gay into something positive and affirmative. The older gay and lesbian adults at this end of the continuum are psychologically well-adjusted, vibrant, and are growing older successfully. This strategy of managing heterosexism results in the minimization of internalized homophobia, and this group is labeled "Affirmative Older Lesbian and Gay People,"

In the mid-range of Friend's linear identity continuum are the group called "Passing Older Lesbian and Gay People." The lives of these older gay and lesbian people accommodate to heterosexism by conditionally accepting some aspects of homosexuality while still believing that heterosexuality is inherently superior to homosexuality. These individuals have not challenged the prevailing heterosexist belief system and still experience moderate levels of internalized homophobia; they are motivated by a strong investment in passing as heterosexual or "at least" not appearing to be stereotypically lesbian or gay. Heightened levels of anxiety and self-consciousness are generated by the fear of being "found out"; the emotional costs of needing to "pass" can be high. The compartmentalization used by the individuals in this group often leads to a fragmented sense of self and a lack of authenticity in interpersonal relationships. Especially for men, it may lead to a splitting off of sexual and emotional relationships. For some men, other men are used for sex, with little or no emotional attachment, while heterosexual families or marriages are used for intimacy.

Friend's second continuum is a set of affective responses that correspond to the cognitive/behavioral continuum.[20] For example, Friend sees feelings of self-hatred, low self-esteem, and minimal acceptance of self as corresponding to the negative evaluation of homosexuality and associated with the "Stereotypic" group. Feelings of increased self-acceptance, high self-esteem, personal empowerment, and self-affirmation correspond with the "Affirmative" group. The "Passing" group has to cope with heightened levels of anxiety generated by the possibility of their sexual orientation being discovered, as well as with conditional self-acceptance and the absence of emotional supports during crises and times of need.

Older gay and bisexual men in the "Affirmative" group may experience some discrimination in their everyday lives and difficulties with some medical, nursing and other health care professionals; for example, they may not be permitted in the intensive care unit of hospitals in some locations that only allow next of kin to visit loved ones. But for those in the "Passing" and "Stereotypic" groups, nondisclosure of their sexual identity or behaviors may impact the quality of care they receive. For example, those gay and bisexual men who do not inform health care providers of their receptive oral or anal sexual behaviors are hiding information that would lead to a more comprehensive sexual history and physical examination. Further, the effects of race, ethnicity, culture, and socioeconomic class may add other burdens and stressors related to health education and care.[21]

According to Friend, published scholarly writings tend to portray the vast majority of older gay and lesbian people as attaining high levels of self-acceptance and psychological adjustment to growing old.[20] These findings may be a result of members of the "Affirmative Older Lesbian and Gay People" group being more willing and accessible to participate in research projects. Furthermore, having experience in reframing the meanings of homosexuality and bisexuality from negative to positive, these individuals may be more likely to use a similar process in transforming negative societal views of older people into positive identities of themselves. Along the continuum of unsuccessful to successful aging, they challenge myths that most people do not age successfully, for example, are senile, dependent, unproductive, asexual, unhealthy. At the same time they provide models that include older people as active, productive, sexual, self-determining, healthy individuals.

What We Currently Know about Older Gay and Bisexual Men

As indicated above, research about older gay and bisexual men has focused almost exclusively on the lives of those who are most visible and who have come forward as research participants for whatever personal and social reasons. These older men have been primarily white, well-educated, of middle socioeconomic status, and willing to be identified as gay or bisexual, while others remain invisible. Using Friend's identity continuum as a reference,[6,20] most of what we know about older gay and bisexual men comes from the "Affirmative" group, but we know almost nothing about members who fall along the continuum at the markers labeled "Passing" and "Stereotypic." Another limitation of the published research studies is that the findings frequently distinguish between homosexual and heterosexual participants, but do not specify results that are specific to bisexuals as they tend to be categorized with the homosexual groups.

Initial Studies

Dorfman and her colleagues[22] reported on a sample of 108 people (55 women and 53 men) between the ages of 60 and 93 years ($M = 69.3$, $SD = 6.8$), of whom 56 were homosexual (23 women and 33 men) and 52 were heterosexual (32 women and 20 men). No significant differences were found between older homosexuals and heterosexuals with regard to depression and social support; as expected, larger social networks were associated with lower depression. However, the sources of social support varied: older gay men and lesbians received significantly more support from friends, and heterosexual elderly people derived more support from their families of origin. Beeler, Rawls, Herdt and Cohler[23] also found that a large majority (89%) of the 160 participants (49 gay men and 51 lesbians, ranging in age from 45–90 years) in their study indicated that they could turn to at least three friends for advice and emotional support if they were dealing with "a serious problem" and that 60% indicated that they had six or more such friends. More than half of the respondents (68%) indicated that they had a "family of choice" with whom they socialized on holidays. Beeler and colleagues concluded that friendship networks were among the most important sources of social support for older lesbians and gay men. Dorfman and colleagues[22] took the implications of their findings a step further, concluding that there is a need to redefine the concept of family to include "friendship families," suggesting that health care professionals need to be aware of the importance of nonfamily relationships among older gay men and lesbians. However, Greene[11] cautions that the absence of legal status of a same-sex relationship may have negative implications for older gay and lesbian couples, especially if one member is ill, hospitalized, disabled, or in need of residential care.

Quam and Whitford[24] studied adaptation and age-related expectations of 80 gay and lesbian adults (41 men and 39 women) over the age of 50 years, living in a Midwestern metropolitan area. Participants reported acceptance of the aging process and high levels of life satisfaction. Being active in the gay community and publicly identifying as gay were found to be assets in accepting one's own aging and in developing positive coping skills. Close to 64% of the participants reported that they had gone to or participated in a lesbian/gay social group; however, only 8.8% reported participating in activities at a general population senior center or club. The investigators also determined that over half of the women reported that most of their closest friends were lesbians, while only 27.5% of the men reported that most of their friends were gay men. Sixty-five percent of the men indicated that their network of close friends included women and men, gay and nongay; while only 38.5% of the women described their friendship network similarly.

From an exploratory study of 71 (17 women and 54 men) self-identified gay men, lesbians, and bisexuals ages 50–80 years ($M = 60.8$, SD 8.31), Jacobs, Rasmussen and Hohman[25] concluded that social support services for the older lesbian/gay population may best be provided in a lesbian/gay environment. Among their findings were that the participants used social and support groups within the gay/lesbian community and that gay/lesbian community services were rated significantly more adequate in meeting needs in times of emotional crises than non–gay/lesbian services. They also found that both men and women indicated that they would be interested in participating in social groups that were segregated by gender.

The Beeler, Rawls, Herdt, and Cohler study[23] of 160 lesbians and gay men in Chicago drew three primary conclusions regarding the planning and provision of services for older gay men and lesbians. First, they indicated that providers needed to recognize the diversity of the population, for example, those single, those partnered, those with children, and those making transitions from a heterosexual lifestyle and becoming more integrated into the gay community. Second, the investigators found that it was important to consider the social context in which services are provided, for example, an agency perceived to be catering to young white gay men will have difficulty in recruiting older gay men and people of color. Also, tensions between competing agencies could obstruct coordination of the delivery of services to all segments of the target population. Finally, the researchers concluded that a community organizing approach appeared to offer more promise in meeting the needs of the population compared to an approach limited to the direct provision of specific services, as community organizing proactively involves older gay men and lesbians in identifying, planning, and implementing a variety of services.

The initial studies focused on the social context of the lives of older gay and bisexual adults. They concentrated on examining sources of social support, including families of choice, friendship families, participation in the social groups, and being active in the gay community. One of their major conclusions was that lesbian, gay, and bisexual older adults use friendship families as vital sources of support, while their heterosexual counterparts use families of origin. The absence of the legal status of these relationships has negative implications for older gay and bisexual men in the institutions comprising the health care delivery system. More recent studies, reported in the next section, focus on the mental health (e.g., self-esteem, internalized homophobia, loneliness, substance abuse, happiness) and physical health (e.g., chronic illnesses, safe sexual activity, physical decline, exercise) of older gay and bisexual adults, and the effects of disclosing their sexual orientation to primary care providers. They also examined the frequency of sexual orientation victimization and its effects.

Recent Studies

Recruiting a sample of 105 gay men 65 years or older (range = 65–87 years), Mostade[26] explored two specific health care choices of older gay men: self-disclosure of sexual orientation to a physician, and completion of a Durable Power of Attorney for Health Care (DPAHC). The majority of the men were from the Midwestern region of the United States, with smaller percentages from the Eastern and Western regions. Approximately three-fourths were fully or partially retired, and approximately one-half lived alone. More than 85% were of European ethnicity and more than two-thirds had earned a bachelor's or higher degree. Among the sample, 37% of the participants reported having one or more chronic health conditions limiting their mobility or otherwise causing a burden. Mostade found that older gay men who had self-disclosed their sexual orientation to physicians showed a lower discomfort with their gay identity than nondisclosers. Those who disclosed their orientation were also more likely to have completed a DPAHC. His findings indicated that increased discomfort with a gay identity was associated with decreased likelihood of disclosure of sexual orientation to a physician.

Cruz[27] conducted a study of 125 gay and bisexual men in Texas, collecting data between 2000 and 2001. The mean age of the men was 65, ranging from 55–84 years. The men were primarily white (92%), homosexual/gay (92%), and highly educated (72% with bachelor's or higher degree). Nearly half of the participants (46%) reported being in a committed relationship, and 43% reported being single. Almost two-thirds of the participants (64%) had no experience with heterosexual marriage earlier in their lives.

With regard to their physical health, 80% of the men reported it to be "good" or "excellent." Sixty-nine percent of the men participated in exercise frequently, with 72% exercising 2 or more times per week, primarily in aerobic/cardiovascular activity. Although 89% of the men did not smoke, 71% reported regular drinking behavior, mostly wine and liquor. More than three-fourths of the men (79%) reported taking physician-prescribed medications for hypertension, cholesterol, diabetes, depression, or cancer (prostate and other types). With regard to HIV/AIDS, 83% were previously tested and 95% reported a negative HIV status. More than two-thirds reported that HIV/AIDS had an impact on their lives, mainly through the loss of friends, family members, or previous partners to conditions association with HIV infection.[27]

Cruz[27] found that 81% of the 125 men in his study described themselves as "fairly happy" or "very happy." Those who were in committed relationships perceived themselves as happier than those who were single or casually dating. When those who described themselves as "not very happy" or "not at all happy" were asked "what would make them happier," they indicated things such as having a partner, better health, more money, more travel, and a better job. Approximately one-half of the men (48%) had received some form of counseling or psychological therapy, but only 5% were currently seeing a therapist. One-fourth of the men reported experiencing depression, due to such causes as aging, physical decline, health problems, and their financial situations. Additionally, 48% of the men reported experiencing loneliness at least some of the time. Those who were in committed relationships reported experiencing less depression and less loneliness than those who were single or casually dating.

When asked about stigma associated with being homosexual, 49% indicated that they had experienced stigma related to being gay, while 49% had not. When asked about the ways in which they had experienced stigma, the men reported job discrimination (e.g., not being promoted or being denied work), loss of friends, or being shunned by family. Over half of the men (54%) reported stigma related to aging, while 44% did not. Those men who reported experiencing age-related stigma indicated that it occurred mainly in the work environment and in being shunned by younger gay men.[27]

Orel[28] reported findings about 10 gay, 13 lesbian, and 3 bisexual elders who participated in three focus groups conducted in Ohio and Michigan. Participants ranged in age from 65 to 84, with a mean age of 72 years. Groups were diverse with regard to ethnicity (6 African Americans, 17 European Americans, 1 Asian American, and 2 Latinos) and socioeconomic status (5 low-income, 15 middle-income, and 6 upper-income). During discussions, several themes of major importance to gay, lesbian, and bisexual elders emerged: physical health, mental health, legal rights, housing, spirituality, family, and social networks. Their findings related to men's physical and mental health are reported here.

In the area of physical health, the older adults discussed concerns related to rising health care costs and to failing health. Chronic illnesses were reported by participants, including arthritis, hypertension, diabetes, heart disease, emphysema, and cancer; however, they all rated their current health status as good and did not report any medical needs for which they were not receiving care. Most interestingly, Orel[28] found distinct differences between the experiences of those older adults who "disclosed" their sexual orientation compared to those who did not. A heightened sense of frustration with the health care system was reported by those elders who did not share their sexual orientation with their health care providers. She also noted that more than half of the participants indicated that their physicians never discussed the issue of sexual activity, suggesting that many physicians may assume that older adults are not sexually active. The men in the focus groups included not practicing "safe sex" as a health risk, with all 10 of the male respondents saying they were sexually active and not practicing safe sex. Other specific health risks reported by the older adults included over-indulging in alcohol and nicotine, and over-indulging in high-calorie foods.

The majority of the focus group participants in Orel's study[28] perceived themselves as being healthy, happy, well-adjusted, and able to negotiate the challenges of aging, saying that the psychological resiliency necessary for "coming out" prepared them for the psychological issues related to aging. Half of the participants indicated that they had previously utilized formal mental health services, being treated for substance abuse, anxiety, and depression. At the time of the study, two of the participants were seeing therapists for issues related to bereavement.

Grossman, D'Augelli, and O'Connell[7] surveyed older lesbians, gays, and bisexuals they recruited from 18 groups or agencies (17 in the US and 1 in Toronto) providing social and recreational services to older gay, lesbian, and bisexual adults. Of their sample of 416 participants, most (297) individuals self-identified as gay and bisexual men, which makes it the largest North American study to date focusing on elderly gay and bisexual men. The men ranged in age from 60 to 91 years ($M = 68.9$ years). Despite efforts to diversify the sample by ethnicity and race, most of the participants (92%) identified themselves as Caucasian/white; 1% described themselves as African American/black, and 2% as Hispanic/Latino. The remaining 5% indicated "mixed race" or "other" on the list of choices. One-third (34%) of the men lived in a major metropolitan area; approximately another third (35%) lived in a small city. Of the remaining men, 10% lived in a suburb, 13% in a small town or a rural area, and 8% named other areas, for example, a province. The majority of men (61%) reported living alone, 30% lived with a partner; 3% lived with friends, 2% lived with relatives, and 4% identified other living arrangements. Thirty-five percent of the men indicated that they had children. Reporting their highest educational level, 20% of the participants had earned a high school diploma, and 70% had a bachelor's or higher degree; the other 10% had obtained associate degrees or various types of certificates. Most of the men (78%) were retired. However, 14% said they were still working; 2% received disability payments, and 6% continued to work even though they had retired from other work. With regard to personal yearly income, 12% of the men earned less than $15,000, 47% between $15,000 and $35,000, and 41% more than $35,000. When asked the current percentage of people who knew that they were gay or bisexual, 43% of the men reported that 50% or less knew, and the other 57% reported that more than 50% knew.

Three-quarters of the men (74%) in the Grossman et al. study[7] described their physical health as good to excellent, 22% said fair, and only 4% reported their physical health status to be poor or very poor. Although 61% of the older adults stated that their physical health never or seldom stood in the way of their doing the things they wanted to do, the remaining 39% of the men indicated that it sometimes, often, or very often did. More than half of the men

(60%) indicated that they regularly participated in exercise activities (e.g., walking, hiking, jogging, biking or swimming), while 24% did sometimes, and 16% seldom or never exercised.

Regarding their ability to perform physical activities (such as walking, shopping, working around the house), more than half of the men (59%) indicated that their ability had not changed in the past five years. However, 35% of the men said it was somewhat or much worse, and only 6% indicated that it was somewhat or much better. Thirty-four percent of the men reported having a physical disability or handicap, and 14% of those indicated that they required an assistive device.[7]

While the large majority of the men (93%) in the Grossman et al. study[7] had known people diagnosed as HIV-positive or with AIDS, an equally large percentage of participants (87%) said that they were very unlikely or unlikely to be infected with HIV. However, only 71% of the men said they had ever been tested for HIV, and 27% indicated that they did not expect to be tested. Further, 47% of the men indicated that they knew 3 or more people who had died from HIV/AIDS, and 2 percent reported being HIV-infected. The physical realities of HIV as well as the developmental process of aging can become complex for older gay men as both impact issues of physical attraction and the connected affirmation of sexual desirability.[29]

Most of the gay and bisexual men (85%) in the Grossman et al. study[7] reported that their mental health was good or excellent, while 13% said fair, and 2% poor. Ten percent of the men described themselves as having a mental disability or illness, and 18% of those indicated that they were required to take medication for the mental disorder. Regarding their mental health, 61% of the men indicated that their status had not changed in the past five years. However, 11% of the men said it was somewhat or much worse, and 28% indicated that it was somewhat or much better. In other words, over four-fifths of the men saw themselves as mentally healthy. These findings are similar to those found by Cruz,[27] who found that 85% of the 125 gay and bisexual men (mean age of 65 years) were not currently in psychological therapy for mental health problems, and 81% reported that were very happy or fairly happy. When Cruz asked the participants what makes a man adjust well to growing old, the majority indicated self-acceptance of age and sexual orientation, friends, romantic/sexual relationships, meaningful social groups, financial security, and good health. While these states could be said to be beneficial for all aging persons, one must be reminded of the challenges of accepting one's sexual orientation and finding romantic/sexual relationships and meaningful social groups for gay and bisexual men in a society that embraces heterosexuality as the norm.

Most gay and bisexual men in the Grossman et al. study[7] reported a slightly higher than average level of self-esteem on the Rosenberg Self-Esteem Scale ($M = 24.6$, $SD = 2.2$), which is a 10-item scale with total scores ranging from 4 to 40. Those with a lover or partner reported higher self-esteem than those who did not have a partner, and those men with higher self-esteem reported less victimization. Loneliness was experienced by many of the men, as indicated by a mean score of 23.3 ($SD = 3.1$) on the UCLA Loneliness Scale; it is an 8-item scale with total scores ranging from 4 to 32. Not surprisingly, men who lived with a lover or partner reported less loneliness and viewed their physical and mental health more positively than those living alone. Cruz[27] reported similar findings, with three-fourths of his participants who were in committed relationships reporting no loneliness. What is unique to older gay men, when compared to their heterosexual male counterparts, is that fewer of them cohabit with a partner, that is, 30% in the Grossman et al. study and 50% in the Cruz study.

In the Grossman et al. study,[7] feelings of isolation were reported by 10% of the men, and 26% reported that they felt a lack of companionship. Only 11% ($n = 33$) of the men reported using alcohol to the extent that they could be currently classified as "problem drinkers" on the AUDIT, achieving scores at or above the cut-off score of eight. However, eleven other men added comments that they were "recovering alcoholics." No significant differences were found in alcohol consumption between those men who encountered verbal and physical abuse over their lifetimes and those who did not. Ten percent of the men reported using "drugs [not including alcohol] other than those required for medical reasons" in the last year.

The men reported significant rates of internalized homophobia or a negative view of one's own sexual orientation ($M = 24.2$, $SD = 6.50$) on twelve items from the Revised Homosexuality Attitude Inventory (total scores ranging from 12 to 48), with those who were older reporting more internalized homophobia.[30] However, less internalized homophobia was reported by those men having more supportive people in their networks and having more involvement with lesbian, gay, and bisexual organizations. More than three-quarters of the men (77%) said that they were "glad to be gay or bisexual," while only 10% reported being depressed about their sexual orientation and 11% said they had received counseling to stop their same-sex feelings. However, 28% said they wished that they were heterosexual.

Over their lifetimes, approximately two-thirds of the men in the Grossman et al. study[7] (65%) reported experiencing verbal abuse based on their sexual orientation. Many men reported having been victims of violence (32%) and assault (16%). Eleven percent had had objects thrown at them, while 15% of the men reported being assaulted with a weapon. Ten percent of the men reported being sexually attacked or raped. Twenty-one percent experienced discrimination in employment, and 8% of the men reported housing discrimination. A significant percentage of the men (28%) reported being victimized by someone who threatened to disclose their sexual orientation. Older men reported less victimization; however, those men who attended lesbian, gay, and bisexual organizations reported more victimization. Self-reports of poor health were associated with more victimization experiences.

Nine percent of the men said that they had sometimes or often considered suicide, and 11% said they had considered committing suicide in the last year.[30] Of those who had ever thought of suicide, 15% said those thoughts were related to their sexual orientation. Past suicide attempts were reported by 12% of the men, with those reporting suicide attempts being more likely to report sexual orientation victimization. While there was a strong relationship between victimization and attempted suicide, suicidal ideation on its own was not found to be related to experiences of harassment.

With regard to support networks, gay and bisexual men in another study conducted by Grossman and colleagues[18] reported an average of 6 people in their networks ($M = 6.3$, $SD = 3.5$; permitted to list a maximum of 10), 67% of whom were men, and of those 54% were gay and bisexual men.[17] Of the people listed in the men's support networks, 87% were described as being aware of the respondents' sexual orientation, and the men were more satisfied by the support from those who knew of their sexual orientation. Also, the more satisfied they were with their support networks, the less lonely they were. Networks have the potential to ward off and buffer the effects of exclusion, discrimination, victimization, and the morbidity associated with such negative experiences.[31]

Higher measures of current self-assessed physical and mental health were significantly associated with higher current income, higher self-esteem, more positive views of one's sexual orientation, and being less lonely among the men in the Grossman et al. study.[7] Analyses comparing the men living alone with those who lived with partners found that those living with partners reported better overall current physical and mental health.[30]

Older Gay and Bisexual Men: Barriers to Accessing and Receiving Health Care

Society's continuing heterosexism and homophobia, together with the reactions of older gay and bisexual men who have experienced them for many years, have created barriers to providing and receiving optimal health care (and other human services).[2] Many of these men are those who would fall along that part of Friend's[6,20] continuum that comprises the stereotypic and passing older gay people. These barriers are usually compounded for older gay and bisexual men of color, as a range of other factors have to be considered in determining the impact of ethnic and racial identities and their ongoing, dynamic interactions with sexual orientation.[32]

Perhaps the greatest barrier is the one stated at the beginning of this chapter: the invisibility of older gay and bisexual men. Living in Western cultures in which youth and youthful attractiveness are esteemed and privileged, these barriers are accentuated for older gay and bisexual men living in a gay culture with its emphasis on youthful looks, physical attractiveness, and desirability.[33] Furthermore, invisibility allows stereotypes to persist, for example, gay and bisexual men are stereotyped to be focused on sex, to be feminine, to be significantly different from the "normal healthy adult," to wear

jewelry, and to be creative.[34] Although some men may fit each of these stereotypes, the majority do not act in stereotypical ways. Stereotypes on the
other end of the continuum consider older gay and bisexual men as asexual
or otherwise no longer having romantic attractions or sexual desires, which
are also erroneous.[11] Additionally, gay and bisexual men of traditional religious and ethnic groups in which homosexuality is not acceptable remain
invisible as they opt to be immersed in the realities of the extended family as
they age; therefore, being openly gay or bisexual is not an option for them.[35]
To some professionals, older men who self-identify as gay or bisexual are
considered oddities or curiosities whose existences are atypical, and who can
therefore be dismissed. All of these portraits, however, lead to the same result:
inadequate health needs assessment, health prevention education, and health
care delivery for older gay and bisexual men.

Lack of visibility leads to a second barrier in the provision of and accessibility to health care services for older gay and bisexual men, and that is the
persistence of negative myths about them. The existing myths are that older
gay and bisexual men are predators of young boys; or that they become hy-
persexual and alcoholics or drug users because they live unhappy, lonely, and
sad lives; and that substance use dulls their feelings of shame and embar-
rassment.[31] These negative myths can provoke intense anxieties among some
health care providers, prohibiting them from establishing needed health
outreach and care services for older gay and bisexual men, to avoid being
associated with them and the stigmas connected to their lives.

A third set of barriers consists of fears. The primary fears of many older gay
and bisexual men are related to their sexual orientation or behaviors being
discovered, or to their being rejected when others learn about them. Some of
these fears are based on internalized homophobia, resulting from decades of
hearing negative views about same-sex attractions and behaviors.[33] Other fears
emanate from having experienced rejections and other negative consequences, for example, verbal victimization and inferior health care, because
they disclosed their sexual orientation or same-sex behaviors.[36,37] Some older
gay adults fear forms of discrimination such as forced separation of long-term
partners in nursing homes, prejudicial comments made by some staff and
other residents of retirement communities, and the failure of some senior
centers to provide information or support for gay-specific issues. Additionally,
partners who may have had long-term relationships are frequently not officially recognized in the medical centers, including hospitals, nursing homes,
inpatient hospice centers, retirement homes, assisted-living facilities, and
adult day care programs. Providers may directly or indirectly create barriers
between life partners, such as biased behavior to outward signs of affection
between same-sex couples.[38]

Although hiding one's sexual orientation may lead to feelings of isolation
and alienation, it may also foster a sense of security that disclosing one's same-
sex attractions or behaviors tends to jeopardize. While the stress of hiding may
lead to self-destructive behaviors such as substance abuse or unsafe sex, having

to cope with the ongoing consequences of stigmatization and victimization may make men prone to similar outcomes.[32] Some gay and bisexual men have created a family of friends to combat isolation and to nurture and support them as they age. Over time, however, they lose some of these loved ones, and that circle of support shrinks. They become secluded and isolated, as there is not a significant social or health-related network for older gay and bisexual men in most areas.[35] By establishing advocacy programs and creating safe health care spaces for older gay and bisexual men, health care professionals can allay their clients' fears.

Old age leads some gay and bisexual men to become dependent when infirmities take their toll in later life. After having spent most of their lives fighting societal stigmas and living independently, this hard-fought battle is not easy to give up. Others have never succeeded in fighting the social stigma associated with being gay or bisexual, and they come to see themselves as not worthy or decent. Some of these individuals embrace the concept of self-neglect, believing that they are unworthy people who deserve to be forgotten. This barrier of self-neglect "creates a downward spiral leading to poor health, poor living conditions, depression, and in some cases a gloomy hope for death." [35[p172]] Finally, these older people do not ask for help, and some of them refuse assistance.

A significant barrier related to the health care of older gay and bisexual men is the lack of end-of-life care programs. While end-of-life care programs for gay people with AIDS tend to be excellent, an older gay or bisexual man dying of some other disease or condition is not likely to find end-of-life care that supports his identity.[39] Cahill, South, and Spade[33] reported that 90% of all care for frail elderly people is done by family, but 65% of older gay people do not receive care from their families: 90% do not have children and may be estranged from their families of origin. Some older gay and bisexual men may refuse home health care because they are afraid that home health workers will harm them or treat them disrespectfully when they find out about their sexual orientation. A 1994 study by the Gay and Lesbian Medical Association reported that 52% of gay doctors in the study saw colleagues deny or reduce care to patients based on their sexual orientation.[37]

A major barrier to providing quality health education and care to older gay and bisexual men is the absence of education about them in most professional preparation programs for health care professionals and a similar lack of training in continuing education. This is not a new observation, and studies have repeatedly concluded that homophobic attitudes are prevalent among a significant proportion of health professionals.[37] While HIV/AIDS has brought attention to young gay and bisexual men, health issues related to older members of these groups tend to remain neglected, even though there is some evidence that among older gay and bisexual men, HIV may have elevated the risk of cancers, cognitive impairment, and mortality.[35] The US Centers for Disease Control and Prevention (CDC)[40] estimated that 441,380 cumulative deaths of persons with AIDS (i.e., from the beginning of the epidemic through 2004) were among men who reported male-to-male contact, and another 64,833 deaths were among men who reported male-to-male contact and injection drug use. Six percent of all people who died were 55 years of age or older, so we can assume that at minimum 6% percent of those who had been in one of the two transmission categories were older men who had sex with men. Additionally, the CDC estimated that of 462,792 persons living with HIV/AIDS in 2004 (in the 35 areas with confidential name-based HIV infection) 222,422 (48%) were among persons who reported male-to-male sexual contact (some with injection drug abuse).

Health care administrators, policy-makers, and educators must support education and training about older gay and bisexual men so that providers are competent to provide sensitive preventive care and treatment that is inclusive of the older gay and bisexual man. In addition to advocating for the necessity of nondiscrimination and confidentiality policies that include sexuality, health care professionals must be trained to assist those individuals with HIV in reconciling successful aging and living with the disease. Many aspects of HIV overlap with similar aspects of the aging process. For example, individuals in both groups are stigmatized and vulnerable to rejection and ostracism. Additionally, they face issues of mortality, deal with physical debilitation, and find themselves susceptible to infectious diseases. The unique differences of this cohort of older gay and bisexual men, including their not revealing their sexual orientation after a lifetime of living in the closet, limits the efforts of prevention, education, and treatment. Many of these older gay and bisexual men do not feel tainted and unacceptable, but they have experienced verbal and physical sexual orientation victimization, entrapment, discrimination, and oppression. Therefore, they do not want to reexperience the same negative feelings in terms of HIV/AIDS; so they avoid HIV testing and AIDS treatment. They attribute their symptoms to aging, and unfortunately, some of their health providers support this attribution.[41,42] Vance and Robinson[43] found that a synthesis of topics related to both phenomena of aging and HIV disease reveal unique influences on disease prognosis, which affect the social, psychological, and medical well-being of persons aging with this disease.

Another substantial barrier to providing high-quality clinical prevention and treatment services to older gay and bisexual men is the limited knowledge base about them. For the most part, health professionals and researchers have not asked this group about their unique needs, and the population seldom makes requests of health care services in ways that make their personal lives known. Gerontologists and other researchers studying older people need to include questions that will assess the behaviors and health needs of older gay and bisexual men. Among those who disclose their sexual orientation, there may be a tendency to overemphasize sexual health at the expense of other health needs.[44] On the other hand, nondisclosure of sexual orientation can lead to examinations that tend to be no more than cursory, as the health care professional is constrained in his or her ability to treat the patient holistically.[46] Disclosure in a safe and nonprejudicial environment is optimal for increasing a health care professional's capacity to understand and support older gay and bisexual men as consumers of medical care.

Discussion, Interventions, and Recommendations

What we know about older gay and bisexual men derives from studies conducted with opportunistic samples of these men. These men mainly fall on the end of the continuum that Friend[6, 20] identified as "Affirmative," and they tend to be well-educated, white, and of middle to higher socioeconomic status. Consequently, there are significant gaps in our current knowledge base; we need to study the needs and behaviors of older gay and bisexual men across class, race, ethnicity, and culture. Also, we need to include romantic attractions, sexual identities, and sexual behaviors in population surveys of health, so that we obtain accurate data about the physical and mental health statuses, concerns, and needs, from representative samples of all older gay and bisexual men. Additionally, evaluations of existing services for older gay and bisexual men are sorely needed. Furthermore, there is a great need for enhanced training of health care professionals so that they can deliver sensitive and competent care to older gay and bisexual men. This training should target both clinical and management personnel. Legislation is needed to extend the prohibition of discrimination based on sexual orientation to the entire health care delivery system, including physicians' offices, hospitals, nursing homes, long-term care facilities, and home care services. Laws need to be enacted so that older gay and bisexual men do not feel they are vulnerable to rejection, discrimination, or reduced quality of service because of their sexual identity and behaviors or age. Prevention education and health care services need to be expanded to include all older gay and bisexual men, and appropriate social services should be provided to informal caregivers of same-sex partners and close friends of older gay and bisexual men.[33]

Public health activities related to the mental and physical health issues of older gay and bisexual men must be created, targeted and delivered, for example, HIV/AIDS and other sexually transmitted diseases, chronic diseases, mental health problems, hate crimes and domestic violence. Older gay and bisexual men must be included in trials for new drugs, including HIV/AIDS medications. Education campaigns and outreach programs should be conducted to encourage older gay and bisexual men to disclose their sexual orientation and behaviors to mental health and other health care professionals, and to sensitize providers to the existence and needs of older homosexual men so that their clients will receive appropriate services. Successful public health measures must fight age discrimination and ethnic/racial inequality in order to undertake meaningful work for the improvement of mental and physical health care of older gay and bisexual men. Battling homophobia with determination throughout one's life can seriously affect one's health and quality of life as an older gay or bisexual man because of the continuing impact of "minority stress."[16,17] Consequently, it is vitally important to understand that public policy and services that affect the lives of young and middle-aged gay and bisexual men will have an impact on their aging experiences.[33]

Research on aging needs to explore the life-course perspective of older gay and bisexual men with an appreciation of the fact that they are people who lived their lifetimes as men in a society with rigid gender role expectations for men and women. If the life-course view of older men's health emphasizes the effects of childhood and early adult experiences as essential to understanding how people come to have different degrees of functioning in old age, it is imperative that we recognize the nature of the experiences of men who diverged from normative expectations of heterosexuality. As Lee and Owens[47] pointed out, men who have sex with men may have many health concerns and needs that overlap with those of other men; however, they are also affected by a history of homophobia and marginalization. Research on male aging can no longer remain silent on the experiences of gay and bisexual men.

As stated at the beginning of this chapter, older gay and bisexual men not only have to cope with the heterosexism of mainstream society, but they also have to endure intensified ageism within the gay and bisexual community (or communities) in which being old means one is less attractive, less worthy of attention, less important, less useful, and less worthy of resources.[30] As younger gay people began to form their own social, political, and activist organizations in metropolitan communities and on college and university campuses in the late 1960s,[45] older gay and bisexual men became increasingly ignored, dismissed, and excluded from the communities' decision-making processes.[30] Unlike many of the older gay adults, the younger gay adults were not only focused on ensuring the elimination of discrimination (e.g., in the workplace, in housing, and in public accommodations), but they also established an agenda to obtain equal rights (e.g., to same-sex marriage, to gay parenting, to equal access to societal institutions such as health care and military services).[48,49] When gay and bisexual men born after the Stonewall Riots become older adults, they are not likely to internalize the gay community's ageism and let themselves be seen as less desirable, capable, important, or "on the way out."[50] They will expect to remain an integral part of their gay community and demand that the community embrace them in its continuing fight for equal rights; they will insist on their part of the social contract with mainstream society.

Concluding Remarks

Older gay and bisexual men confront many of the same concerns that their heterosexual peers confront when they are aging, for example, psychological well-being, economics, housing, and health.[31] For both, the main barrier to successful aging is the phenomenon of ageism that has fueled a kind of

pejorative image or stigmatization.[51] Ageism intervenes in assessments of individual capacity; aging adults "are viewed through a stereotypic lens, sub-
verting personal characteristics to the point of invisibility. . . . cultural practices have set older people apart from their younger counterparts . . . older
age is cast as a territory apart, a country of old, so to speak."[52[pp5–6]] This
separation is further exacerbated in the gay community as most events are
stratified by age, especially for gay and bisexual men who age out of a youth-
focused gay life.[10]

Older gay and bisexual men face a number of additional concerns as they
age due to institutionalized heterosexism; they often cannot access adequate
health care, affordable housing, and other social services.[30] Looking "old"
(e.g., wrinkles, gray hair, hearing aids) interacts with isolation and invisibility
in the gay community to contribute to an appalling combination "causing
debilitating health and emotional struggles."[10[p13]] These barriers indicate
that older gay and bisexual men may not fare as well in terms of their health as
their heterosexual peers. Research findings tell us that many have limited
access to health care and experience discrimination and bias.[35] Others are
uninsured, underinsured, or geographically far from a gay-friendly source of
care.[53]

A number of observations suggest that gay and bisexual men do not fare as
well as their heterosexual counterparts: a lack of a coordinated health infrastructure to support and direct funded initiatives on lesbian, gay, bisexual,
and transgender (LGBT) health; barriers to communication between health
care professionals and LGBT consumers; institutional barriers to quality
health services, such as denial of benefits to same-sex partners or their children by insurers and employers; lack of a say in the disposition of an inca-
pacitated partner in most cities unless advanced directives (such as health care
proxies and powers of attorney) have been completed; and emergency rooms
and inpatient units that restrict or deny access to partners and nonbiological
parents.[31]

Only the elimination of ageism, heterosexism, and sexual orientation
prejudice, and the addressing of societal structures that perpetuate inequality
in the provision of health services will reduce the disparities in the provision of
health services between older gay and bisexual men and their heterosexual
counterparts. A society that espouses equality and an individual's right to live a
healthy life can accept nothing less.

References

1. Vacha K. *Quiet Fire: Memoirs of Older Gay Men.* Trumansburg, NY: The Crossing
   Press; 1985.
2. Grossman AH. Homophobia and its effects on the inequitable provision of health
   and leisure services for older gay men and lesbians. In: Brackenridge C, Howe D,
   Jordan F, eds. *JUST Leisure: Equity, Social Exclusion and Identity.* Eastbourne, UK:
   LSA, 2000:105–118.

3. Smith DM, Gates, GJ. *Gay and Lesbian Families in the United States: Same-Sex Un-married Partner Households: A Preliminary Analysis of 2000 United States Census Data.* Washington, DC: Human Rights Campaign Report; August 22, 2001.
4. Kertzner R, Meyer I, Dolezal C. Psychological well-being in midlife and older gay men. In: Herdt G, deVries B, eds. *Gay and Lesbian Aging: Research and Future Directions.* NY: Spring Publishing Company; 2004;97–115.
5. Rice FP. *Human Development: A Life-Span Approach.* 4th ed. Upper Saddle River, NJ: Prentice Hall.
6. Friend RA. Older lesbian and gay people: responding to homophobia. *J Homosex.* 1989; 14(3–4): 241–263.
7. Grossman AH, D'Augelli AR, O'Connell TS. Being lesbian, gay, bisexual and 60 or older in North America. *J Gay Lesb Soc Serv.* 2001;13(4):171–179.
8. Belsky JK. *The Psychology of Aging: Theory, Research and Interventions.* Pacific Grove, CA: Brooks/Cole Publishing; 1999.
9. Bayer R. *Homosexual and American Psychiatry: The Politics of Diagnosis.* New York: Basic Books; 1981.
10. Altman C. Shining light on the golden years. *In the Fam.* 2004;9:8–14.
11. Greene B. Beyond heterosexism and across the cultural divides: developing an inclusive lesbian, gay and bisexual psychology. A look to the future. In: Greene B, Croom GL, eds. *Education, Research and Practice in Lesbian, Gay, Bisexual and Transgender Psychology: A Resource Manual.* Thousand Oaks, CA: Sage, 2000:1–45.
12. Pope M, Schulz R. Sexual attitudes and behavior in midlife and aging homosexual males. *J Homosex.* 1990;20:169–177.
13. Orel, N. Community needs assessment: documenting the need for affirmative services for LGB older adults. In: Kimmel D, Rose T, David S, eds. *Lesbian, Gay, Bisexual and Transgender Aging: Research and Clinical Perspectives.* New York, NY: Columbia University Press; 2006:227–246.
14. Bohan JS. *Psychology and Sexual Orientation: Coming to Terms.* New York, NY: Routledge; 1996.
15. Meyer IH. Minority stress and mental health in gay men. *J Health Soc Behav.* 1995;7:9–25.
16. DiPlacido J. Minority stress among lesbians, gay men, and bisexuals: a consequence of heterosexism, homophobia, and stigmatization. In: Herek G, ed. *Stigma and Sexual Orientation: Understanding Prejudice against Lesbians, Gay Men, and Bisexuals.* Thousand Oaks, CA: Sage; 1998:138–159.
17. Meyer I. Prejudice, social stress and mental health in lesbian, gay, and bisexual populations: conceptual issues and research evidence. *Psychol Bull.* 2003;129:674–694.
18. Grossman AH, D'Augelli AR, Hershberger SL. Social support networks of lesbian, gay and bisexual adults 60 years of age and older. *J Gerontol B Psychol Sci.* 2000;55B(5):P1–P9.
19. D'Augelli AR, Grossman, AH, Starks MT. Childhood gender atypicality, victimization, and PTSD among lesbian, gay, and bisexual youth. *J Inter Viol.* 2006;21: 1462–1482.
20. Friend RA. Older lesbian and gay people: a theory of successful aging. *J Homosex.* 1990;20(3–4):99–118.
21. Greene B. Lesbians and gay men of color: the legacy of ethnosexual mythologies in heterosexism. In: Bonet, LA, Rothblum, ED, eds. *Preventing Heterosexism and Homophobia.* Thousand Oaks, CA: Sage; 1996:59–70.

22. Dorfman R, Walters K, Burke P, Hardin L, Karanik T, Raphael, et al. Old, sad, and alone: the myth of the aging homosexual. *J Gerontol Soc Wk.* 1995;24:29–44.

23. Beeler JA, Rawls TD, Herdt G, Cohler BJ. The needs of older lesbians and gay men in Chicago. *J Gay Lesb Soc Serv.* 1999;9:31–49.

24. Quam JK, Whitford, GS. Adaptation and age-related expectations of older gay and lesbian adults. *The Gerontologist.* 1992;32:367–374.

25. Jacobs R, Rasmussen L, Hohman M. The social support needs of older lesbians, gay men, and bisexuals. *J Gay Lesb Soc Serv.* 1999;9:1–30.

26. Mostade SF. *Components of Internalized Homophobia, Self-Disclosure of Sexual Orientation to Physician, and Durable Power of Attorney for Health Care Completion in Older Gay Men* [dissertation]. Kent, OH: College of Education, Kent State University; 2004.

27. Cruz JM. *Sociological Analysis of Aging: The Gay Male Perspective.* New York, NY: Harrington Park Press; 2003.

28. Orel NA. Gay, lesbian and bisexual elders: expressed needs and concerns across focus groups. *J Gerontol Soc Wk.* 2004;43:57–77.

29. Halkitis PN, Wilton L. The meanings of sex for HIV-positive gay and bisexual men: emotions, physicality, and affirmations of self. In: Halkitis PN, Gomez CA, Wolitski RJ, eds. *HIV+ Sex: The Psychological and Interpersonal Dynamics of HIV-Seropositive Gay and Bisexual Men's Relationships.* Washington, DC: American Psychological Association; 2005:21–37.

30. D'Augelli AR, Grossman AH, Hershberger SL, O'Connell TS. Aspects of mental health among older lesbian, gay, and bisexual adults. *Aging Ment Health.* 2001;5(2):149–158.

31. Wilkinson R, Marmot M. *Social Determinants of Health: The Solid Facts.* 2nd ed. WHO Regional Office for Europe. http://www.who.dk/document/e81384pdf. Accessed July 15, 2005.

32. Cabaj, RP. Clinical issues with gay male clients. In: *A Provider's Introduction to Substance Abuse Treatment for Lesbian, Gay, Bisexual, and Transgender Individuals.* Rockville, MD: US Department of Health and Human Services, Substance Abuse and Mental Health Services Administration; 2001:79–85.

33. Cahill S, South K, Spade J. *Outing Age: Public Policy Issues Affecting Gay, Lesbian, Bisexual and Transgender Elders.* New York, NY: The Policy Institute of the National Gay and Lesbian Task Force; 2004.

34. Simon A. The relationship between stereotypes of and attitudes toward lesbians and gays. In: Herek GM, ed. *Stigma and Sexual Orientation: Understanding Prejudice Against Lesbians, Gay Men, and Bisexuals.* Thousand Oaks, CA: Sage; 1998:62–81.

35. Shankle MD, Maxwell CA, Katzman ES, Landers JD. An invisible population: older lesbian, gay, bisexual and transgender individuals. *Clin Res & Regul Aff.* 2003;20:159–182.

36. Hunter S. *Midlife and Older LGBT Adults: Knowledge: Knowledge and Affirmative Practices for the Social Services.* New York, NY: The Haworth Press; 2005.

37. O'Hanlan K, Cabaj RP, Schatz, JD, Lock J., Nemrow P. A review of the medical consequences of homophobia with suggestions for resolution. *J Gay Lesbian Med Assoc.* 1997;1:25–39.

38. Claes JA, Moore WR. Issues confronting lesbian and gay elderly: the challenge for health and human services providers. *J Health Hum Serv Adm.* 2001;23:181–202.

39. End-of-life issues and the gay community. *State Initiatives in End-of-Life Care.* April, 2005: 8.

40. Centers for Disease Control and Prevention. *HIV/AIDS Surveillance Report, 2004; 16.* Atlanta, GA: US Department of Health and Human Services, Centers for Disease Control and Prevention; 2005.

41. Grossman, AH. At risk, infected, and invisible: older gay men and HIV/AIDS. *J Assoc Nurses AIDS Care.* 1995;6(6):13–19.

42. Grossman, AH. Older adults. In: Ungvarski P, Flaskerud, JH. *HIV/AIDS: A Guide to Primary Care Management.* 4th ed. Philadelphia, PA: WB Saunders Co., 1999;296–298.

43. Vance DE, Robinson FP. Reconciling successful aging with HIV: a biopsychosocial overview. *J HIV/AIDS Soc Serv.* 2004;3:59–78.

44. Taylor I, Robertson A. The health needs of gay men: a discussion of the literature and implications for nursing. *J Adv Nurs.* 1994;20:560–566.

45. Loughery J. *The Other Side of Silence—Men's Lives and Gay Identities: A Twentieth Century History.* New York, NY: Henry Holt & Co.; 1998.

46. Keogh P, Weatherburn P, Henderson L, Reid D, Dodds C, Hickson F. *Doctoring Gay Men: Exploring the Contribution of General Practice.* London: Sigma Research. www.sigmaresearch.org.uk/downloads/report04d.pdf. Accessed July 15, 2005.

47. Lee C, Owens RG. *The Psychology of Men's Health.* Philadelphia, PA: Open University Press; 2002.

48. Vaid U. *Virtual Equality: The Mainstreaming of Gay & Lesbian Liberation.* New York, NY: Anchor Books; 1995.

49. Nava M, Dawidoff R. *Created Equal: Why Gay Rights Matter to America.* New York, NY: St. Martin's Press; 1994.

50. Jones BE. Is having the luck of growing old in the gay, lesbian, bisexual, and transgender community good or bad luck? *J Gay Lesbian Soc Sev.* 2001;13:13–14.

51. Butler R. Age-ism: another from of bigotry. *Gerontologist.* 1969;9:301–318.

52. Hendricks, J. Ageism: Looking across the margin in the new millennium. *Generations.* 2005:29:5–7.

53. Mail, PD. The case for expanding educational and community-based programs that serve lesbian, gay, bisexual, and transgender populations. *Clin Res Regul Aff.* 2002;19:223–273.

12

Social Discrimination and Health Outcomes in African American, Latino, and Asian/Pacific Islander Gay Men

Rafael M. Díaz, John L. Peterson, and Kyung-Hee Choi

The overrepresentation of gay and bisexual men in negative health indicators—the subject matter of this edited volume—echoes the health disparities observed across ethnic and racial minority groups in the United States; African American and Latino populations in the United States, for example, show higher rates of chronic and infectious diseases, ranging from childhood asthma and diabetes to HIV/AIDS[1,3]. Disparities across ethnic minority groups are also found in a wide range of mental health problems, with documented higher rates of depression, suicide, violence. and substance abuse among poor communities of color.[4] These disproportionate rates of physical and mental health problems remind us that social oppression in the shape of poverty, racial discrimination, and forced patterns of migration has a detrimental, often devastating, impact on the health and well-being of affected communities.[5,6] The US Department of Health and Human Services, in the year 2000, declared the elimination of health disparities as the top priority in the nation's health plan for the current decade.[7] It is thus crucial and timely that we examine health disparities that might be associated with the compounding effects of social discrimination on the basis of sexual orientation, ethnicity, and race.

The present chapter explores issues of social discrimination and health outcomes among men who are self-identified members of ethnic and racial minority groups, and who also report a homosexual, bisexual, or other non-heterosexual orientation (e.g., "queer," "pansexual"), subsequently referred to as "gay men of color." Where scientific evidence is available, we present data that indicate differential rates of health outcomes for specific ethnic and racial minority groups. More importantly, we will examine and document, for African American, Latino and Asian/Pacific Islander (API) gay men, the fact that their physical and mental health is seriously impacted by discrimination on the basis of race, class, and sexual orientation. In this chapter, the descriptors *African American* and *black* are used interchangeably to refer to men of African descent. We have not included data on Native American gay— Two-Spirited—men, due to the fact that the authors' expertise and research is on the three ethnic groups stated in the chapter title. It is important to note, however, that studies of Native American gay men are necessary to gain a full understanding of health disparities among men of color who have sex with men in the United States.

As members of both sexual minority and ethnic minority groups, gay men of color experience discrimination on the basis of their sexual orientation (homophobia) as well as on the basis of their race and ethnicity (racism), with multiple incidents of racial discrimination happening in the context of gay community and same-sex relationships. Many gay men of color also suffer the impact of financial hardship as a result of poverty, and others are often the target of anti-immigration sentiments in the United States on account of their looks and linguistic variations. It is thus not surprising to find that in studies of men who have sex with men (MSM), for example, African Americans and Latinos show disproportionate rates of HIV prevalence and incidence, higher morbidity and mortality rates related to HIV/AIDS, and higher rates of depression.[1,8,9]

Because social discrimination is known to negatively impact health, particularly mental health,[4,5] it is expected that the triple oppressive experiences of gay men of color—poverty, racism, and homophobia—would produce serious health consequences for this population. However, beyond studies concerning their increased HIV risk and a few studies on substance use and mental health outcomes, little is known about the health of gay men of color. Moreover, only a handful of studies have systematically tested specifically the relationship between poverty, racism, and homophobia and health outcomes among gay men of color.

In this chapter we present the relevant data known to date. First, we present what we currently know about experiences of homophobia and racism for African American, Latino, and Asian/Pacific Islander (API) men, including data on poverty and financial hardship whenever available. Second, we present what is known about mental health, substance use/abuse, and HIV risk, including studies that document actual relationships between experiences of discrimination and health among gay men of color, calling for further study on the health impact of multiple minority status, particularly factors of resiliency that must be taken into account and strengthened in future intervention work.

Experiences of Homophobia and Racism

In this section, we present the available data on both perceived negative attitudes toward homosexuality and reported experiences of discrimination on the basis of sexual orientation and gender nonconformity among African American, Latino, and API gay and bisexual men in the US.

African American Men

Research has shown that the majority of African American teenagers, like adolescents from other ethnic groups who engage in homosexual behavior, perceive their friends and neighbors as unsupportive of their homosexuality.[10,11] Similarly, studies of adult MSM show that African Americans are more likely than whites to think their friends and neighbors disapprove of homosexuality, to have sex with women, and to identify as heterosexual.[11] In a study of gay men who attended black gay pride festivals, one-fifth or more of respondents reported negative experiences in black heterosexual organizations, in their families, and in churches or religious institutions.[12] Such perceptions may explain why black adolescents have reported less involvement in gay-related social activities, less comfort with others knowing their sexual identity, and less disclosure of their identity than white adolescents.[13]

While African American adolescent and adult gay males perceive strong anti-gay attitudes in the black community, it must be noted that studies of racial differences in heterosexual attitudes toward homosexuality have yielded mixed results. For example, one study found that blacks were more willing than whites to restrict gay people's civil liberties,[14] while another study found that blacks' attitudes on the morality of homosexuality did not differ from that of whites[15]. A number of studies have found that blacks have significantly more negative attitudes toward homosexuality than whites[16–20]; however, a study conducted more than three decades ago[21] found the opposite effect. Some studies have found no significant racial differences in attitudes toward homosexual populations,[22,23] while other studies have found more positive attitudes among blacks, in comparison to whites, expressing greater approval for the civil rights of gays, lesbians, and transgender persons.[15,19] Most notably, a recent analysis of 31 studies conducted since 1973 shows that blacks are more supportive of gay civil liberties and markedly more opposed to anti-gay employment discrimination than whites, when religious and educational differences are controlled for.[20] To date, it is not clear why African American gay men perceive stronger anti-gay attitudes in the black community, even when the data do not unequivocally support the expected racial differences in negative attitudes toward homosexuality.

In contrast to multiple articles on homophobia in the black community, we found only one study about experiences of racism among black gay, lesbian, bisexual, and transgender populations in the United States.[12] The study was conducted among 2645 participants who completed self-administered questionnaires at "Black Gay Pride" festivals in nine cities (Philadelphia, Houston, Washington DC, Oakland, Chicago, Los Angeles, Detroit, New York, and Atlanta) in the summer of 2000. Most respondents (43%) resided in the South, similar to most African Americans in the United States, and men comprised the majority (58%) of study respondents. Among males, the most common type of reported discrimination was based on racial/ethnic identity (57%), particularly within the mainstream (mostly white) gay community.

Between one-fourth and one-third of male respondents reported negative experiences with white lesbian, gay, bisexual, and transgender (LGBT) people in gay bars and clubs, in white LGBT organizations, at LGBT community events, and in their personal relationships.

Latino Men

The most comprehensive data on experiences of homophobia and racism among Latino gay and bisexual men come from a time/location probability sample of 912 men drawn from Latino gay social venues in three US cities (a study named "Nuestras Voces"[24]). The study was conducted from 1996–2000 in the cities of Miami, Los Angeles, and New York; the three cities were chosen not only because of their obvious regional diversity, but also because they represent the three largest Latino ethnic subgroups in the United States, namely, Cubans in Miami, Puerto Ricans in New York, and Mexicans in Los Angeles. The survey was preceded by a qualitative focus group study ($n = 298$) and, based on the qualitative data, survey items were created that quantitatively measured past experiences of social discrimination on account of race, class, and sexual orientation. The main focus of the study was to document experiences of social discrimination and oppression, and to test their impact on the health and well-being of Latino gay and bisexual men in the United States, particularly their HIV risk.

In the focus group meetings, men spoke about experiencing both verbal and physical abuse, police harassment, and decreased economic opportunities on account of their being gay and/or perceived as effeminate. They spoke about powerful messages—both explicit and covert—in their communities, telling them that their homosexuality made them "not normal" nor truly men; that they would grow up alone without children or families; and that their homosexuality is dirty, sinful, and shameful to many of their families and loved ones. Some men mentioned having to opt for exile and migration in order to live as gay men, away from their families, whom they worried they would hurt if they opted to live openly. And many others admitted that they had to live double lives, pretending to be straight in order to maintain social connections and employment opportunities.

Similarly, men reported multiple instances of discrimination, verbal and physical violence, police harassment, and decreased sexual and social opportunities on account of their being Latino, immigrant, Spanish-speaking, and/or of a darker skin color. Similar to Battle and colleagues' findings[12] with African-American gay men, a great deal of racism was experienced in the context of gay community and gay venues, where men reported not feeling at ease, not feeling welcomed, and some even reported being "escorted out" of venues on account of their different looks, color, or accent. Some men felt sexually objectified by white boyfriends and lovers, who stereotypically paid more attention to their skin color or Spanish accents than to their personal selves. Many of these men felt invisible, that they were just being used as fantasy material, rather than being part of a more authentic and equitable relationship. Many others encountered overt racist rejection in the context of sexual and lover relations.

Many focus group participants also reported experiencing poverty both while growing up and in the present. Men talked about difficulties meeting their day-to-day living expenses and often struggled with inconsistent employment and sources of income. Many reported not having health insurance or access to decent health care. Others reported that they did not have their own place to live and had to rely on friends or relatives for temporary housing. Anger often surfaced among those who were children of Mexican migrant farm workers when remembering the poor conditions of their families of origin, in the face of obvious social inequality. Others had to face the harsh reality of extreme poverty and misery in the inner city, with a deep sense of lack of control and unsettled resignation. Voices from the South Bronx, one of the poorest and more devastated areas in the country, often made an implicit connection between the poverty of the neighborhood and the seeming inevitability of HIV infection.

The subsequent Nuestras Voces quantitative survey confirmed that the overwhelming majority of Latino gay men have experienced homophobia personally and quite intensely: approximately two-thirds of the men (64%) were verbally insulted as children for being gay or effeminate; 70% felt that their homosexuality hurt and embarrassed their family; 64% had to pretend to be straight in order to be accepted; 71% heard as a child that gays would grow old alone; 29% had to move away from their family on account of their homosexuality; and 20% reported instances of police harassment on account of their homosexuality.

Similarly, the data showed that about one-third of Latino gay men have experienced racism in the form of verbal harassment as children (31%) and by being treated rudely as adults on account of their race or ethnicity (35%). One out of four men (26%) have experienced discomfort in white gay spaces because of their ethnicity, and more than one out of five (22%) have experienced racially related police harassment. Interestingly, the majority (62%) reported experiencing racism in the form of sexual objectification from other gay men. The quantitative data also revealed that, within a one-year period, more than half of the sample ran out of money for basic necessities (61%) and had to borrow money to get by (54%). With unemployment rates around 30%, close to one-half of the men (45%) had to look for work in the past year.

Asian/Pacific Islander Men

Research has consistently shown that homosexuality is highly stigmatized by most Asian families and communities.[25–28] In this population, homosexuality is equated with rejection of fundamental cultural values that emphasize the importance of the continuation of the family name by sons; homosexuality is considered a form of social deviance that brings family disorder and shame.

These views are evident in the following quotes by API gay men who were interviewed in the context of two HIV prevention "needs assessment" studies.[26,29]

"Homosexuality is a real stigma, and certainly not to be dealt with openly unless you have been desensitized to it. . . . I don't know how you would deal with it, with a gay son, probably very badly."

"Asian families are not able to acknowledge sexual identity. [This stems from] Asian value of loyalty to family, saving face, and honor."

"I'm the most closeted with the straight Asian Pacific Islander community. There's that whole cultural thing of just feeling like I'm not supposed to be this way."

"The majority of them do not accept these young men and don't care about them. It makes them feel not accepted, he does not belong anywhere in the Asian community."

Although API gay and bisexual men are likely to face homophobic attitudes in their ethnic/racial communities and, if they come out, risk shaming their families, little is known about their experiences of homophobia. Similarly, empirical data on experiences of racism among API gay and bisexual men are scarce. In one of the few studies that document experiences of discrimination within the API gay community, Wilson and Yoshikawa[30] conducted in-depth interviews with 23 API gay and bisexual men in New York City. Participants reported a total of 166 episodes of discrimination experiences, of which 16% were related to homophobia, and almost half (45%) were related to racism.

Beyond Wilson and Yoshikawa's study,[30] additional focus group data[31] reveal qualitative information on experiences of racism among API gay and bisexual men. The majority of focus group participants felt that the mainstream gay community had inaccurate stereotypes of API gay men such as being smart, asexual, and "bottoms" (being an anal receptive sexual partner). Also, all focus group participants reported having been objectified by "rice queens" (a colloquial term used for white men who prefer Asian men as their sexual partners), or exoticized, or reduced to "bodies without souls" by white gay men in general.

The only study to quantitatively assess experiences of homophobia and racism in API gay men was done by Yoshikawa and colleagues[32] in New York City; the study is unique in that it also assessed experiences of anti-immigrant discrimination as well as coping mechanisms to deal with them. Because the study showed strong correlations between experiences of racial discrimination and depression, this study is discussed in more detail under the "mental health" heading below. The published study did not report prevalence rates of experiences of discrimination; however, we were able to obtain from the lead author Hiro Yoshikawa and his collaborator David Chae the rates obtained in the study, which are briefly described in the following paragraph.

The majority of the sample reported experiences of homophobia in childhood, with 77% reporting verbal mockery and ridicule on account of being gay or effeminate at least once in their lifetime (22% reported it happened "many times").[32] One in five men (21%) reported having been physically assaulted on account of their homosexuality as they were growing up. Very notably, close to 90% of the sample reported feeling that their homosexuality hurt and/or embarrassed their family, with 42% feeling that way "many times." Experiences of racism were also frequently reported by study participants, such as being teased or laughed at on account of their race or ethnicity (75%), and on account of their use and/or pronunciation of the English language (42%). Experiences of racism were quite prevalent in the context of the gay community, with 61% reporting being made to feel uncomfortable in a mostly-white gay bar, and 80% reporting racially based sexual objectification in the context of sexual relationships with other men. More than two-thirds (69%) of the men reported that their race and/or ethnicity had been an obstacle to finding boyfriends or developing intimate relationships. It is difficult to compare these results to other studies of MSM of color because of differences in sampling methods and survey questions used to ascertain experiences of discrimination. However, available data suggest that API men may be more likely than African American and Latino men to experience discrimination, especially racism within the white gay community. The percentage of men reporting sexual objectification by white gay men was higher among API respondents (80%) in Yoshikawa and colleagues' study[32] than among Latino respondents (62%) in Díaz and Ayala's study.[24] In Battle and collegaues' study of African American gay men,[12] 57% of the sample reported negative experiences in the mainstream (mostly white) gay community.

Mental Health

African American Men

Evidence is available regarding the effects of gay-related psychological distress on the mental health of African American gay men, including some studies that examined the additional effects of HIV status. The data show a strong relationship between gay-related stressors and negative mental health outcomes for both adolescents and adults, independent of HIV status. For example, in their sample of 136 gay and bisexual predominantly black and Hispanic teenage males, Rosario and colleagues[33] found that stressful life events related to their homosexual or bisexual orientation were related to current levels of emotional distress. In another study with 311 HIV-negative African American adult men—including heterosexual, homosexual, and bisexual men—Richardson and colleagues[34] found that gay/bisexual orientation was a primary predictor of anxiety disorder. Later, the same investigators found high rates of depression or dysthymia (11.5%) in a sample of 243 black gay and bisexual men, noting no significant relationship between HIV status and depression or dysphoric mood.[35]

The negative effects of homophobia on mental health have also been documented among African American HIV-infected men. In their study of

HIV-positive gay men in New York City, Siegel and Epstein[10] reported racial/ethnic differences among 144 HIV-infected black, Hispanic, and white gay men on psychological stressors related to their sexual orientation. African American and Puerto Rican men experienced significantly greater frequency and severity of daily hassles associated with their gay identity than white men, suggesting that psychological stressors related to a homosexual orientation may have more negative consequences for HIV-infected gay men of color, when compared to their white HIV-infected counterparts.

Studies of African-American gay men to date have shown negative mental health outcomes associated with the development of HIV-related symptoms, but not simply in relation to a positive HIV status. For example, a study of 234 black MSM found that HIV-positive status, regardless of disease stage, was not associated with increased risk for anxiety or depressive disorders.[36] On the other hand, Cochran and Mays[9] found that men with symptomatic HIV disease were significantly more distressed than men who were HIV-infected but asymptomatic, HIV-antibody negative, or whose HIV status was unknown. These differences may be due to differences in life stressors and the lack of social support among African American men who experience stigma across multiple social statuses.

Other studies have documented multiple factors of resiliency among African American homosexuals, such as positive social psychological attitudes and effective survival skills that protect men from experiences of homophobia and racism.[37] A few studies of black HIV-positive MSM have examined the association between social support and HIV risk behavior or social support and mental health. A pilot study[38] of 40 HIV-positive MSM found that social support was inversely correlated with mental health problems among black MSM, but not for white MSM. Similar results were reported in a small comparative study[39] of 16 white and 17 black MSM in Detroit, which found marginally significant inverse relationships between material social support from family or friends and mental health outcomes among black MSM, in contrast to strong positive relationships for white men. The authors suggest that their measures of social support may less adequately reflect the social support systems of African American men than those of white men. Peterson, Folkman, and Bakeman[40] examined the associations between stress, physical health, psychosocial resources, coping, and depressive mood in a community sample of 139 African American gay, bisexual, and heterosexual men. Results revealed that psychosocial resources buffered the adverse effects of social and physical stressors, including health symptoms, daily hassles, and life events, on depressive mood.

Latino Men

In their study of 912 Latino gay men in three US cities, Díaz et al[41] measured the frequency of five symptoms of psychological distress, including symptoms related to anxiety and depression, experienced during the last six months prior to the survey. The most frequently reported symptoms were depressed mood and sleep difficulties. During the last six months, an estimated 80% of Latino gay men experienced feelings of sadness and depression at least once or twice during the time period, with 22% experiencing a depressed mood at a relatively high ("many times") frequency. Close to two-thirds of the sample (61%) suffered sleep problems at least once or twice during the previous six months, with 20% experiencing sleep problems many times. Feelings of anxiety (i.e., experiences of fear and/or panic with no apparent reason) and a general feeling of being sick or not well were experienced by about half of the sample, at least once or twice during a six month period. The most serious symptom of psychological distress—thoughts of taking one's own life—was experienced by 17% at least once or twice during a six-month period, with 6% having suicidal ideation a few times or more.

More importantly, the authors showed that psychological symptoms among Latino gay men were strongly predicted by experiences of homophobia, racism, and financial distress. The authors reported strong associations between suicidal ideation and specific experiences of homophobia, racism, and financial hardship within the last six months. Of the 24 Chi-square analyses conducted to test the bivariate association between specific items of social discrimination and suicidal thoughts, 18 (or 75%) were statistically significant; of the remaining six tests, three had marginally significant probabilities between .06 and .10. The multivariate analysis showed that homophobia, racism, and poverty had independent and cumulative effects on symptoms of psychological distress, and that those effects were partially mediated by their negative impact on self-esteem and social support.

More recently, Zea and colleagues[42] studied the relationship between HIV disclosure and mental health outcomes in a sample of 301 HIV-positive Latino gay and bisexual men. Very appropriately, the researchers measured HIV disclosure separately to specific targets (mother, father, closest friend, and main male partner) and to target groupings (family members and close friends). While rates of HIV disclosure to main male partner and closest friend were relatively high (78% and 85%, respectively), disclosure rates to mother (37%) and to father (23%) were very low, controlling for having parents alive after diagnosis. Because HIV status is associated with homosexuality in Latino as well as other communities, the investigators commented that the low level of family disclosure is likely related to homophobia experienced in the context of the immediate family. Because nondisclosure is strongly related to a sense of isolation (47% of the sample reported that after disclosing they felt "less lonely than before"), nondisclosure to family members can have a very negative consequence for Latino men who strongly value family ties and family support. Not surprisingly, the researchers found that HIV disclosure was strongly related to greater quality of social support, higher self-esteem, and lower levels of depression. Further mediational analyses confirmed that quality of social support mediates the effect of HIV disclosure on both depression and self-esteem.

The prevalence of two important markers of mental health problems—childhood sexual abuse (CSA) and intimate partner violence (IPV)—is particularly high among Latino gay men. Data for the Urban Men's Health Study[43] a random-digit telephone probability survey of 2881 adult men who have sex with men (MSM) residing in four US cities, show that Latino MSM were twice as likely to report sexual abuse before age 13 than did non-Latino MSM (22% vs.11%). Similarly, overall rates for different types of IPV in the Nuestras Voces study of Latino gay men are consistently higher than the reported overall (across all ethnic groups) IPV rates for the Urban Men's Health Study. Greenwood et al[44] reported rates of intimate partner "battering" as 34% for psychological/symbolic, 22% for physical, and 5% for sexual battering among all 2881 MSM studied in the Urban Men's Health Study. More recently, Feldman and Díaz[45] reported rates of intimate partner victimization of 45% for psychological, 33% for physical, and 9.5% for sexual victimization among the sample of 912 Latino gay men. Although neither the IPV survey items nor the studies' sampling strategies are exactly comparable, the data from these two probability studies suggest that Latino MSM have much higher rates of different types of IPV, a finding that parallels findings about CSA. Because histories of both childhood sexual abuse and intimate partner violence are strongly correlated with anxiety, depression, and substance-related problems, these data suggest the presence of important disparities in some mental health outcomes for Latino MSM in comparison to those from other ethnic groups.

Asian/Pacific Islander Men

To our knowledge, only two studies have examined API gay and bisexual men's psychological well-being. Choi et al.[46] surveyed 150 API gay and bisexual men in San Francisco and found high rates of psychological distress. Almost all ($n = 146$) reported having ever suffered from depression; of these 146 respondents, 47% reported having been depressed about being gay and some ($n = 7$) reported having had suicidal thoughts. In addition, more than two-thirds (70%) of respondents reported having ever being stressed about being gay.

In a more recent study, Yoshikawa and colleagues[32] found high levels of depressive symptoms in their sample of 192 API gay and bisexual men in New York City. Close to half of the sample (45%) were at risk for clinical depression (scoring above the clinical cutoff of 16 on the Center for Epidemiological Studies-Depression, or CES-D scale) and 29% were at high risk for depression (scoring above the cutoff of 23 on the CES-D scale). The proportion of API men at risk for clinical depression was comparable to that reported in Peterson and colleagues' study (1996)[40] of African American gay and bisexual men (50%), but higher than that reported in Perdue and colleagues' study[47] of white gay and bisexual men (22%). Yoshikawa and colleagues[32] further analyzed their data to investigate the influence of experiences of racism, homophobia, and anti-immigrant discrimination on depressive symptoms. They found a significant association between experiences of racism and higher rates of depressive symptoms, but did not detect such an association for homophobia or anti-immigrant discrimination, even though all three types of discrimination were related to HIV risk, as discussed below.

Substance Use and Abuse

African American Men

Few studies have examined the prevalence of substance use among African American gay or bisexual men or homosexually active men separate from studies of HIV/AIDS. The available studies reveal contradictory findings regarding substance use between African American and other MSM. Some studies[48,49] found comparable or less use of amphetamines, barbiturates or LSD, nitrites, tranquilizers, and powdered cocaine in black than non-black MSM. Other evidence revealed that African American MSM have comparable use of marijuana or heroin as other MSM.[49] Some studies[50,51] found no ethnic differences in hard drug use (i.e., crack, cocaine, heroin, speed) or use of opiates, cocaine, hallucinogens, and other drugs (e.g., ecstasy) between African American MSM and other MSM. In contrast, other studies[52,53] have found that African American MSM were significantly less likely than other MSM to use Diazepam, hallucinogens, or nitrites. There is also mixed evidence regarding ethnic differences in alcohol use between African American MSM and other MSM. Some studies found no differences between African American MSM and other MSM in the prevalence of alcohol use,[54] alcohol-related problems,[51,55] and alcohol use during sexual intercourse.[56] However, other studies found that African American MSM report similar or less alcohol consumption and less dependency on substance use than other MSM.[49,57]

Studies of injection drug use yield equally contradictory evidence regarding ethnic differences in substance use between African American MSM and other MSM. Some studies reported greater injection drug use in African American MSM than in white MSM.[50,52] However, several other studies reported that African American MSM were either equally, or less, likely to use injection drugs in comparison with white MSM.[48,59,60,61] However, African American MSM report substantially greater use of non-injected crack cocaine than white MSM,[52,56] although this may be more apparent for older men, since young African American MSM were either as likely or significantly less likely to report that they ever used crack cocaine in comparison with other young MSM.

Also, despite few ethnic differences, one study[62] found that lifetime substance use, as well as quantity of use and abuse symptoms, was prevalent and frequent across race among gay, lesbian, and bisexual youth. Both number of substances and abuse symptoms were associated with drug use to cope with psychological issues as sexual minorities.

Latino Men

Two studies that involved venue-based probability samples of Latino gay men in large US urban centers (Miami, Los Angeles, New York, and San Francisco) estimate the prevalence of "illicit" substance use at approximately 50%, with over one-third of men reporting regular marijuana use and between 15% and 20% reporting recent use of stimulants, including cocaine, methamphetamine, ecstasy, and amyl nitrate inhalants (poppers). Prevalence data, however, are not yet published and have only been reported in the context of scientific presentations.[63,64] The prevalence data from San Francisco show that rates of substance use in the past six months, particularly stimulants and other so-called "party" or "club" drugs, vary significantly according to the type of venues where men were recruited. Those recruited in mainstream (mostly white) gay venues show higher rates of drug use than those recruited in Latino-identified gay venues (50% versus 37%), suggesting increased use of drugs as a function of increased acculturation and participation in mainstream gay culture.

By far, the highest rates of drug use, particularly stimulants, within Latino MSM populations were found among men who were recruited from Internet sex chat rooms and sex phone lines; of these, 62% reported recent methamphetamine use, 53% recent use of poppers, and 39% recent use of ecstasy. The data also showed that stimulant use and Internet-mediated unprotected casual sexual encounters were strongly related among Latino gay men, as it is often found in studies of (mostly white) gay men. The high prevalence of drug use among Internet users is also reported by Fernández et al[65] in a study of club drug use and risky sex among Latino MSM recruited on Internet chat rooms in Miami. The researchers reported that close to half (48.5%) of those recruited in the Internet study used "club drugs" defined as cocaine (15.8%), crystal meth (11.7%), poppers (31.6%), ecstasy (14%), gamma-hydroxybutyrate (GHB, 3.5%), ketamine (3.5%), and Viagra (19.3%). In multivariate analyses, the use of club drugs was associated with higher number of partners, unprotected receptive anal intercourse, and social isolation. The lower rates of stimulant use found among Miami users in comparison to San Francisco users must be interpreted with caution, given the different recruitment procedures and aims of the two studies, the different Internet sites sampled, and possible cultural differences between East and West Coast drug users.

Latino nationality has been found to be a predictor of illicit drug use during sexual activity, with Puerto Rican MSM showing the highest prevalence (60%) as compared to Dominican (46%), Mexican (40%), and Colombian (31%).[66] The study, including MSM of four different Latino ethnic subgroups residing in New York, showed that difference in illicit drug use among the groups was mostly due to the increased use of stimulants (cocaine/crack and nitrates) by Puerto Rican MSM in the city. The study also showed significant correlations between alcohol and drug use and unprotected anal intercourse with casual partners.

In a recent study of 300 Latino stimulant-using gay men, randomly selected from social and sexual venues in San Francisco, 51% reported methamphetamine, 44% reported cocaine, and 5% reported crack as their most frequently used stimulant.[67] The investigators assessed reasons for use for the participant's specific most frequently used stimulant. Reasons for stimulant use clustered by five main factors, including, in order of reported frequency: energy, sexual enhancement, social connection, coping with stressors, and focused work productivity. Methamphetamine users gave reasons more frequently related to sexual enhancement (to have better sex, more sex, and more anal sex), while cocaine users gave reasons more often related to social connections (to be more sociable and to fit in with other gay men). The findings suggest that Latino gay men use stimulants for reasons that are important in their social, emotional, work, and sexual lives. However, there is no empirical evidence to suggest that reasons or motivations for stimulant use among Latino gay men are qualitatively or quantitatively different from reasons reported by men from other ethnic groups. In fact, similar to studies of non-Latino whites, Latino gay men were found to rely on methamphetamine for reasons related to sexual enhancement, possibly to meet cultural expectations and norms of sexual prowess and sexual success in the gay community.

It is important to note that the most important and most frequently cited reason reported for stimulant use is "energy." Qualitative data from the same study suggest that many Latino gay men rely on stimulants to meet the demand of heavy work schedules and to deal with the exhaustion of highly stressed lives. Stimulant use, particularly the use of methamphetamine and cocaine, plays an important and "functional" role for men who, exhausted by work demands, use the drug in order to participate in the joys of social and sexual life in the context of gay community. Unfortunately, particularly in the case of highly addictive substances like methamphetamine, the "functional" use often becomes "dysfunctional," resulting in a host of negative consequences, including loss of employment, estrangement from partners and friends, physical depletion, and psychological symptoms such as severe depression and paranoia.[68] While increased frequency of use is related to increased acculturation and participation in the mainstream gay community, it is not clear at this time how experiences of social discrimination (both inside and outside the gay community) may play a role in the frequency and patterns of substance use or abuse among Latino gay men.

Differences between Latino MSM and MSM from other racial and ethnic groups regarding illicit drug use can be estimated only indirectly, given that few studies has focused directly on examining racial and ethnic differences in substance use and abuse among MSM. Moreover, most of the studies that provide comparisons tend to have relatively few (less than 10%) Latino MSM in their samples The best comparative data on substance use to date come from the baseline survey of the Community Intervention Trial for Youth (CITY), a multi-ethnic study of 3075 young MSM, ages 15–25 years, recruited in 13 US urban centers through time-location sampling procedures[69,70]; in this study, Latinos comprised the largest proportion (36.6%) of the sample. In Thiede and colleagues'[70] analysis, white MSM showed the highest (71%) prevalence of illicit drug use, closely followed by Latino (67%) MSM, who had the highest rate of the other three ethnic minority groups studied. In a different analysis of the data set, even though Latinos in the sample were more likely than other MSM (OR$=1.76$, $p < .06$) to report unprotected anal intercourse with casual partners, no ethnic or racial differences were found on being "high" during the last sexual encounter with a casual partner.[69] On the other hand, studies of alcohol use among multi-ethnic samples of MSM have shown that Latino young gay and bisexual men show the highest rates of frequent-heavy alcohol consumption[57] and that Latino adult MSM have the highest prevalence of alcohol-related problems.[55]

Asian/Pacific Islander Men

We are aware of only three published papers[70,71,72] that describe the extent of substance use among API gay and bisexual men. The first two papers report data from the Asian Counseling and Testing (ACT) Study that assessed HIV prevalence and related risk factors in the sample of 496 young API gay and bisexual men aged 18–29 years. The ACT study was conducted in San Francisco from 2000 and 2001. The paper by Operario and colleagues[71] shows strikingly high prevalence of substance use among young API gay and bisexual men: during the past six months, 89% used alcohol and 63% used illicit drugs. Ecstasy was the most popular drug reported (47%), followed by marijuana (44%), crystal methamphetamine (20%), ketamine (20%), gamma-amino-butyric acid (GHB; 18%), inhalant nitrites (poppers; 16%), lysergic acid diethylamide (14%), and powder or crack cocaine (10%). The Operario et al. study[71] also showed that 44% of their sample used three or more different types of drugs and 26% used drugs at least once a week in the same six-month time period. Choi et al.[72] reported a high prevalence of substance use during sex among young API gay and bisexual men. Approximately one-third of study participants reported using alcohol (32%) or drugs (34%) during sex in the past six months, respectively. The most frequently used drugs during sex were ecstasy (19%), marijuana (14%), inhalant nitrites (11%), and crystal methamphetamine (10%).

Thiede and colleagues[70] reported findings from the Young Men's Survey, which was a multi-ethnic study of MSM aged 15–22 recruited from seven US cities from 1994 to 1998. According to the Thiede et al. study, use of illicit drugs during the prior six months was lower among APIs (48.5%) compared to African Americans (57.1%), Latinos (66.9%), and whites (70.9%). A similar pattern was observed for frequent use of illicit drugs (at least once a week in the past six months) with 14.2% of APIs, 22.3% of African Americans, 29.7% of Latinos, and 32.5% of whites reporting such a behavior. Polydrug use (using three or more different types of drugs in the past six month) among APIs (18.6%), on the other hand, was higher than among African Americans

(7.4%), but lower than among Latinos (29.9%) and whites (36.4%). The comparison of the Young Men's Survey[70] and the Asian Counseling and Testing (ACT) Study[71] indicates that illicit drug use, polydrug use, and frequent drug use were more prevalent among older API MSM aged 18–29 relative to younger API MSM aged 15–22.

Operario and colleagues[71] examined the correlates of polydrug and frequent drug use using data from the ACT Study. Increased frequency of drug use was associated with having no college degree, disclosing homosexuality to more people, and having had sex under the influence of a substance in the past six months. The researchers also found that polydrug use was associated with being 18 to 24 years old (versus 25 to 29 years old), disclosing homosexuality to more people, going to dance clubs more than once a month in the past six months, having ever attended a "circuit party," having had sex under the influence of a substance in the past six months, and having had unprotected anal sex in the past six months. Similar to the data from Latino gay men, the data on API men suggest that polydrug use is related to greater acculturation and participation in mainstream gay community, a finding that must be explored in more detail.

HIV Risk and Its Predictors

African American Men

In 2005, the Centers for Disease Control and Prevention (CDC) reported that 46% of black MSM in five US cities are estimated to be infected with HIV.[1] However, most studies with large, racially diverse samples of MSM have found that black MSM report comparable, if not lower, rates of UAI and fewer male sex partners than other MSM.[8,50,59,73,74,75,76] Given the puzzling evidence that black MSM show the highest prevalence of HIV infection, but not necessarily the highest prevalence of HIV risk behaviors, there is an urgent need to understand the reasons for these contradictory findings. In their critical review, Millett, Peterson, Wolitski and Stall[77] consider several possible factors—demographic, biomedical, behavioral, interpersonal, sociocultural, and structural—that may combine to influence racial disparity in rates of HIV infection among white and black MSM.

Studies have reported inconsistent results regarding the association between demographic factors (e.g., age, education, income) and HIV risk behaviors.[76,78,79,80] However, some research suggests that seropositive HIV status may reduce unprotected anal intercourse. For example, an earlier study found that black HIV-positive MSM were more likely than black HIV-negative MSM to seek help for risky sexual behavior.[81] A more recent study found that HIV-positive men engaged in fewer sexual risks than HIV-negative men.[80] Similarly, another study found that more black HIV-positive MSM (100%) than black HIV-negative MSM (33%) reported that they used condoms consistently during anal sex with another man.[82] However, the protective influence of HIV-positive status on risk behavior seems less effective among men who have experienced incarceration. A separate report from Wohl's study[83] found that the majority (59%) of the black HIV-positive men in the study had previously been incarcerated, and one-fourth (23%) had engaged in anal sex with men while in custody. Although history of incarceration was unrelated to HIV status, HIV-positive men were significantly less likely than HIV-negative men to use condoms during anal sex while incarcerated, and HIV-positive men reported more sexual partners and more episodes of coercive sex in prison than HIV-negative men. However, since this was a retrospective study, it is unclear if these differences in risk behavior occurred before or after diagnosis with HIV.

Substance use has been studied as a behavioral factor of HIV risk in black MSM. Injection drug use has been associated with unprotected anal intercourse in black gay and bisexual men.[84] Older (50+ years old) black HIV-positive gay and bisexual men were significantly more likely than older white HIV-positive gay and bisexual men to report unprotected vaginal/anal intercourse and a history of intravenous drug use.[58] Black HIV-positive MSM who were aware of their HIV status were significantly less likely than black HIV-negative MSM to report alcohol or drug use during sex.[82] In addition, black gay and bisexual male adolescents who reported alcohol use were more likely to engage in risky sexual behavior.[85]

Men who have sex with men (MSM) now account for the highest rates (49%) of new cases among black men and the highest proportion (46%) of MSM infected with HIV.[95] Also, black men constitute a sizeable proportion (27%) of all MSM diagnosed with AIDS.[95] HIV testing appears to promote a reduction of HIV risk behavior in black MSM. For example, black gay and bisexual men who had taken an HIV test were more likely than those who had never been tested for HIV to seek help (e.g., emotional, social, and tangible assistance) for high-risk sexual behavior.[81] However, many black men who are infected with HIV do not know their status and/or obtain HIV testing long after their HIV infection.[1,86] Moreover, HIV testing has been associated with specific contextual influences—geographic location of the testing site, comfort with the place of testing—in a three-city (Atlanta, Birmingham, and Chicago) sample of black MSM.[87] These findings suggest that the likelihood of structural and sociocultural barriers to HIV testing.

Latino Men

Latino gay men constitute a vulnerable group in the United States for the transmission of HIV, showing disproportionately high rates of HIV infection and unprotected anal intercourse.[88,24] Latino gay men represent over half of all AIDS cases among Latino males in the United States. This percentage is much larger in the Western states, where Latino gay men represent 80% to 90% of all AIDS cases among Latino males. By the end of 2003, a total of

112,595 AIDS cases among Latinos in the United States were attributed to male-to-male sexual contact.

Two large studies that involve probability samples suggest that approximately 20% of Latino gay men of all ages in large US urban centers may be infected with HIV. In a recent household probability sample (Urban Men Health Study; $n = 2,881$) of geographic areas with high concentration of MSM in four different US cities (San Francisco, Los Angeles, Chicago, and New York), a substantial number of Latinos ($n = 246$, or 10% of the sample) were included. In this study, 19% of the Latino sample reported an HIV-positive status.[89] In a second study, a probability sample (Nuestras Voces; $n = 912$) of Latino gay/bisexual men who attend Latino gay venues in the cities of Los Angeles, Miami, and New York yielded a somewhat similar, though slightly higher prevalence of 22%.[63] From these two studies, and taking into account the limitations of self-reporting a stigmatized status, it can be said with some confidence and conservatively that about one in five Latino gay and bisexual men in large US urban centers are infected with HIV.

The latest CDC HIV surveillance data, reported in June 2005, reported the prevalence of HIV among Latino MSM at 17%, this prevalence is lower than the prevalence reported for African American (46%) and white (21%) MSM. However, about 50% of those Latino MSM who were infected did not know their HIV status, similar to the data reported for black gay men. In the largest study to date of young MSM in the United States, CDC researchers reported an HIV prevalence of 14% among Latinos ages 23–29, double the HIV prevalence (7%) of their white same-age counterparts.[8] Also, in the same study, the overwhelming majority (about 70%) of young Latino gay men who were infected did not know their HIV status.

In the Nuestras Voces study, involving a venue-based probability sample of Latino gay men in three US cities, rates of unprotected anal intercourse were 28% (estimated by sexual activity in the last two months) and 37% (estimated by sexual activity with the last two sexual partners within a 12-month period). However, the data from the last two partners suggest that only about half of the 37% of men who report unprotected anal intercourse (or 18% of the sample) do so with a nonmonogamous partner. Thus, it must be noted that a large majority of Latino gay men are genuinely attempting to be safe in their sexual activity, by either condom use and/or monogamy practices.

In Latino gay men, high-risk sexual practices occur in the presence of substantial knowledge about HIV/AIDS and in the presence of relatively strong personal intentions and skills to practice safer sex.[91] HIV risk behavior tends to occur within particular contexts and situations—such as sexual activity aimed to alleviate exhaustion and depression, sexual activity within relationships of unequal power, or sexual activity under the influence of drugs and/or alcohol—where it is subjectively difficult to act according to personal intentions for health and sexual safety.[92] Men, who are knowledgeable, capable of, and skillful at safer sex practices, confess certain helplessness and inability to be safe is those situations that we have labeled "risky." Because the same individual can act safely in some situations and unsafe in others, Díaz and his collaborators have conceptualized "risk" as a property of contexts and situations, rather than as an intra-individual characteristic.

In the Nuestras Voces study, the strongest predictor of unprotected anal intercourse among Latino gay men is participation in those high-risk situations. Furthermore, participation in those difficult and risky situations are strongly predicted by individual and group histories of social discrimination and financial hardship, and to the negative impact of such discrimination and hardships on men's social connectedness and sense of self-worth.[41,24,92] Other studies have shown that histories of childhood sexual abuse and intimate partner violence—highly prevalent among Latino MSM, and closely connected to histories of discrimination based on gender nonconformity and sexual orientation—are also strong predictors of HIV risk in this population.[92,63,94]

Sex under the influence of drugs, particularly methamphetamine, is a high-risk context for HIV transmission among Latino gay men, as is true for MSM of all ethnic and racial groups. In a qualitative study comparing protected and unprotected sexual episodes among Latino, African American, and non-Latino white gay/bisexual men, unprotected anal intercourse was more likely to occur while under the influence of drugs, particularly methamphetamine; this finding was true for all three ethnic groups studied.[88] In a quantitative study, conducted in New York City with a sample of Colombian, Dominican, Mexican, and Puerto Rican MSM, Dolezal et al[66] found strong correlations between drug use and unprotected anal sex among three of the four ethnic subgroups studied. Drug use was predictive of unprotected sex, particularly with casual sexual partners. However, among men who engaged in both protected and unprotected anal sex episodes, substance use was *not* more common on their unprotected episodes. On the other hand, Díaz[68] reports that 72% of methamphetamine users had at least one instance of unprotected anal intercourse in the last six months, which constitutes the highest HIV risk rate ever reported for any Latino MSM subgroup studied to date. Rates of unprotected anal intercourse under the specific most frequently used stimulant were also high, particularly for methamphetamine users in contrast to cocaine users (53% vs. 32 %). The data on self-perceptions of risk confirm the fact that men are well aware that methamphetamine use is closely connected to their risk for acquiring or transmitting HIV.

Asian/Pacific Islander Men

According to the CDC,[95] men who have sex with men (MSM) account for 69% of all cumulative AIDS cases reported through December 2004 among API men in the United States. This figure is comparable to the 73% reported for whites, but is substantially higher than for African Americans (37%) and Latinos (43%). API MSM have relatively lower HIV prevalence compared to other MSM groups. A seven-city survey of MSM aged 15–22 years reported the same 3% HIV prevalence for APIs and whites, but a lower prevalence for APIs relative to Latinos and African Americans (3% vs. 7% and 14%, respectively[8]). A Los Angeles survey[60] of MSM aged 23–29 years reported a similar pattern, in which HIV prevalence was almost equal for APIs and whites (6% vs. 7%), but was lower for APIs compared to Latinos and African Americans (6% vs. 15% vs. 26%). Data from older MSM (aged 18 or over) in four US cities show APIs having the lowest HIV prevalence (9%), followed by whites (16%), Latinos (19%), and African Americans (29%).[89]

Although API MSM have much lower rates of HIV infection compared to African American, Latino, and possibly white MSM, they engage in unprotected anal intercourse at very high rates, some of which are similar or greater than those reported for other ethnic groups. A survey[60] of MSM aged 23–29 years in Los Angeles found equivalent rates of unprotected insertive anal intercourse in the past six months among APIs, Latinos, and African Americans (38%, 39%, and 33%, respectively) and similar rates of unprotected receptive anal intercourse among APIs and African Americans (29% vs. 24%). A four-city study[96] of MSM aged 17–25 years found comparable rates of unprotected anal intercourse during the six-month time period for APIs and whites (39% vs. 36%), but a higher rate for APIs relative to African Americans (39% vs. 30%). A 13-city survey[76] of MSM aged 15–25 years showed similar patterns of unprotected anal intercourse in the past three months (28% APIs, 24% whites, 17% African Americans).

Studies show that individual characteristics affect HIV risk among API gay and bisexual men. Being American-born is strongly associated with HIV infection.[97] Being more comfortable about disclosing homosexual behaviors to others[46] and self-identifying as gay or bisexual were related to having unprotected anal intercourse.[99] These data are consistent with the finding that greater risk for HIV and substance use is correlated with increased acculturation and participation in the mainstream gay community. Similar to data on black gay men, having never been tested for HIV is another predictor for having unprotected anal intercourse among API gay men.[99]

Substance use has a powerful influence on sexual risk for HIV among API gay and bisexual men.[29,46,73,100] Choi and colleagues[46] identified using alcohol or drugs during sex as the most significant independent factor associated with risky sex in their study of API men. Respondents who used substances during sex were five times more likely to engage in unprotected anal intercourse than those who did not use substances during sex. A more recent study of young API gay and bisexual men revealed that having unprotected anal intercourse varies by substance choice.[72] Using ecstasy or inhalant nitrites during sex is associated with unprotected anal intercourse, whereas using marijuana, GHB, and crystal methamphetamine during sex was not. Moreover, data from the same study[97] showed a significant association between HIV seropositivity and attending multiday large MSM gatherings or "circuit parties" where "club" drugs such as ecstasy, GHB, and crystal methamphetamine are widely used. HIV infection was more than six times higher among respondents who had ever attended a "circuit party" than among those who had not, even after controlling for demographic characteristics and number of sexual partners.

Characteristics of sexual partnerships influence HIV risk among API gay and bisexual men. An HIV prevalence survey of API men aged 18–29 years found that having 51 or more lifetime sexual partners was associated with HIV infection.[97] A study of API men aged 15–25 years found that having a larger number of sexual partners and having sex with a steady partner were associated with having unprotected anal intercourse.[99] In a study of older API men aged 18–39 years, however, having one or two sexual partners (versus four or more partners) and having a steady partner were related to having unprotected anal intercourse.[101] In addition to number of sexual partners and relationship status, sexual partners' age and ethnicity were linked to having unprotected anal intercourse among API men aged 18–39 years.[101]

Several sociocultural factors have been shown to affect HIV-related risk behaviors among API gay and bisexual men. One qualitative study of API MSM aged 18–25 years found that the lack of communication about sex and support around homosexuality within API families as well as sexual norms and attitudes perceived in the gay and API communities (e.g., sexual freedom, stereotypes, and homophobia) contribute to sexual risk-taking in young API MSM.[100] In one quantitative study of older API gay and bisexual men (aged 18 years or older)[32] respondents who had experienced anti-immigrant discrimination were more likely to engage in unprotected anal intercourse with nonsteady partners, and those who had never talked to their family about discrimination were more likely to engage in unprotected anal intercourse with their steady partner. Safer sex peer norms were another factor associated with unsafe sexual practices. A study of young API MSM aged 15–25 years found that those who perceive that their friends endorse safer sex were less likely to engage in unprotected anal intercourse.[99] The same association between safer sex peer norms and unprotected anal intercourse was observed among older API gay and bisexual men (aged 18 years or over).[46]

Conclusion

In this chapter, we have presented an overview of what is currently known, both from qualitative and quantitative studies, about experiences of social discrimination and health outcomes among gay men of color in the United States. The data show that gay men of color do in fact report extensive experiences of discrimination on the basis of sexual orientation, race/ethnicity, and immigration status. The findings regarding experiences of racism in the gay community, particularly in the context of social, sexual, and romantic relationships, is troubling, considering that many gay men of color who participate in the gay community are looking for a welcoming and accepting environment to express and live their same-sex desires. Because of the additive and cumulative effects of multiple sources of discrimination, it is not surprising that cross-ethnic comparisons tend to show increased rates of depression and HIV infection among gay men of color. The available evidence suggests that increased rates of physical and mental health problems may be partially explained by factors commonly related to ethnic minority status, such as racial discrimination, financial hardship, and lack of access to care.

The relation between social discrimination and disease is typically inferred from differences in health statistics *between* groups who are differentially disadvantaged, discriminated and oppressed, such as the observed health disparities among African-American and Latino populations in the United States. Seldom have studies measured and examined specific factors of discrimination as they impact the health, behavior, and risk of individuals *within* the most affected groups. Such analyses within specific groups affected by social discrimination are essential to understand both the specific lived experiences and the specific mechanisms by which oppression impacts the most affected individuals within those groups. In this chapter, we have presented not only between-ethnic group differences in health indicators, when available, but also data from three studies that have shown direct relationships between experiences of homophobia, racism, poverty, and a number of health indicators, particularly symptoms of psychological distress and HIV risk.[41,91,33,32] However, data from three studies are certainly not enough to understand the complexity and diversity regarding the impact of social discrimination on the health of gay men of color. We need more within-ethnic group studies, particularly studies that can focus on ways that social discrimination may result in the observed negative health disparities.

Our review of the literature reveals some important convergent findings, as well as gaps in our understanding of the issues at hand. The gross overrepresentation of African American and Latino men who have sex with men (MSM) in the HIV epidemic, for example, is an issue of extreme concern to all of us. However, there is little understanding of why this is the case. Perhaps the most important unanswered question in this field of investigation is why black and Latino MSM have such high rates of HIV infection in comparison to their white and API counterparts when, in fact, the rates of HIV risk behavior do not seem to consistently differ across ethnic groups. Current thinking suggests that different patterns of sexual mixing—that is, the different characteristics of sexual partners and the patterns of relation to them—may account for the disparities, and that such patterns of sexual mixing might be predicted by factors of social and racial inequality. However, Millett and colleagues[77] review the available research and examine 12 hypotheses to identify potential explanations for this racial disparity and conclude that there is insufficient evidence to explain it.

A major gap in the literature is the lack of studies regarding sources of resiliency and strength. How are gay men of color coping with experiences of discrimination? What seems to help? What does not? Beyond some studies regarding the importance of social support, as demonstrated among African

American men by Peterson and colleagues,[40] little is known about resiliency factors. Among API men, Yoshikawa and colleagues[32] have shown that specific conversations with family and friends about experiences of discrimination can serve as a protective factor. Díaz and colleagues[41] measured factors of resiliency among Latino gay men, including family acceptance, social and sexual satisfaction, and participation in social activism. All these factors predicted increased self-esteem and a greater sense of social connection, which are in turn important predictors of better mental health and lower HIV risk (see also Ramírez-Valles and Díaz[102]). Above all, we believe that interventions are most likely to succeed when they are designed to support and enhance naturally occurring sources of resiliency and strength in the given communities. The lack of information about resiliency among gay men of color is thus a very serious gap that hinders our current and future efforts to intervene. In addition, the striking scarcity of evaluated interventions for non-white MSM[103] raises the need for an expansion of intervention trials, especially at the community level. Structural and environmental interventions offer a greater possibility to address the effects of social networks and social norms on HIV risk reduction[78] and the pervasive influence of stigma and discrimination that impede behavior change.

References

1. Centers for Disease Control and Prevention. HIV prevalence, unrecognized infection, and HIV testing among men who have sex with men—five US cities, June 2004-April 2005. *MMWR.* 2005;54:597–601.
2. Kington RS, Smith JP. Socioeconomic status and racial and ethnic differences in functional status associated with chronic diseases. *Am J Public Health.* 1997;87: 805–810.
3. Williams DR, Collins C. U.S. socioeconomic and racial differences in health: patterns and explanations. *Annu Rev. Sociol.* 1995;21:349–386.
4. Williams DR, Neighbors HW, Jackson JS. Racial/ethnic discrimination and health: findings from community studies. *Am J Public Health.* 2003;93:200–208.
5. Krieger N. Embodying inequality: a review of concepts, measures, and methods for studying health consequences of discrimination. *Int J Health Serv.* 1999;29: 295–352.
6. Krieger N. Discrimination and health. In: Berkman L and Kawachi I, eds. *Social Epidemiology.* New York, NY: Oxford University Press; 2000:36–75.
7. US Department of Health and Human Services. *Healthy People 2010.* Vol I. Washington, DC: US Government Printing Office; 2000.
8. Valleroy L, MacKellar D, Karon J et al. HIV prevalence and associated risks in young men who have sex with men. *JAMA.* 2000;284:198–204.
9. Cochran S, Mays V. Depressive distress among homosexually active African American men and women. *Am J Psychiatry.* 1994;151:524–529.
10. Siegel K, Epstein JA. Ethnic-racial differences in psychological stress related to gay lifestyle among HIV-positive men. *Psychol Reports.* 1996;79:303–312.
11. Stokes JP, Vanable PA, McKirnan DJ. Ethnic differences in sexual behavior, condom use, and psychosocial variables among Black and White men who have sex with men. *J Sex Res.* 1996;33:373–381.

12. Battle J, Cohen CJ, Warren D, Fergerson G, Audam S. Say it loud: I'm Black and I'm proud. Black pride survey, 2000, Policy Institute of the National Gay and Lesbian Task Force. 2000;41–47.

13. Rosario M, Schrimshaw EW, Hunter J. Ethnic/racial differences in the coming-out process of lesbian, gay, and bisexual youths: a comparison of sexual identity development over time. *Cultur Divers Ethnic Minority Psychol.* 2004;10: 215–228.

14. Dejowski EF. Public endorsements of restrictions on three aspects of free expression by homosexuals: socio-demographic and trends analysis, 1973–1988. *J Homosex.* 1992;23:1–18.

15. Bonilla, L, Porter J. A comparison of Latino, Black and non-Hispanic White attitudes toward homosexuality. *Hispanic J Behav Science.* 1990;12(4):437–452.

16. Hudson WW, Ricketts WA. A strategy for the measurement of homophobia. *J Homosex.* 1980;5:357–372.

17. Schneider W, Lewis IA. The straight story on homosexuality and gay rights. *Public Opinion.* 1984;7:16–20, 59–60.

18. Ernst FR, Nevels FH, Lemeh C. Condemnation of homosexuality in the Black community: a gender-specific phenomenon? *Arch Sex Behav.* 1991;20:579–585.

19. Loftus J. America's liberalization in attitudes toward homosexuality: 1973–1998. *Am Soc Rev.* 2001;66:762–782.

20. Lewis GB. Black-White differences in attitudes toward homosexuality and gay rights. Public *Opinion Quart.* 2003;67:59–78.

21. Levitt EE, Klassen AD. Public attitudes toward homosexuality: part of the 1970 National Survey by the Institute for Sex Research. *J Homosex.* 1974;1:29–43.

22. Alcalay R, Sniderman PM, Mitchell J, Griffin R. Ethnic differences in knowledge of AIDS transmission and attitudes towards gays and people with AIDS. *Intl Quart Community Health Educ.* 1990;10:213–222.

23. Herek GM, Capitanio JP. Black heterosexuals' attitudes toward lesbians and gay men in the United States. *J Sex Res.* 1995;32:95–105.

24. Díaz, R.M., Ayala, G. *Social Discrimination and Health: The Case of Latino Gay Men and HIV Risk.* New York, NY: The Policy Institute of the National Gay and Lesbian Task Force; 2001

25. Aoki B, Ngin CP, Mo B, Ja DU. AIDS prevention models in Asian-American communities. In: Mays VM, Albee GW, Schnedier SF, eds. *Primary Prevention of AIDS.* Hanover, NH: University of New England Press; 1989:290–308.

26. Choi K, Yep G, Kumekawa E. HIV prevention among Asian and Pacific Islander American men who have sex with men: a critical review of theoretical models and directions for future research. *AIDS Educ Prev.* 1998;10(Supplement A):19–30.

27. Wong FY, Chng CL, Ross MW, Mayer KH. Sexualities as social roles among Asian and Pacific Islander American gay, lesbian, bisexual, and transgender individuals: Implications for community-based health education and prevention. *J Gay Lesbian Med Assoc.* 1998;2:157–166.

28. Chng CL, Wong FY, Park RJ, Edberg MC, Lai DS. A model for understanding sexual health among Asian American/Pacific Islander men who have sex with men (MSM) in the United States. *AIDS Educ Prev.* 2003 Feb;15(1 Suppl A):21–38.

29. Nemoto T, Operario D, Soma T, Bao D, Vajrabukka A, Crisostomo V. HIV risk and prevention among Asian/Pacific Islander men who have sex with men: listen to our stories. *AIDS Educ Prev.* 2003;15(1 Suppl A):7–20.

30. Wilson PA & Yoshikawa H. Experiences of and responses to social discrimination among Asian and Pacific Islander gay men: their relationship to HIV risk. *AIDS Educ Prev.* 2004;16:68–83.

31. Ona FF, Cadabes C, Choi K. [Focus groups with gay Asian and Pacific Islander men in San Francisco]. Unpublished data, 1996.

32. Yoshikawa H, Wilson PA, Chae DH, Cheng JF. Do family and friendship networks protect against the influence of discrimination on mental health and HIV risk among Asian and Pacific Islander gay men? *AIDS Educ Prev.* 2004;16:84–100.

33. Rosario M, Rotheram-Borus, MJ, Reid H. Gay-related stress and its correlates among gay and bisexual male adolescents of predominantly Black and Hispanic background. *J Community Psychol.* 1996;24:136–159.

34. Richardson M, Myers, H, Bing E, Satz P. Substance use and psychopathology in African American men at risk for HIV infection. *J Community Psychol.* 1997;25: 353–370.

35. Richardson MA, Satz P, Meyers HF, Miller EN, Bing EG, Fawzy FI, Maj M. Effects of the depressed mood versus clinical depression on neuropsychological performance among African American men impacted by HIV/AIDS. *J Clin Exp Neuropsychol.* 1999;21:769–783.

36. Myers, HF, Durvasula RS. Psychiatric disorders in African American men and women living with HIV/AIDS. *Cult Diversity Ethnic Minority Psychol.* 1999;5:249–262.

37. Edwards W. A sociological analysis of an invisible minority group: male adolescent homosexuals. *Youth Soc.* 1996;27:334–355.

38. Ostrow DG, Whitaker RE, Frasier K, Cohen C, Wan J, Frank C, Fisher E. Racial differences in social support and mental health in men with HIV infection: a pilot study. *AIDS Care* 1991;3:55–63.

39. Grant LM, Ostrow DG. Perceptions of social support and psychological adaptation to sexually acquired HIV among White and African American men. *Soc Work.* 1995;40:215–224.

40. Peterson JL, Folkman S, Bakeman R. Stress, coping, HIV status, psychosocial resources and depressive mood in African American gay, bisexual and heterosexual men. *Am J Community Psychol.* 1996;24:461–487.

41. Díaz RM, Ayala, G, Bein E, Henne J, Marin BV. The impact of homophobia, poverty and racism on the mental health of gay and bisexual Latino men: findings from 3 U.S. cities. *Am J Public Health.* 2001;91:927–932.

42. Zea MC, Reisen CA, Poppen P.J., Bianchi F. T., Echeverry JJ. Disclosure of HIV status and psychological well-being among Latino gay and bisexual men. *AIDS Behav.* 2005;9:15–26.

43. Arreola SG, Neilands TB, Pollack LM, Paul JP, Catania J.A. Higher prevalence of childhood sexual abuse among Latino men who have sex with men than non-Latino men who have sex with men: Data from the Urban Men's Health Study. *Child Abuse Negl.* 2005;29:285–290.

44. Greenwood GL, Relf MV, Huang B et al. Battering victimization among a probability sample of men who have sex with men. *Am J Public Health.* 2002;92:1964–1969.

45. Feldman MB, Díaz RM. Intimate partner violence and HIV sexual risk in Latino gay men: the role of sexual self-efficacy and participation in difficult sexual situations. Paper presented at the conference of the Society for Social Work and Research, San Antonio, TX. January 2006.

46. Choi K, Coates TJ, Catania JA, Lew S, Chow P. High HIV risk among gay Asian and Pacific Islander men in San Francisco. *AIDS.* 1995;9:306–308.

47. Perdue T, Hagan H, Thiede H, Valleroy L. Depression and HIV risk behavior among Seattle-area injection drug users and young men who have sex with men. *AIDS Educ Prev.* 2003;15:81–92.

48. Harawa NT, Greenland S, Bingham TA, et al. Associations of race/ethnicity with HIV prevalence and HIV-related behaviors among young men who have sex with men in 7 urban centers in the United States. *J Acquir Immune Defic Syndr.* 2004;35: 526–536.

49. McNall M, Remafedi G. Relationship of amphetamine and other substance use to unprotected intercourse among young men who have sex with men. *Arch Pediatr Adolesc Med.* 1999;153:137–154.

50. Siegel K, Scrimshaw EW, Karus D. Racial disparities in sexual risk behaviors and drug use among older gay/bisexual and heterosexual men living with HIV/AIDS. *J Natl Med Assoc.* 2004;96:215–223.

51. Irwin TW, Morgenstern J. Drug-use patterns among men who have sex with men presenting for alcohol treatment: differences in ethnic and sexual identity. *J Urban Health.* 2005;82(Suppl 1):i127–i133.

52. Sullivan PS, Nakashima AK, Purcell DW, Ward JW. Geographic differences in non-injection and injection substance use among HIV-seropositive men who have sex with men: western United States versus other regions. *J Acquir Immune Defic Syndr Hum Retrovirol.* 1998;19:266–273.

53. Halkitis PN, Green KA, Mourgues P. Longitudinal investigation of methamphetamine use among gay and bisexual men in New York City: findings from Project BUMPS. *J Urban Health.* 2005;82:18–25.

54. Heckman TG, Kelly JA, Bogart LM, Kalichman SC, Rompa DJ. HIV risk differences between African-American and White men who have sex with men. *J Natl Med Assoc.* 1999;91:92–100.

55. Stall R, Paul JP, Greenwood G, et al. Alcohol use, drug use and alcohol-related problems among men who have sex with men: the Urban Men's Health Study. *Addiction.* 2001;96:1589–1601.

56. McKirnan DJ, Vanable PA, Ostrow DG, Hope B. Expectancies of sexual "escape" and sexual risk among drug and alcohol-involved gay and bisexual men. *J Subst Abuse.* 2001;13:137–154.

57. Greenwood GL, White EW, Page-Shafer K, et al. Correlates of heavy substance use among young gay and bisexual men: the San Francisco Young Men's Health Study. *Drug Alcohol Depend.* 2001;61:105–112.

58. Siegel K, Scrimshaw EW, Karus D. Racial disparities in sexual risk behaviors and drug use among older gay/bisexual and heterosexual men living with HIV/AIDS. *J Natl Med Assoc.* 2004;96:215–223

59. Easterbrook PJ, Chmiel JS, Hoover DR, et al. Racial and ethnic differences in human immunodeficiency virus type 1 (HIV-1) seroprevalence among homosexual and bisexual men. *Am J Epidemiol.* 1993;138:415–429.

60. Bingham T, Hawara N, Johnson E, Secura G, MacKellar D, Valleroy L. The effect of partner characteristics on HIV infection among African American men who

have sex with men in the Young Men's Survey, Los Angeles, 1999–2000. *AIDS Educ Prev.* 2003;15:39–52.

61. Kunawararak P, Beyrer C, Natpratan C, et al. The epidemiology of HIV and syphilis among male commercial sex workers in northern Thailand. *AIDS.* 1995;9:517–521.

62. Rosario M, Hunter J, Gwadz M. Exploration of substance use among lesbian, gay, and bisexual youth: prevalence and correlates. *J Adoles Res.* 1997;12:454–476.

63. Díaz RM, Ayala G, Bein E. Substance use and sexual risk: findings from the national Latino gay men's study. Presentation at the seminar Sexual Scripts Revisited: International and Interdisciplinary Perspectives in Sexuality and HIV/AIDS Research. HIV Center for Clinical and Behavioral Studies, New York, NY. March 1999.

64. Díaz RM, Heckert AL, Sánchez J. Fabulous effects, disastrous consequences: stimulant use among Latino gay men in San Francisco. Presentation at the National Institute on Drug Abuse, Washington DC. March 2004.

65. Fernández MI, Perrino T, Collazo JB, et al. Surfing new territory: club-drug use and risky sex among Hispanic men who have sex with men recruited on the Internet. *J Urban Health.* 2005;82, No. 1, Supplement 1.

66. Dolezal C, Carballo-Diéguez A, Nieves-Rosa L, Díaz F. Substance use and sexual risk behavior: understanding their association among four ethnic groups of Latino men who have sex with men. *J Subst Abuse.* 2000;11:323–336.

67. Díaz RM, Heckert A L, Sánchez J. Reasons for stimulant use among Latino gay men in San Francisco: A comparison between methamphetamine and cocaine users. *J Urban Health.* 2005;82 (Supplement 1):i71–i79.

68. Díaz RM. Methamphetamine use and its relation to HIV risk: data from Latino gay men. In: I. Meyer and M. Northridge, eds. *The Health of Sexual Minorities: Public Health Perspectives on Lesbian, Gay, Bisexual and Transgender Populations.* New York, NY: Springer, 2006.

69. Stueve A, O'Donnell L, Duran R, San Doval A, Geier J. Being high and taking sexual risks: findings from a multisite survey of urban young men who have sex with men. *AIDS Educ Prev.* 2002;14: 482–495.

70. Thiede H, Valleroy LA, MacKellar DA, Celentano DD, Ford WL, Hagan H, et al. Young Men's Survey Study Group. Regional patterns and correlates of substance use among young men who have sex with men in 7 US urban areas. *Am J Public Health.* 2003;93:1915–1921.

71. Operario D, Choi KH, Chu PL, et al. Prevalence and correlates of substance use among young Asian Pacific Islander men who have sex with men. *Prev Sci.* 2006;7:19–29.

72. Choi K, Operario D, Gregorich SE, McFarland W, MacKellar D, Valleroy L. Substance use, substance choice, and unprotected anal intercourse among young Asian and Pacific Islander men who have sex with men. *AIDS Educ Prev.* 2005;17:418–429.

73. Lemp GF, Hirozawa AM, Givertz D, et al. Seroprevalence of HIV and risk behaviors among young homosexual and bisexual men: the San Francisco/Berkeley young men's survey. *JAMA.* 1994;272:449–454.

74. Mansergh G, Marks G, Colfax GN, Guzman R, Rader M, Buchbinder S. Barebacking in a diverse sample of men who have sex with men. *AIDS.* 2002;14:653–659.

75. Montgomery JP, Mokotoff ED, Gentry AC, Blair JM. The extent of bisexual behaviour in HIV-infected men and implications for transmission to their female sex partners. *AIDS Care.* 2003;15:829–837.

76. Peterson J, Bakeman R, Stokes J. The community intervention trial for youth study team: racial/ethnic patterns of HIV sexual risk behaviors among young men who have sex with men. *JGLMA.* 2001;5:155–162.

77. Millett G, Peterson JL, Wolitski RL, Stall R. Greater risk for HIV infection of black men who have sex with men (MSM): a critical literature review. *Am J Public Health.* 2006;96:1007–1019.

78. Hart T, Peterson J. Predictors of risky sexual behavior among young African-American men who have sex with men. *Am J Public Health.* 2004;94:1122–1123.

79. Crawford I, Allison KW, Zamboni BD, Soto T. The influence of dual-identity development on the psychosocial functioning of African-American gay and bisexual men. *J Sex Res.* 2002;39:179–189.

80. Myers HF, Javanbakht M, Martínez M, Obediah S. Psychosocial predictors of risky sexual behaviors in African-American men: implications for prevention. *AIDS Educ Prev.* 2003;15:66–79.

81. Peterson JL, Coates TJ, Catania JA, Hilliard B, Middleton L, Hearst N. Help-seeking for AIDS high-risk sexual behavior among gay and bisexual African-American men. *AIDS Educ Prev.* 1995;7:1–9.

82. Wohl AR, Johnson DF, Lu S, et al. HIV risk behaviors among African-American men in Los Angeles County who self-identify as heterosexual. *J Acquir Immune Defic Syndr.* 2002;31:354–360.

83. Wohl AR, Johnson D, Jordan W, et al. High-risk behaviors during incarceration in African-American men treated for HIV at three Los Angeles public medical centers. *J Acquir Immune Defic Syndr.* 2000;24:386–392.

84. Peterson JL, Coates TJ, Catania JA, Middleton L, Hilliard B, Hearst N. High-risk sexual behavior and condom use among gay and bisexual African-American men. *Am J Public Health.* 1992;82:1490–1494.

85. Rotheram-Borus MJ, Rosario M, Meyer-Bahlburg HFL, Koopman C, Dopkins SC, Davies M. Sexual and substance use acts of gay and bisexual male adolescents in New York City. *J Sex Res.* 1994;31:47–57.

86. Centers for Disease Control and Prevention. HIV/STD risks in young men who have sex with men who do not disclose their sexual orientation—six U.S. cities, 1994–2000. *MMWR.* 2003;52:581–586.

87. Mashburn AJ, Peterson JL, Bakeman R, Miller RL, Clark LF. Community Intervention Trial for Youth Study Team. Influences on HIV testing among young African-American men who have sex with men and the moderating effect of geographic setting. *J Community Psychol.* 2004;32:45–60.

88. Díaz RM. Trips to Fantasy Island: contexts of risky sex for San Francisco gay men. *Sexualities.* 2;1:89–112.

89. Catania JA, Binson D, Dolcini M, et al. The continuing HIV epidemic among men who have sex with men. *Am J Public Health.* 2001;91:907–914.

90. Díaz RM. *Latino Gay Men and HIV: Culture, Sexuality and Risk Behavior.* New York, NY: Routledge; 1998.

91. Díaz RM, Ayala G, Bein E. Sexual risk as an outcome of social oppression: data from a probability sample of Latino gay men in three US cities. *Cult Divers Ethnic Minority Psychol.* 10;3:255–267.

92. Caraballo-Diéguez A, Dolezal C. Association between history of childhood sexual abuse and adult HIV-risk sexual behavior in Puerto Rican men who have sex with men. *Child Abuse Negl.* 1995;19:595–605.

93. Díaz RM, Morales E, Bein E, Dilán E, Rodríguez R. Predictors of sexual risk in Latino gay/bisexual men: the role of demographic, developmental, social cognitive and behavioral variables. *Hisp J Behav Sci.* 1999;21:480–501.

94. Nieves-Rosa LE, Carballo-Diéguez A, Dolezal C. Domestic abuse and HIV-risk behavior in Latin American men who have sex with men in New York City. *J Gay Lesbian Soc Serv.* 2000;11:77–90.

95. Centers for Disease Control and Prevention. *HIV/AIDS Surveillance Report, 2004.* Atlanta, GA: US Department of Health and Human Services, Centers for Disease Control and Prevention; 2004;16:1–46.

96. Ruiz J, Facer M, Sun R. Risk factors for human immunodeficiency virus infection and unprotected anal intercourse among young men who have sex with men. *Sex Transm Dis.* 1998;25:100–107.

97. Choi K, McFarland W, Neilands T, et al. An opportunity for prevention: prevalence, incidence, and sexual risk for HIV among young Asian and Pacific Islander men who have sex with men, San Francisco. *Sex Transm Dis.* 2004;31:475–480.

98. Choi K, Cortes J, Lew S, Chow P, Coates TJ. AIDS risk, dual identity, and community response among gay Asian and Pacific Islander men in the United States. In: Herek GM, Greene B, eds. *AIDS, Identity, and Community: The HIV Epidemic and Lesbians and Gay Men.* Thousand Oaks, CA: Sage; 1995:115–134.

99. Choi K, Han C, Hudes ES, Kegeles S. Unprotected sex and associated risk factors among young Asian and Pacific Islander men who have sex with men. *AIDS Educ Prev.* 2002;14:472–481.

100. Choi K, Kumekawa E, Dang Q, Kegeles SM, Hays RB, Stall R. Risk and protective factors affecting sexual behavior among young Asian and Pacific Islander men who have sex with men: implications for HIV prevention. *J Sex Educ Ther.* 1999;24:47–55

101. Choi K, Operario D, Gregorich SE, Han L. Age and race mixing patterns of sexual partnerships among Asian men who have sex with men: implications for HIV transmission and prevention. *AIDS Educ Prev.* 2003;15:53–65.

102. Ramírez-Valles J, Díaz RM. Public health, race, and the AIDS movement: the profile and consequences of Latino gay men's community involvement. In: Omoto A, ed. *Processes of Community Change and Social Action.* Mahwah, NJ: Lawrence Erlbaum Associates; 2005:51–66.

103. Johnson WD Semaan S Hedges LV, Ramirez G Mullen PD Sogolow E. A protocol for the analytical aspects of a systematic review of HIV prevention research. *J Acquir Immune Defic Syndr* 2002;30(Suppl 1):S62–72.

13

Access to Optimal Care among Gay and Bisexual Men: Identifying Barriers and Promoting Culturally Competent Care

Rajeev Ramchand and Claude Earl Fox

Optimal health care can be defined as "providing the right service at the right time in the right place."[1] As the previous chapters of this book have indicated, gay and bisexual men have unique health care needs; what is considered optimal for their straight peers might not be optimal for them.

In this chapter, we provide an in-depth description of the barriers facing gay and bisexual men's access to optimal health care in the United States and identify key practices that health care providers can adopt when caring for these men and actions that policymakers can pursue to remove certain barriers. We begin with a discussion of unequal access to health insurance for gay and bisexual men and then highlight the impact that HIV and AIDS, as well as current legislative policies that do not recognize same-sex relationships, can have on this access. We then turn to the health care relationship and identify barriers that prevent gay and bisexual men from accessing optimal care in medical settings, as well as strategies that health care providers can employ to ensure that their gay and bisexual patients do receive optimal care. We also highlight the unique issues that both younger and elder gay and bisexual men face in accessing optimal health care, as well as health care access issues faced by black/African American men who have sex with men (MSM).

Access to Health Insurance Coverage

In the United States, health insurance is one of the most crucial elements impacting access to health care. People who lack health insurance are less likely to receive preventive medical care, more likely to be hospitalized for avoidable health problems, and more likely to be diagnosed with diseases at their later stages.[2] According to analyses conducted by the Kaiser Commission on Medicaid and the Uninsured, 45 million Americans, or 18% of people under age 65, lacked health insurance in 2004.[2] Recent analyses of data from six years (1997–2003) of the National Health Interview Survey indicated that men in same-sex relationships ($n = 316$) were less likely to have health insurance than men in opposite-sex relationships ($n = 42,856$). This difference approached, but did not achieve, statistical significance (OR = 0.70, 95% confidence interval [CI] = 0.50, 1.06).[3] Somewhat paradoxically, men in same-sex relationships had equal or greater access to care than did men in opposite-sex relationships. Although this study was based on a large representative sample, the number of men in same-sex relationships was relatively small. In addition, this finding can not be generalized to men who are not involved in relationships or to those who do not identify themselves in surveys in this way.

Gay and bisexual men may face particular challenges when attempting to access health insurance. In 2000, the Kaiser Family Foundation conducted a telephone survey of 405 self-identified gay, lesbian, and bisexual respondents in 15 major metropolitan areas. Their report highlighted that almost 50% of respondents reported that they were either discriminated against when attempting to obtain insurance because of their sexual orientation or that they knew someone else who was.[4]

As will be discussed in the section that follows, gay and bisexual men may face impediments to accessing health insurance for a variety of reasons. Since the 1980s, the costs associated with treating patients with HIV and AIDS, combined with the disease's increased prevalence among gay and bisexual men compared to the general population, has negatively impacted the abilities of some gay and bisexual men, including those living with HIV and AIDS, to obtain health insurance. Many gay and bisexual men in committed relationships are also prevented from accessing health insurance benefits from their partners' employer-sponsored health plans, an option that is often available for their married, heterosexual counterparts. Finally, gay and bisexual men may be unable to access health insurance because, like their heterosexual counterparts, they may be members of families for whom health insurance is not available at the workplace or is unaffordable.

The Impact of HIV and AIDS on Gay and Bisexual Men's Access to Health Insurance

Risk classification, defined as the practice of classifying individuals for insurance coverage based on their disease risk potential, emerged in the US health insurance market in the 1940s when commercial coverage policies entered the market.[5] In response to this practice, by the 1960s every US state and the District of Columbia had passed an Unfair Trade Practices Act. Although designed to prohibit unfair discrimination, the Acts "have been interpreted not only as a protection against differential treatment for individuals of the same risk but also as justification for differential treatment among individuals of different risk."[5]

The practice of risk classification by insurers has impacted many gay and bisexual men's ability to access health insurance. The AIDS epidemic began in the early 1980s, heralded by increased reports of gay men presenting with unusual cancers and pneumonia.[6] Almost as soon as the epidemic began, researchers and advocates became concerned about how individuals with the disease would pay for the required medical care. Others turned their attention to the impact that the HIV epidemic would have on those individuals considered to be at greatest risk of becoming infected, including gay and bisexual men.

There are three broad means by which most individuals in the United States access health insurance: privately, through an employer, or from a government-subsidized health program. Under each category, gay and bisexual men may face discrimination due to their perceived risk of HIV infection, which can adversely affect their ability to obtain health insurance.

In general, individuals in the United States with the greatest risk of facing insurance discrimination are those people who access private individual insurance coverage. In the individual insurance market, consumers' protections from discrimination vary widely and "very much depend on where they live, their coverage history, and other factors."[7] As will be discussed below, individual insurance is generally unavailable for persons with HIV and AIDS. Private individual insurers have also been shown to discriminate against people whom they believe to be gay men. In her 1996 legal analysis, Li highlighted cases in which insurance companies refused coverage to individuals suspected to be gay men because of their perceived higher risk of HIV infection.[8] In one of the legal cases Li referenced, which was settled in 1990, an insurance company had instructed its salespeople to ask only single male applicants without dependents in nonphysically demanding occupations (specifically noting waiters and hairdressers) whether they had experienced significant weight gain or loss, "deviations" from good health, or whether they had been treated or tested for any sexually transmitted disease or immune disorder during the past 12 months.[8]

Individuals who access health insurance by means of a group health plan provided by their employers are generally protected from discrimination based on their health or "risk status" because individuals with preexisting conditions may not be excluded from group coverage.[5] On the other hand, gay and bisexual men are not as systematically protected from discrimination due to their sexual orientation when obtaining the jobs themselves. As of June 2006, only 16 states and the District of Columbia (though many more cities and counties) prohibited discrimination on the basis of sexual orientation in employment. According to the National Gay and Lesbian Task Force, in 2005, 53% of the US population lived in areas where employers were legally permitted to discriminate against gay, lesbian, and bisexual individuals when making hiring decisions, thereby affecting these individuals' ability to access employer-sponsored insurance.[9] In one survey, close to 50% of lesbians, gay men, and bisexuals living in metropolitan areas of the United States reported either experiencing discrimination themselves because of their sexual orientation, or knowing somebody who was discriminated against when applying for or maintaining employment.[4]

Small businesses, especially those that insurers deem more likely to employ gay men, have also been found to face obstacles when attempting to obtain insurance coverage for their employees. For example, in a 1991 survey of insurance companies and agents, respondents indicated that hair salons were often ineligible for or restricted from being offered small group health insurance because they posed a "triple threat—high employee turnover with little interest in long-term employment, a high proportion of women of child-bearing age, and a high proportion of homosexual men."[10]

Gay men may also face barriers to accessing government-subsidized health insurance. In general, non-elderly adults who access government-subsidized health insurance rely primarily on Medicaid. Although eligibility requirements vary across states, the Medicaid program generally covers three groups of non-elderly, low-income individuals: children, their parents, and persons with disabilities.[3] In other words, adults in the United States most likely to qualify for Medicaid are low-income individuals with children. Gay and bisexual men are less likely to have children than their heterosexual counterparts, thereby creating another impediment in their ability to access health insurance, even if they have a low income.

Health Insurance for Persons with HIV/AIDS

HIV/AIDS has had and continues to have a profound impact on the lives of many gay and bisexual men. In 2004, approximately half of the reported prevalent HIV/AIDS cases in the United States were attributed to men who have sex with other men.[11] From 2000 to 2004, the estimated number of HIV/AIDS cases transmitted through male-to-male sexual contact increased.[11] It would be remiss not to discuss the coverage challenges facing persons with HIV/AIDS today.

Much progress has been made since the start of the AIDS epidemic in treating patients, including the introduction of the first antiretroviral, AZT, and the subsequent development of several medications that have resulted in highly active antiretroviral therapy (HAART). In 2004, the current average annual cost of treating a person with HIV/AIDS in the United States ranged from $18,000 to $20,000 and could be even higher for individuals with advanced HIV-related illnesses.[12] The patchwork of policies designed to care for individuals with the disease highlights the insurance industry's unwillingness to provide coverage to patients with HIV/AIDS.

Title I of the Americans with Disabilities Act of 1990 prohibits employers from discriminating against persons with HIV/AIDS in hiring, firing, and other employment-related decisions. In addition, if HIV-infected individuals leave their jobs involuntarily (for reasons other than gross misconduct) or voluntarily (e.g., become too sick to work), they are entitled to continue their health insurance coverage via the Consolidated Omnibus Budget Reconciliation Act (COBRA) passed in 1996. Generally, COBRA guarantees individuals access to continuation of their health insurance for 18 months after they leave their jobs or reduce their work hours. This coverage can be extended beyond 18 months if individuals can prove that they became disabled within the first 60 days of their insurance coverage. If they cannot extend their COBRA coverage, the only available options are private insurance and Medicaid. In a 2001 report, the Kaiser Family Foundation found that persons with HIV/AIDS have little to no hope of accessing individual private insurance.[7] Medicaid benefits, on the other hand, only become available to patients if they are "poor enough" and disabled.

For persons with HIV/AIDS, both the COBRA extension policy and Medicaid qualification policies present a "Catch-22" situation. For each plan, an individual is considered disabled only if he meets the Supplemental Security Income (SSI) definition of disability, which is the inability to engage in any "substantial gainful activity by reason of a medically determined physical or medical impairment expected to result in death, or that has lasted or can be expected to last for a continuous period of at least 12 months"; as of 2004, eleven states impose even more stringent criteria.[12] However, much of the current treatment for HIV-infected persons is designed specifically to impede or delay the onset of such disability. Furthermore, starting HAART late in the course of HIV infection has resulted in worse health outcomes and reduced survival.[13,14] In other words, an economically disadvantaged individual with HIV may not be able to receive the treatments designed to maintain his otherwise good health or prevent disability until he is actually very sick or disabled.

Because of the gaps in health care coverage for HIV-infected persons living in the United States, the federal government authorized the Ryan White Care Act in 1990, and reauthorized the program in 1996, 2000, and 2006. This is an insurance program administered by states designed specifically for uninsured or underinsured individuals living with HIV, and it is estimated that more than 500,000 HIV-infected individuals and their families fill the gap in their insurance coverage by using Ryan White funds.[15] Eligibility requirements for the Ryan White program vary widely across states, and because client-level data are generally not reported, it is unclear whether gay and bisexual men with HIV/AIDS have disproportionate access to these funds. However, it is clear that statewide variation in Ryan White Programs results in unequal access to care across the country. The primary example is differences in the AIDS medications available through the Ryan White AIDS Drug Assistance Programs (ADAP) in various states.

Marriage and Domestic Partner Benefits

As mentioned above, employer-sponsored health insurance is currently the most common source of health insurance in the United States for both employees and their family members. National estimates indicate that 62% of non-elderly American adults with health insurance are covered by employer-sponsored plans. Approximately half of these adults are covered by their own employer, while the other half are covered by virtue of being dependents of a worker.[2] Although there is no legislation that requires employers to provide or offer health insurance to their employees, in 2004, 99% of firms with over 200 employees and 63% of firms with fewer than 200 employees did so.[16]

In 1996, the so-called Defense of Marriage Act (or DOMA) defined marriage as exclusively heterosexual and proclaimed that states are not required to recognize same-sex marriages performed in other states.[17] Although no same-sex marriages had yet been performed in the United States, this legislation barred individuals in committed same-sex relationships from being defined as their partners' dependents in the future. As such, gay men and lesbians in committed relationships are denied access to health insurance that may be offered to their heterosexual married counterparts through one member of the family's workplace.

Some employers have confronted this systematic discriminatory practice by establishing domestic partner benefits. Although these benefit plans vary, they generally extend fringe benefits, including health insurance, to unmarried same-sex partners. In a 2004 survey of 1,925 randomly selected employers, 14% of all firms offered health benefits to same-sex couples, with larger firms (over 5,000 workers) more likely to offer these benefits than smaller firms.[16] According to proprietary research methods developed by the Human Rights Campaign, as of 2006, over 9,000 employers in the United States offered same-sex domestic partner benefits. A little over half of the Fortune 500 companies, 8695 private sector companies, 13 state governments, 139 city and county governments, and 298 colleges and universities also offered domestic partner benefits to their employees.[18]

Although domestic partner benefits may alleviate some of the barriers to accessing health insurance experienced by gay and bisexual men, they differ from the employer-sponsored benefits available to heterosexual workers' dependents in certain ways. Most importantly, for heterosexual couples who are married, contributions made by an employer or employee to cover an employee's dependents are considered tax-free for both state and federal income taxes. In comparison, if an individual opts to have his partner covered as a domestic partner, the premium contribution is typically treated as taxable income. However, in California, Massachusetts, Vermont, Oregon, and the District of Columbia, contributions from an individual's gross income to cover domestic partner premium contributions are exempt from state income taxes. Additionally, New Jersey now permits an additional personal exemption for state taxes for a registered domestic partner, and parties to a civil union in Connecticut are also exempt from state income taxes for moneys used to access domestic partner benefits.

The Uninsured: A Large and Diverse Group

Close to 45 million people, or approximately 18% of Americans under age 65, lack health insurance. The uninsured come largely from families that are poor or nearly poor yet who have one or more full-time workers. Most uninsured are adults, American citizens, and minorities.[2] The policies and processes that impede poor working families from accessing health insurance also affect gay and bisexual men who are members of these disadvantaged groups. In a qualitative study of black men who have sex with men in New York and Georgia, insurance coverage was a commonly mentioned barrier to health care, with one respondent stating "[T]hat's been my goal, to get a job with insurance. Because if you don't have insurance, it's like you don't exist."[19]

Recommendations for Removing/Reducing Barriers to Health Insurance Coverage

There are a variety of policy responses that could address the barriers in access to health insurance coverage faced by many gay and bisexual men in the United States. These range from policies that expand health insurance coverage generally to research designed to more specifically define barriers to coverage. In addition, policies that prevent employment discrimination and that recognize same-sex couples would also positively impact gay and bisexual men's ability to access health insurance.

Reform the Health Insurance Market

Advocates have proposed a variety of policy options and ideas to fill the gaps in insurance coverage that currently leave 45 million individuals in the United States without health insurance. These range from a single plan that covers all Americans to plans that build on the current mix of privately and publicly funded insurance coverage. In its 2006 report, the Kaiser Commission on Medicaid and the Uninsured highlighted three different strategies being proposed that all aim to extend coverage to the uninsured.[2] They are: (1) expanding coverage for low-income populations by building on programs like Medicaid, particularly by offering coverage to low-income adults without children; (2) bolstering employer-sponsored insurance plans, including offering financial incentives to employers who offer insurance coverage; and (3) subsidizing the cost of private individual health insurance, including offering tax credits or deductions to help with costs.

In the recent past, the number of employers offering health insurance for their employees has fallen from 69% to 60%.[16] As workplace health insurance coverage becomes less available, individuals may increasingly rely on private individual insurance, especially if current policies that promote participation in these markets (e.g., tax credits and deductions) are adopted. In the current private individual insurance market, the cost of coverage varies with respect to age, sex, and geographic location.[7] As mentioned above, protections against discrimination also vary widely in this market.[7] Future research should monitor this market closely, including studying the extent to which men may be discriminated against based on their likelihood of being gay or bisexual.

Persons with HIV/AIDS face unique hurdles in accessing health insurance and care in the United States. Primary among these is the fact that access to care for these individuals varies widely across states. Researchers and policy makers interested in addressing access to care among persons with HIV/AIDS should thus work within states to identify specific barriers to care as well as differences in the quality of care afforded to individuals, specifically those who are uninsured, publicly insured, and minority Americans. Policy and public health research that looks across states can also identify policies and strategies that states have adopted to promote access to care among persons with HIV/AIDS. Of note, efforts are needed to reduce the variability in access to care across states to ensure that persons with HIV/AIDS face more equitable access to care, including access to medications for HIV/AIDS, across the country.

Prevent Workplace Discrimination

Most people with health insurance in the United States access this insurance as a benefit offered by their employers.[2] In many areas in the United States, employers are legally permitted to discriminate against individuals when making employment decisions; thus lesbian, gay, bisexual, and transgender (LGBT) individuals may have inequitable access to employer-sponsored coverage. Although proposed in 1994, the US Congress failed to pass the Employment Nondiscrimination Act (ENDA) that would have made discrimination in employment based on sexual orientation illegal. Still, organizations such as the National Gay and Lesbian Task Force (the Task Force) are calling for a lesbian, gay, bisexual, and transgender Civil Rights Law that would make discrimination against LGBT individuals in employment and other areas (housing, education, public accommodations, and credit) illegal. Until this occurs, the Task Force recommends that the US Equal Employment Opportunity Commission monitor complaints in which individuals claim to have been discriminated against based on their sexual orientation and gender identity.[20]

Recognize Same-Sex Couples

Federal and most state policies currently impede same-sex couples from civil marriage, thereby denying these couples' ability to access social security benefits and taxing any contributions made to their partner's health benefits. In 1996, Congress passed the so-called Defense of Marriage Act (DOMA), which "allows" states the ability to not recognize same-sex marriages performed in other states.[17] In addition, DOMA defines marriage as being between members of the opposite sex, meaning that the federal government does not recognize a same-sex marriage performed in a state. In June 2006, the US Senate voted on legislation that aimed to amend the US constitution to define marriage as between a man and woman, though this legislation was defeated.

In spite of these discriminatory federal policies, same-sex couples are continuing to pursue their right to marry, though this is occurring primarily within states. As of June 2006, one state (Massachusetts) issued marriage licenses to same-sex couples, and four states (New Jersey, New Mexico, New York, and Rhode Island) and the District of Columbia did not have laws prohibiting marriage between same-sex couples. On the other hand, most other states have passed laws or even amended their state constitution to define a marriage as between a man and woman, and many states have explicit laws that prohibit recognition of same-sex marriages performed in other states.[21] However, many of these laws are being challenged in the courts. For example, in Maryland, the Baltimore City Circuit Court ruled in January 2006 that the state's ban on marriage for same-sex couples violated the state constitution's equal rights amendment.[22]

In the absence of civil marriage benefits between same-sex couples, civil rights groups should continue to advocate for fair treatment for the costs that LGBT individuals incur when accessing health insurance on behalf of their partners. In fact, there is momentum across states to exempt contributions made toward domestic partner contributions from state taxes. Since January 2006, the District of Columbia has enacted a law to this effect. On the other hand, state bills in Maryland and New York that would allow individuals to take deductions on their state taxes for health insurance and other medical expenses incurred on behalf of a same-sex domestic partner did not pass.[23]

The Health Care Relationship

Even if a gay or bisexual man has health insurance, he may face additional challenges in receiving optimal care from his health care provider. Gay or bisexual men may be wary of disclosing their sexuality to their health care providers, and/or their providers may be unknowledgeable about, or unwilling to provide, the type of care that their patients require.

Disclosure of Sexual Identity

By disclosing their sexual orientation to health care providers, gay or bisexual men present their providers the opportunity to better tailor health care. Though limited in scope, most research indicates that around two-thirds of adult gay men report that their primary health care providers know of their sexual orientation. In the Kaiser Family Foundation's 2001 survey of lesbian, gay, and bisexual respondents from 15 US metropolitan areas, 44% of respondents reported that their health care providers had asked about their sexual orientation, and 64% said that they had voluntarily revealed this information to their providers.[4] In 2002, a survey revealed that bisexual men and women were much less likely to disclose their sexual orientation to their health care providers than were lesbians or gay men.[24] Young gay and bisexual men are also less likely to report their sexual orientation to their providers than are older gay and bisexual men: 78% of a group of approximately 100 gay men, lesbian women, and bisexual men and women between the ages of 18 and 23 years reported having never discussed their sexual orientation with their health care providers when they were between the ages of 14 and 18.[25]

Gay and bisexual patients withhold information about their sexuality from their health care providers for a variety of reasons. Like everyone else, gay and bisexual men pass through developmental stages when establishing their own personal identities, and acceptance of their sexuality will vary during these periods. Gay and bisexual men also typically pass through stages unique to the process of "coming out." At the beginning of this process, a boy or man begins to develop vague feelings of attraction to people of the same sex, which is usually followed by actual sexual behaviors with other boys or men. The process continues as the man labels himself as homosexual, discloses his sexual identity to others, has a same-sex relationship, and eventually integrates his homosexuality into his personality.[26] During this process, some men may experience feelings of internalized homophobia, which "occurs when homophobic cultural messages are incorporated into the LGBT person's own self-concept."[27] Internalized homophobia is likely to influence the information that gay and bisexual men choose to reveal to their health care providers, and may even impede their willingness to seek care. Some gay and bisexual men fear a negative judgmental response from their health care providers or the provision of substandard care. Such fears may be justified—a survey of members of the Gay and Lesbian Medical Association (GLMA) found that 67% of physicians reported witnessing a gay or lesbian patient receiving substandard care because of his or her sexual orientation (we discuss the topic of providers' attitudes toward gay and bisexual patients in more detail in the following section).[28]

Health care providers serve both themselves and their patients well by notating all relevant information with respect to a patient's health and care in that patient's medical record. The privacy offered to these records, however, varies widely by state and legal jurisdiction. In general, these records might be shared with other health care providers in the case of a referral, to an individual's health insurance company, and even to an employer if a company self-insures.[29] Records may also be subpoenaed or requested in the event of a civil lawsuit or criminal investigation. Parents also typically have the right to review their child's medical record if the child is under the age of 18. If gay and bisexual men are worried about the privacy of their records or the possibility of a disclosure of information, they might also be less likely to report their sexual orientation to their health care providers.

Provider Attitudes

Provider attitudes toward their gay and bisexual patients are likely to influence not only their patients' willingness to disclose their sexual orientation, but also the care that providers offer to these patients. In a 1989 study of provider attitudes toward gay patients, only 33% of physicians reported feeling comfortable with gay men.[30] More recently, however, results from the Kaiser Family Foundation's 2001 National Survey of Physicians indicated that 92% of physicians reported that they would be "comfortable" treating a patient who was openly gay or lesbian, and only 6% said that they would be uncomfortable caring for a patient who identified him- or herself this way.[31]

The relatively low prevalence of anti-gay sentiment among physicians noted above is also seen in health care providers' attitudes toward their gay and lesbian colleagues. For example, in a 1996 survey of New Mexico physicians, only 4% said that they would deny accepting openly gay men and lesbians to medical schools.[32] On the other hand, there is some evidence of increased prevalence of anti-gay sentiment when physicians are probed about whether gay men and lesbians should pursue certain medical specialties. In the same survey of New Mexico practitioners referenced above, 10% said that gay men and lesbians should be discouraged from seeking obstetrics/gynecological training, and 11% said that they would discontinue referring patients to obstetricians/gynecologists, pediatricians, and urologists who they learned were gay or lesbian.[32] Furthermore, in a 1996 survey of family practice residency directors, one-quarter reported that they might rank an applicant lower if they knew that he or she was homosexual.[33]

An unfortunate episode at one US medical school suggests that some administrators may still hold anti-gay attitudes that are likely to affect the training that future health care providers receive. In 2004, the New York Medical College (NYMC) revoked the charter of the school's group, NYMC Lesbian, Gay, Bisexual and Transgender People in Medicine. Although the president of the student senate reported that the revocation did not reflect that the school was "against education related to homosexual medical issues/medical concerns/medical care," the student asserted that the club's proposed activities "would be in conflict with the Catholic Church."[34] The Gay and Lesbian Medical Association (GLMA) publicly decried the school's decision to revoke the charter, and the college later reinstated the group.[34–36]

Recommendations

In order to better care for gay and bisexual patients, providers can adopt strategies to foster open discussion between themselves and their patients.

These strategies include creating safe physical spaces for gay and bisexual patients and adopting terms and phrases that are unassuming and nonjudgmental. In addition, the training of health care professionals regarding the unique needs of their lesbian, gay, bisexual, and transgender patients will ultimately benefit the care that these individuals receive.

Improve the Health Care Environment

In its "Provider's Handbook on Culturally Competent Care: Lesbian, Gay, Bisexual and Transgender Population," Kaiser Permanente advises health care providers and their staff that "any person who walks into a provider's office could self-identify as LGBT and/or have a history of relationships with members of the same sex."[27] With this in mind, it is important that providers create environments that facilitate open and frank discussions between themselves and their patients. For gay and bisexual patients, this could mean providing physical cues in the office and/or waiting room, training staff, and creating intake and record forms sensitive to LGBT issues.

Health care providers' practice spaces can include visible cues that indicate to gay and bisexual patients that providers are accepting of all sexual orientations. The Gay and Lesbian Medical Association (GLMA) suggests that waiting rooms and examining rooms can display posters showing same-sex couples or brochures on health-related topics pertinent to gay and bisexual men. In addition, a visible nondiscrimination statement that emphasizes equal care to all patients, regardless of age, race, ethnicity, physical ability or attributes, religion, sexual orientation, and gender identity can also help achieve more welcoming environments.[37] Prominently displayed LGBT symbols, such as pink triangles or rainbow flags, can also help promote open dialogue between health care providers and gay and bisexual men, and may be particularly important in school-based and university health clinics.

Members of health care providers' staffs are vital components of the health care team and should also be trained to be mindful of the respect necessary to provide optimal care for gay and bisexual patients. For example, providers and their staff should be instructed to avoid telling insensitive jokes and using derogatory language. Providers and their staff should also be mindful of the media (radio and television programs) that are audible to patients within the health care environment and should make efforts to minimize the likelihood of a patient hearing inappropriate comments through these media outlets. Providers and staff should also be very sensitive to the families of gay and bisexual patients. For example, same-sex partners should be treated with the same respect given to the spouses of heterosexual patients, and same-sex couples who have children should be given the same respect offered to heterosexual parents.

Intake forms can also be tailored to foster an atmosphere of openness and respect. These forms should avoid using gender-specific pronouns limited to heterosexual relationships. Instead of the terms *husband* or *wife*, providers can use the terms *partner*, *life partner*, or *spouse*. For young patients, the terms "*parent*" or "*parents*" can be used instead of the gender-specific terms *mother* or *father* to accommodate gay families. Providers should also use terms that show respect for gay couples. For example, forms can be written to include the terms *partnered* or *other* (with a space for explanation) in addition to traditional marital status categories such as single, married, divorced, or widowed. Finally, GLMA indicates that providers might want to consider including on intake forms a question about sexual identity, and lists as potential options: straight/heterosexual, lesbian, gay, bisexual, queer, other (leave space for patient to fill in), not sure, and "don't know."[37]

Foster Communication and Ensure Confidentiality

As with the intake forms described above, health care professionals should be mindful of the language that they use when communicating with all of their patients. When talking about sexual behaviors and/or relationships, health care providers should use gender-neutral terms and pronouns. Providers should take cues from their patients about how the patients describe themselves, and use terms such as *gay* or *bisexual* only when the patient has already used the term to describe himself first.

Health care providers should also make it a priority to inform patients of their privacy rights at both patient intake as well as during the patient interview. In a study of 100 gay, lesbian, and bisexual youth, those informed of their right to medical confidentiality were more than three times more likely to have discussed their sexual orientation with their providers.[25] Providers should develop a protocol for handling information concerning their patients' sexual orientation and should inform their patients—particularly their young patients—of their procedures for documenting and protecting such information. Providers should also be aware of the confidentiality rights to which patients are entitled under the Health Insurance Portability and Accountability Act (HIPAA) of 1996. Like all patients, LGBT patients should also be aware of their privacy rights under HIPAA, and can access resources such as those created by the Health Privacy Project (www.healthprivacy.org) to learn about these rights.

Improve Sexual Histories and Risk Assessment

For preventive purposes, it is important that health care providers incorporate sexual risk assessment into routine patient visits. However, the frequency with which physicians perform risk assessments varies. In one study that videotaped interactions between physicians and patients, physicians often exhibited uneasiness or discomfort and changed the topic of conversation when patients made statements or cues related to HIV risk.[38] Health care providers' performance of sexual risk assessments is also related to their patients' presenting symptoms, with providers more likely to take comprehensive sexual histories when patients report symptoms associated with HIV-related disease (e.g., prolonged diarrhea, dyspnea and fever, sore throat with white spots on the tongue).[39]

When taking sexual histories, health care providers should again reflect those terms used by their patients. Most medical schools suggest a pattern of questioning such as asking first whether the patient is sexually active, and if the patient responds "yes," asking whether the patient has sex with men, women, or both.[40] Providers are then encouraged to discuss specific sexual behaviors. Providers should become familiar and comfortable with terms (including colloquial references) related to sexual practices for both their homosexual and heterosexual patients and should be prepared to answer questions about the risks associated with specific behaviors and strategies to minimize these risks. Health care providers should also be prepared to apologize to patients who seem upset or offended by certain questions, particularly those regarding their sexual orientation. If patients are upset by these questions, providers should be ready to explain why this information is pertinent to the provision of optimal patient care. The use of computers to assist in taking sexual histories, such as audio computer-assisted self-interviews (ACASI) in health clinics, may also elicit more frequent reporting of sensitive behaviors.[41]

Improve Education for Health Professionals

It was acknowledged in the early 1990s that medical schools were doing a poor job in teaching future health care providers about treating gay and bisexual men, as well as lesbians and bisexual women. In 1991, US medical schools spent, on average, four hours training their students on homosexuality, most of which was taught in lectures on human sexuality and not integrated throughout the entire curriculum.[42] In a 1998 study, close to half of all US medical schools with departments of family medicine reported spending no time training their medical students on homosexuality or bisexuality.[43]

In 1996, the American Medical Association advocated that medical schools devote more attention to training their students on the health care needs of gay men and lesbians.[44] Medical schools that have begun to educate their students about the needs of their LGBT patients have used a variety of methods to do so. Members of the University of Massachusetts Medical School and Tufts University of Medicine created a cross-clerkship (internal medicine, family medicine, pediatrics, and psychiatry) curriculum for third-year medical students that covered a variety of topics in sexuality.[45] Another medical school saw benefits in sexual history taking and HIV counseling among students who participated in a four-hour standardized patient workshop teaching these skills, which was incorporated into the ambulatory internal medicine clerkship.[46] Seminars for residents on the unique health care needs of lesbians and gay men have also yielded promising findings.[47]

It is important that all future health care providers are trained about the health care needs of lesbian, gay, bisexual, and transgender clients. This includes not only physicians, but also nurses, dentists, paramedics, emergency medical technicians, residential and occupational therapists, psychologists and other mental health counselors, and medical/nursing assistants.

Encourage the Government to Promote Access to Care

Government can play an active role in improving access to care for gay and bisexual men in the United States. The June 2001 American Journal of Public Health described both state and federal programs to improve access to care for LGBT individuals.[48] In Massachusetts, the Department of Public Health funded a project that developed standards of practice for the health care services provided to LGBT patients and a training curriculum that was offered to providers to help implement these standards.[49] The US Substance Abuse and Mental Health Services Administration's (SAMHSA) Center for Substance Abuse Treatment not only created a primer on LGBT substance abuse treatment, but also conceived a dissemination plan to accompany the document, including training and technical assistance and program evaluation tools such as intake forms. In addition, the agency created both an internal and external work group on LGBT issues.[50]

Access to Care for Unique Gay and Bisexual Populations

Other chapters of this book provide a thorough evaluation of the unique experiences and health needs of gay and bisexual young adults (Chapter 10), older men (Chapter 11), and men of color (Chapter 12). Here, we provide a brief overview of the issues in access to care that are unique to these populations. To help address the barriers to care that these men, and often their lesbian, bisexual female, and transgender counterparts might face, we provide general recommendations for policy makers and health care providers.

Young Gay and Bisexual Men

Adolescent gay and bisexual men are a unique group of young men who face a great deal of both familial and societal adversity. Such adversity is likely to affect these young men and their health behaviors. In many ways, adolescent gay and bisexual men are no different from their peers, though they may be at increased risk for certain adverse health events.[51] In the United States, rates of HIV infection are disproportionately higher among men under the age of 25 years, many of whom report homosexual contact as the primary exposure category.[52] Gay, lesbian, bisexual, and transgender youth have an increased risk of suicide ideation and attempts, the third leading cause of adolescent mortality.[53] Gay and bisexual youth are also more likely to report use of alcohol and illegal substances, including marijuana, cocaine, inhalants, and hallucinogens.[54,55]

Recommendations

Providers face a challenge when attempting to meet the health needs of gay and bisexual youth. Youth may be at very different stages of their own self-discovery and coming-out process, thereby affecting the likelihood that they will disclose their sexual orientation to their health care providers. Still, providers can surmount this obstacle by adopting some useful clinical tools similar to those recommended for their adult patients.

Providers should not assume that their young patients are heterosexual and should avoid posing their questions to male patients about female partners or using terms such as *girlfriends*. In addition, health care providers may consider asking their young patients whether they are attracted to females, males, or both. This question could be followed by asking patients to rate, on a scale, their level of attraction to males and females. The use of a scale could provide health care providers with the opportunity to discuss sexual feelings and attractions while avoiding using terms such as *gay* and *bisexual*, which could make the young patient uncomfortable.[27]

When a gay or bisexual adolescent patient reveals his sexual orientation to his health care provider, it presents the provider with the opportunity to provide tailored care. With this entree, the health care provider can address the risks that gay and bisexual young men may face, and can facilitate the adoption of strategies to prevent suicide, sexually transmitted infections, and drug use. Providers may want to suggest support services that may exist for gay youth in the area, and warn their patients about the potential dangers of meeting other gay men on the Internet or using false identification to enter gay clubs or bars.[27] Providers should also remember that if the youth does not appear to be in immediate danger, providers should avoid disclosing the patient's sexual orientation to any other adult.

Parents may respond in a variety of ways to their children who reveal themselves as gay, lesbian, bisexual, or transgender. Some parents may show complete acceptance, others may wonder "what they have done wrong." Others may react in ways that will adversely affect the health of their children, from considering "reparative therapy," hormone treatment, shock therapy, or boot camps that claim to "change" young people's sexual orientation. Some parents also force their children out of the home; these children often become homeless and resort to unsafe sexual behaviors, such as prostitution, to survive.[27]

Providers should be able and willing to talk with parents whose children reveal that they are gay, bisexual, lesbian, or transgender. Providers should assist and support parents whose children come out and, if need be, offer or suggest counseling. Providers should also be familiar with support services for families and friends of lesbian, gay, and bisexual individuals, such as Parents, Friends and Families of Lesbians and Gays (PFLAG).

Elderly Gay and Bisexual Men

As the US population ages, there will be a parallel increase in the number of older gay and bisexual men. The National Gay and Lesbian Task Force estimates that there are one to three million LGBT Americans over age 65 and that by 2030, roughly four million elderly Americans will be gay, lesbian, bisexual or transgender.[56]

Evidence provided in this book indicates that the health care needs of gay and bisexual men can differ from those required by their heterosexual counterparts. Elderly gay and bisexual men will benefit from health care that is tailored to their specific needs, such as care required for elderly men with HIV/AIDS as well as preventive care, such as anal pap smears to detect rectal carcinoma. Current policies that deny same-sex couples civil marriage rights can affect the quality of life of many older LGBT individuals. This is most evident in the benefits available through the Social Security program that are denied to same-sex couples. Among these benefits, same-sex partners are not eligible for survivor benefits, which are afforded to heterosexual widows and widowers, and spousal benefits, which entitle one spouse up to one-half of his or her spouse's Social Security benefit if it is larger than his or her own. Outside the Social Security program, a same-sex couple's assets and homes are not protected by Medicaid regulations when one partner enters a nursing home or long-term care facility. Individuals who are same-sex partners of people who have died are also subject to withholding taxes of their same-sex partners' 401(k) plans (married heterosexual couples are exempt from these taxes) and are not likely to qualify for hardship withdrawals from these plans that are generally available to legally married couples. Pension plans are also not required to make payments to anyone but a legally defined spouse.[57]

Not all LGBT individuals are in committed relationships; LGBT adults are actually more likely to live alone than their heterosexual counterparts.[58] While nursing homes, assisted living facilities, and other long-term care settings typically encourage socialization among older adults, LGBT adults may fear placement in these facilities because their sexual orientation may not be incorporated into the living atmosphere.[58] Many long-term care facilities typically inhibit sexual expression among all residents, and studies have also indicated specific anti-gay sentiments among nursing home staff.[59,60]

Recommendations

Current policies can negatively affect the quality of life of older LGBT individuals. This is most evident in the way that the term *spouse* is defined by the Social Security program, Medicaid regulations, and 401(k) and pension policies. Ultimately, same-sex civil marriages would address the negative impact these policies have on same-sex couples. In the short-term, however, policies should be revised to extend the definition of *spouse* or to otherwise extend the benefits that these programs afford to married heterosexual couples to same-sex couples. The definition of *spouse* should also be amended in the 1993 Family Medical Leave Act to ensure that employers provide up to 12 weeks of unpaid leave to employees in the event that the employee's partner has or experiences a serious medical condition.[57]

Nursing homes and other long-term care facilities should take appropriate steps to create environments in which LGBT seniors feel comfortable about expressing their sexuality. This includes adopting and posting nondiscrimination policies and training staff on issues of sexuality. In addition, procedures should be in place to handle staff that mistreat or deny care to residents because of residents' sexual orientation or behavior. Many advocacy groups such as the Senior Action in a Gay Environment (SAGE) are also studying ways to provide LGBT-specific housing communities.[58]

In addition to the recommendations provided above, LGBT individuals should actively prepare for their futures. Central among these preparations, careful financial and estate planning can help protect individuals and their loved ones and can help ensure that they enjoy their older adult age. The American Medical Association also recommends that all elders identify a health care proxy. For LGBT individuals, identifying a health care decision maker is critical because, if one is not otherwise specified, the individual's next of kin—not a same-sex partner or friend—would have legal health care authority.[58]

Gay and Bisexual Men of Color

In recent years, there has been considerable attention in both the mainstream media and in the public health community on the disproportionate affect of HIV/AIDS on black men who have sex with men (BMSM).[61] However, the disparity in the prevalence of HIV infection among these men does not appear to be explained by higher rates of high-risk sexual contact.[62] Among the explanations that have been hypothesized to explain this disparity, limited access to health care among these men may be an important contributor.

In the health care setting, BMSM may experience prejudicial treatment based on both their race and sexuality. Some physicians perceive African Americans as less educated and that those who are HIV-positive are less likely to adhere to HAART.[63,64] In focus groups conducted among BMSM between 2000 and 2001, most respondents indicated that discrimination based on their race was omnipresent and that regardless of sexuality and gender, these men are perceived by the "outside world" first as black men.[19] However, these men reported additional prejudices based on their sexual orientation. One man, for example, spoke of a physician with whom the patient had developed a rapport and his subsequent dismay when the physician invited him to a church service with a pronounced anti-gay theme.[19] Detachment from both the white (including gay) community based on race and from the black community based on sexual orientation may impact the psychology of BMSM and their interactions with health care providers.[19]

The focus groups of BMSM conducted by Dr. David Malebranche and his colleagues reveal additional barriers to medical care experienced by BMSM, which the researchers defined as external and internal barriers. They defined external barriers as money, insurance, privacy/confidentiality, and an impersonal medical system. Internal barriers, on the other hand, include "distrust in the medical system, fear of the health risks of being both black and homosexual, and perceiving healthcare as synonymous with 'bad news' or judgment and discrimination."[19] Additionally, the members of these focus groups indicated preferences for health care providers who reflected their own race and gender.[19] It is important to note, however, that very little research has addressed the needs and experiences of black men who have sex with men, and caution should be exercised when interpreting the results from this single qualitative study.

Recommendations

Many of the recommendations presented in previous chapters will aid in promoting the health care experiences of many BMSM. However, Malebranche and his colleagues advocate for additional recommendations specific to this population. For example, in addition to training health care providers and their staffs on the unique experiences of men who have sex with men, the researchers advocate for additional training on culturally competent care, specifically for foreign-trained physicians who come to practice in the United States. The researchers also indicate that physicians should improve their sexual history–taking, and stress that patients should be screened based on sexual risk behaviors to avoid stigmatizing individuals based on demographic risk groups.[19]

In addition to the recommendations presented above, the focus groups revealed to the researchers the importance of continued recruitment of minority health care providers and placement of these providers in minority communities. Minority providers can foster relationships with BMSM who feel detached from predominantly white gay communities as well as African American communities, based on their race and sexuality, respectively. In addition, minority providers can pursue research on issues pertinent to these men and can collaborate with community-level organizations to "address the roots of social isolation" that BMSM experience in their daily lives.[19]

Conclusion

We began this chapter by stating that optimal health care can be defined as "providing the right service at the right time in the right place."[1] As we have shown, pervasive policies may impede gay and bisexual men from receiving optimal care. Discriminatory practices and policies against gay and bisexual men affect their ability to access health insurance, one of the most basic components of accessing optimal care. Strategies are needed to address discrimination against gay and bisexual men, whether this means making such discrimination illegal or dismantling policies that allow agents to discriminate against this population.

Providers' attitudes and office practices may also impede gay and bisexual men from receiving optimal care. Intake and medical record forms and interview questions that are grounded in the assumption that all patients are heterosexual may prevent gay and bisexual men from disclosing their sexual orientation. While a recent survey holds that most physicians would be comfortable treating gay and lesbian patients, their attitudes regarding their gay and lesbian colleagues reveal that some may harbor significant anti-gay attitudes. The training and policies of some medical schools suggest that some physicians who are responsible for training future physicians may still hold strong anti-gay attitudes.

These challenges aside, providers who want to provide optimal care for their gay and bisexual patients have many ways to do so. Relatively simple actions, such as revising intake forms and interviews to accommodate LGBT patients, can help foster open and accepting environments. Policy makers and advocates can pursue changes at the local, state, and national level that will improve access to health care for all Americans, regardless of their sexual orientation.

Acknowledgments

The authors would like to extend their thanks and appreciation to Dr. Nancy Kass at the Johns Hopkins Bloomberg School of Public Health, Ms. Jennifer Kates at the Kaiser Family Foundation, Ms. Carrie Evans at the Human Rights Campaign, and Dr. David Diemert at the Sabin Vaccine Institute, all of whom provided expert advice and guidance.

References

1. Rogers A, Flowers J, Pencheon D. Improving access needs a whole systems approach. *BMJ.* 1999;319;866–867.
2. Kaiser Commission on Medicaid and the Uninsured. *The Uninsured: A Primer.* Washington, DC: The Henry J. Kaiser Foundation; January 2006.
3. Heck JE, Sell RL, Gorin SS. Health care access among individuals involved in same-sex relationships. *Am J Public Health.* 2006;96:1111–1118.
4. The Kaiser Family Foundation. *Inside-Out: A Report on the Experiences of Lesbians, Gays and Bisexuals in America and the Public's Views on Issues and Policies Related to Sexual Orientation.* Washington, DC: The Henry J. Kaiser Family Foundation; November 2001.
5. Kass NE. Access to insurance and perceived discrimination by homosexual men [dissertation]. 1989.

6. Hymes KB, Cheung T, Greene JB, Prose NS, Marcus A, Ballard H, William DC, Laubenstein LJ. Kaposi's sarcoma in homosexual men; a report of eight cases. *Lancet.* 1981,2:598–600.

7. Georgetown University Institute for Health Care Research and Policy and K.A. Thomas and Associates. *How Accessible Is Individual Health Insurance for Consumers in Less Than Perfect Health?* Washington, DC: The Henry J. Kaiser Family Foundation; June 2001.

8. Li KC. The private insurance industry's tactics against suspected homosexuals: redlining based on occupation, residence, and marital status. *Am J Law Med.* 1996;22:477–502.

9. Cahill S. *The Glass Nearly Half Full: 47% of US Population Lives in Jurisdiction with Sexual Orientation Nondiscrimination Law.* New York, NY: National Gay and Lesbian Task Force Policy Institute; 2005.

10. Zellers WK, McLaughlin CG, Frick KD. Small-business health insurance: only the healthy need apply. *Health Aff.* 1992;11:174–180.

11. Centers for Disease Control and Prevention. *HIV/AIDS Surveillance Report, 2004.* Vol. 16. Atlanta: US Department of Health and Human Services, Centers for Disease Control and Prevention; 2005.

12. The Henry J. Kaiser Family Foundation. *Financing HIV/AIDS Care: A Quilt with Many Holes.* Washington, DC: The Henry J. Kaiser Family Foundation, May 2004.

13. Mauskopf J, Kitahata M, Kauf T, Richter A, Tolson J. HIV antiretroviral treatment: early versus later. *J Acquir Immune Deffic Syndr.* 2005;39:562–569.

14. Jacobson LP, Phair JP, Yamashita TE. Virologic and immunologic response to highly active antiretroviral therapy. *Curr HIV/AIDS Rep.* 2004;1:74–81.

15. Health Resources and Services Administration (HRSA). HIV/AIDS Bureau Web site, Care Act Overview. http://hab.hrsa.gov/programs/factsheets/programfact.htm. Accessed September 1, 2005.

16. The Kaiser Family Foundation and Health Research and Educational Trust. *Employer Health Benefits: 2004 Summary of Findings.* Washington, DC: The Henry J. Kaiser Family Foundation; September 2004.

17. Defense of Marriage Act, Pub L. no. 104–199, 110 Stat 2419 (1996).

18. Human Rights Campaign (HRC). Work Life. Employers that offer domestic partner health benefits. www.hrc.org/Template.cfm?Section=Search_the_Database&Template=/CustomSource/WorkNet/srch.cfm&searchtypeid=3&searchSubTypeID=1. Accessed April 10, 2005.

19. Malebranche DJ, Peterson JL, Fullilove RE, Stackhouse RW. Race and sexual identity: perceptions about medical culture and healthcare among black men who have sex with men. *J Natl Med Assoc.* 2004;96:97–107.

20. National Gay and Lesbian Task Force. The issues: nondiscrimination. http://www.thetaskforce.org/theissues/issue.cfm?issueID=18. Accessed March 6, 2006.

21. Human Rights Campaign. State prohibitions on marriage for same-sex couples and statewide marriage laws. http://www.hrc.org/Template.cfm?Section=Center&Template=/TaggedPage/TaggedPageDisplay.cfm&TPLID=63&ContentID=17353. Accessed June 7, 2006.

22. Brewington K. Gay marriage ban falls. *The Baltimore Sun.* January 21, 2006.

23. 2006 Regular Session Bill Information. House Bill 132. http://mlis.state.md.us/2006rs/billfile/hb0132.htm. Accessed June 12, 2006.

24. Harris Interactive and Witeck-Combs Communications. *Fewer Than Half of All Lesbian, Gay, Bisexual, and Transgender Adults Surveyed Say They Have Disclosed Their Sexual Orientation to Their Health Care Provider.* Washington, DC: Harris Interactive/Witeck-Combs Communications, Inc.; December 2002.

25. Allen LB, Glicken AD, Beach RK, Naylor KE. Adolescent health care experiences of gay, lesbian, and bisexual young adults. *J Adolesc Health.* 1998;23:212–220.

26. Schindhelm RK, Hospers HJ. Sex with men before coming-out: relation to sexual activity and sexual risk-taking behavior. *Arch Sex Behav.* 2004;33:585–591.

27. Kaiser Permanente National Diversity Council and Kaiser Permanente National Diversity. *A Provider's Handbook on Culturally Competent Care: Lesbian, Gay, Bisexual and Transgender Population.* 2nd ed. Oakland, CA: Kaiser Permanente; 2004.

28. Schatz B, O'Hanlan K. *Anti-Gay Discrimination in Medicine: Results of a National Survey of Lesbian, Gay, and Bisexual Physicians.* San Francisco, CA: American Association of Physicians for Human Rights/Gay Lesbian Medical Association; 1994.

29. Health Privacy Project. http://www.healthprivacy.org. Accessed March 21, 2006.

30. Bhugra D, King M. Controlled comparison of attitudes of psychiatrists, general practitioners, homosexual doctors and homosexual men to male homosexuality. *J R Soc Med.* 1989;2:603–605.

31. The Kaiser Family Foundation. *National Survey of Physicians, Part 1: Doctors on Disparities in Medical Care. Highlights and Chartpack.* Washington, DC: The Henry J. Kaiser Family Foundation; March 2002.

32. Ramos MM, Tellez CM, Palley TB, Umland BE, Skipper BJ. Attitudes of physicians practicing in New Mexico toward gay men and lesbians in the profession. *Acad Med.* 1998;73:436–438.

33. Oriel KA, Madlon-Kay DJ, Govaker D, Mersy DJ. Gay and lesbian physicians in training: family practice program directors' attitudes and students' perceptions of bias. *Fam Med.* 1996; 8:720–725.

34. Gay and Lesbian Medical Association (GLMA). GLMA decries decision by new york medical college to ban lesbian gay bisexual transgender people in medicine student group. http://www.glma.org/NYMCPR.shtml. Accessed September 1, 2005.

35. Gay and Lesbian Medical Association (GLMA). Background: New York Medical College's decision to ban Gay Lesbian Bisexual Transgender People in Medicine group. http://www.glma.org/background.shtml. Accessed September 1, 2005.

36. Gay and Lesbian Medical Association (GLMA). GLMA pressure leads NY Medical College to reinstate LGBT student group. http://ce54.citysoft.com/index.cfm?fuseaction=Page.viewPage&pageID=658. Accessed June 16, 2006.

37. Gay and Lesbian Medical Association (GLMA). Guidelines: creating a safe clinical environment for lesbian, gay, bisexual, transgender, and intersex (LGBTI) patients. http://www.glma.org/pub/index.shtml. Accessed March 2006.

38. Epstein RM, Morse DS, Frankel RM, Frarey L, Anderson K, Beckman HB. Awkward moments in patient-physician communication about HIV risk. *Ann Int Med.* 1998;128:435–442.

39. Wenrich MD, Curtis JR, Carline JD, Paauw DS, Ramsey PG. HIV risk screening in the primary care setting: assessment of physicians' skills. *J Gen Intern Med.* 1997; 12:107–113.

40. Nusbaum MR, Hamilton CD. The proactive sexual health history. *Am Fam Physician.* 2002;66:1705–1712.

41. Kurth AE, Martin DP, Golden MR, Weiss NS, Heagerty PJ, Spielberg F, Handsfield HH, Holmes KK. A comparison between audio computer-assisted self-interviews and clinician interviews for obtaining sexual histories. *Sex Transm Dis.* 2004;31:719–726.

42. Wallick MM, Cambre KM, Townsend MH. How the topic of homosexuality is taught in US Medical Schools. *Acad Med.* 1992;67:601–603.

43. Tesar CM, Rovi SL. Survey of curriculum on homosexuality/bisexuality in departments of family medicine. *Fam Med.* 1998;30:283–287.

44. Council of Scientific Affairs, American Medical Association. Health care needs of gay men and lesbians in the United States. *JAMA.* 1996;275:1354–1359.

45. Sack S, Drabant B, Perrin E. Communicating about sexuality: an initiative across the core clerkships. *Acad Med.* 2002;77:1159–1160.

46. Haist SA, Griffith CH, Hoellein AR, Talente G, Montgomery T, Wilson JF. Improving students' sexual history inquiry and HIV counseling with an interactive workshop using standardized patients. *J Gen Intern Med.* 2004;19:549–553.

47. McGarry KA, Clarke JG, Cyr MG, Landau C. Evaluating a lesbian and gay health care curriculum. *Teach Learn Med.* 2002;14:244–248.

48. *American Journal of Public Health.* 2001;91.

49. Clark ME, Landers S, Linde R, Sperber J. The GLBT health access project: a state-funded effort to improve access to care. *Am J Public Health.* 2001;91:895–896.

50. Craft EM, Mulvey KP. Addressing lesbian, gay, bisexual, and transgender issues from the inside: one federal agency's approach. *Am J Public Health.* 2001;91:889–891.

51. Garofalo R, Katz E. Health care issues of gay and lesbian youth. *Curr Opin Pediatr.* 2001;13:298–302.

52. Celentano DD, Sifakis F, Hylton J, Torian LV, Guillin V, Koblin BA. Race/ethnic differences in HIV prevalence and risks among adolescent and young adult men who have sex with men. *J Urban Health.* 2005;82:610–621.

53. Bowowsky IW, Ireland M, Resnick MD. Adolescent suicide and attempts: risks and protectors. *Pediatrics.* 2001 Mar;107(3):485–493.

54. Stall R, Wiley J. A comparison of alcohol and drug use patterns of homosexual and heterosexual men: The San Francisco Men's Health Study. *Drug Alcohol Depend.* 1988;22:63–73.

55. Skinner WF, Otis MD. Drug and alcohol use among lesbian and gay people in a southern U.S. sample: epidemiological, comparative, and methodological findings from the Trilogy Project. *J Homosex.* 1996;30(3):59–92.

56. National Gay and Lesbian Task Force. The issues: seniors. http://www.thetaskforce.org/theissues/issue.cfm?issueID=24. Accessed March 14, 2006.

57. Cahill S, South K, Spade J. *Outing Age: Public Policy Issues Affecting Gay, Lesbian, Bisexual and Transgender Elders.* Washington, DC: The Policy Institute of the National Gay and Lesbian Task Force, 2000.

58. McMahon E. The older homosexual: current concepts of lesbian, gay, bisexual, and transgender older Americans. *Clin Geriatr Med.* 2003;19:587–593.

59. Fairchild SK, Carrino GE, Ramirez M. Social workers' perceptions of staff attitudes toward resident sexuality in a random sample on New York state nursing homes: a pilot study. *J Gerontol Soc Work.* 1996;26:193–96.

60. Cook-Daniels L. Lesbian, gay male, and transgendered elders: elder abuse and neglect issues. *J Elder Abuse Negl.* 1997;9:35–49.

61. Racial/Ethnic disparities in diagnoses of HIV/AIDS—33 states, 2001–2004. *MMWR.* 2006;55:121–125.
62. Malebranche DJ. Black men who have sex with men and the HIV epidemic: next steps for public health. *Am J Public Health.* 2003;93:862–5.
63. Bird ST, Bogart LM. Perceived race-based and socioeconomic status-based discrimination in interactions with health care providers. *Ethn Dis.* 2001;11:554–563.
64. Bogart LM, Catz SL, Kelly JA, Benotsch EG. Factors influencing physicians' judgments of adherents and treatment decisions for patients with HIV disease. *Med Decis Making.* 2001;21:28–36.

14

Moving the Field Forward: A Strategic Framework to Develop Health Research among MSM Communities

Ron Stall, Ronald O. Valdiserri, and Richard J. Wolitski

This volume demonstrates that important health disparities among men who have sex with men (MSM) exist and that these manifest across a range of infectious and chronic, noninfectious diseases and conditions. However, even though the literature on gay men's health disparities is growing, it is also uneven in its focus on specific health problems. It may be that additional epidemics remain uncharacterized and so will be added to the list of health disparities reviewed in this book. It should also be clear to the reader that both the range and the degree to which health disparities exist among MSM suggest that it will require many years to resolve these problems. This fact raises the question of how we can best move forward to address health disparities among MSM. This chapter will outline a schema for health research that culminates in intervention design and suggests a number of strategies that could be pursued to shorten the time that it takes to resolve health disparities among MSM.

A Generations Approach to the Study of Gay Men's Health

At this early stage of development, the study of health and health disparities among MSM is quite complex, addressing as it does questions of definition of the study population, sampling strategies, theoretical development, and substantive findings, to name only some of the most important of these issues. Extreme complexity in a rapidly developing literature can function to impede future progress by making findings difficult to synthesize and can obscure the areas of greatest promise in a field of research. A schema of central research questions could serve a useful purpose by organizing the necessary complexity of an emerging literature and so clarifying how best to move a literature forward. The schema should provide a way of not only organizing questions to be asked by the field but should also suggest a strategy to move basic health research toward the creation of proven public health intervention strategies to promote health in MSM communities.

To this end, we are proposing a schema of "generations" of health research to help organize the emerging literature on health disparities among MSM. The schema that we are proposing outlines different key research questions at each generational research focus, while also suggesting additional research foci that would be productive at each generational level. We note that this schema draws heavily on the history of the development of HIV/AIDS research among gay men—arguably the best developed in the MSM health literature—as well as a recently published conceptual framework to guide the development of health disparities research among racial/ethnic minorities.[1] The primary tasks of the "first generation" of research are those of documentation and description. This first generation of research is defined as that which seeks to document the existence and extent of a health problem within a population and how it may be differentially expressed in MSM populations. Primary examples of such first generation research among MSM include projects that are defined to generate prevalence estimates of specific health problems. Other projects might seek to compare clinical manifestations of a health problem as experienced among MSM to other populations of men, to determine if unique presentations of this disorder need to be addressed as part of a public health response. In addition, descriptions of the distribution of a health problem across MSM populations (i.e., describing its demographic and psychosocial correlates) give a measure of the prevalence of a health problem among distinct MSM subcommunities (e.g., racial/ethnic minorities, age cohorts, etc.) and identify men who may be at particularly high risk for the health problem. In short, the key questions asked by first generation research are defined to document the existence of specific health problems, to measure the prevalence of such problems within MSM communities, and to construct an initial profile of men who are most vulnerable to having those health problems.

The "second generation" of research seeks to explain the distribution of specific health disparities among MSM populations. Examples of such research questions include not only identifying the mediators and moderators of a given health problem but theoretical work that organizes these variables into an explanatory paradigm that could eventually serve as the basis for intervention design. Qualitative research at this level would include work to describe men's conceptualizations of risk for particular health conditions and how they are managing this risk. That said, the core agenda of the second generation work is to generate an explanation for the manifestation of the health problem, which is a necessary component to the design of public health strategies to address the problem.

The primary goals of the "third generation" of research are the design of new interventions that might work to ease health disparities, to test these interventions for efficacy, and to put into public health practice those interventions that have evidence for efficacy. Research at this stage can also include substantial qualitative, formative research to help design interventions to address specific health problems within specific populations. Operational research—to document the best ways to put interventions with evidence of efficacy into the field—is a critical research agenda within this generational level. Research to document and explain, and so circumvent, barriers to the maintenance of proven interventions as part of standard public health practice is also an important component of operational research, and particularly so for culturally marginalized groups such as MSM. In summary, the overarching research task at this generational level is to design and test interventions and translate such interventions to find ways to maintain them in the field as part of standard public health practice to support health among gay men.

Strategies to Move the Field Forward

The use of the term *generations* in presenting the above schemata is not accidental: this agenda is ambitious and will take considerable time and effort to realize. Not only is there a wide variety of health problems to be described among MSM, but the additional work to create empirically tested explanations for the distributions of particular diseases among MSM and to create and test interventions that are proven to manage particular health problems among specific communities of MSM will take many years to complete.

It should be clear from a reading of findings from this volume and the larger literature on health issues that the work that we describe is typically at the first and second generation in terms of the study of most health problems that affect MSM. We are at the start of a very long journey to resolve health disparities among MSM. Accordingly, we should consider strategies that will shorten this journey and will help us achieve our goals more efficiently. We would like to propose several strategies, among others, that could also be proposed, that may be helpful in this regard.

Advocate for Inclusion of Sexual Attraction, Identity, and Sex Behavior Questions in Large-Scale National Health Studies of the American Populace

To advocate effectively for efforts to resolve health disparities among MSM, one must have convincing evidence to demonstrate the extent and distribution of specific health disparities. Although the strongest designs to demonstrate that disparities exist are those that compare MSM and heterosexual men drawn from national probability samples, only a very small number of papers have been able to use this approach to demonstrate health disparities among MSM. While it is theoretically possible to field a large set of studies that focus on specific health issues among MSM (with comparative samples of men drawn from the general population), the costs of this approach to documenting health disparities among MSM would be prohibitive. Hence, it is essential that ongoing large-scale cross-sectional and natural history studies designed to measure the overall health status of Americans include measures of sexual attraction, sexual identity, and same-gender behavior. Recent studies that have included such measures, such as the study conducted by Cochran and colleagues,[2] have already yielded important data to document the extent of health disparities among gay men and lesbians. It should be noted that these studies have been successfully fielded and that earlier fears that the general population of Americans would be offended by the inclusion of sexuality questions in large-scale national health surveys were overstated. It should also be noted that even if some small proportion of the population finds questions about sexuality offensive, that proportion of the population is likely to be far outnumbered by the large number of LGBT (lesbian, gay, bisexual, and transgender) citizens who will directly benefit by having access to rigorous data about the health disparities that affect their communities. Continued efforts to support the inclusion of multiple measures of sexual orientation in large-scale national surveys are essential to the effort to resolve health disparities among MSM.

Create Consensus Statements among Researchers to Describe How Different Sampling Strategies Shape Prevalence and Correlational Findings Concerning Gay Men's Health

MSM are a small minority of the overall male population. Only about 2% to 5% of American men report recent same-gender sexual contacts in general population samples at any given point in time.[3] Because MSM account for such a small proportion of the total male population, sampling issues will probably always be a challenge in generating rigorous data measuring the extent and correlates of health in this population. Furthermore, while large-scale sampling methods of the general population can yield important data using standard measures of health issues that are highly prevalent in the general American population, such strategies are very unlikely to be useful in studying emerging health issues among MSM (as well as health issues that are particularly important among subpopulations of MSM), or to identify unique correlates of health among MSM populations, or to test cutting-edge theories to explain the distribution of health and illness among MSM. Studying small subsets of men within these large-scale national samples also risks confronting significant statistical power problems, particularly if one wishes to study subsets of the MSM population itself, such as racial/ethnic minority MSM.

For all of these reasons, we will probably always need to rely on data measuring health issues among MSM that are drawn from sources other than large-scale population-based samples of the entire American population. Some of these data will be drawn from opportunistic venue samples, some from respondent-driven sampling strategies, and others will come from household-based sampling strategies from neighborhoods rich in gay men, among other possibilities. Our ability to interpret these findings will be strengthened if we conduct analyses to show how a given sampling strategy shapes not only prevalence estimates for health problems among MSM, but also the ability to detect correlations with specific health problems. These analyses may culminate in the production of ongoing consensus statements to guide interpretation of findings regarding health issues among MSM drawn from divergent sampling methods. Such statements should also include attempts to guide interpretation of findings for important subpopulations of MSM, such as racial/ethnic minority MSM.

Improve Understandings of the Determinants of Health Disparities among MSM

Efforts to respond to health disparities among MSM will be more efficient if they address factors have been empirically demonstrated to cause disparities. This "second generation" research agenda will require two components: the creation of testable theoretical models to explain health disparities and empirical testing of these theoretical models. Theory development will serve two important goals in the effort to resolve health disparities. The first of these goals is that of organizing a set of hypotheses to be tested in new data sets; the second of these is to organize a set of empirically supported hypotheses upon which program design can be based. Although challenging, both theory development and testing of new theoretical explanations for health disparities among MSM will ultimately prove most useful if both serve as the basis for innovative health program design.

Study Resilience

Insights about health come from more than the study of disease; they also come from the study of resilience from disease, even among those individuals who have been exposed to unhealthy and even toxic environments. The literature on MSM gives many examples of populations who display considerable variation in vulnerability to disease, even when exposed to comparable insults to health. The usual response to this variation is to focus our primary attention on those segments of a sample that express disease. It also stands to reason that study of those individuals who have been exposed to unhealthy situations and who yet remain healthy are also able to teach us a great deal about health. Thus, study of the considerable strengths that gay men manifest is at least as important as the study of their health vulnerabilities. Continued focus on resilience and strength by gay men in the face of adversity is likely to yield important insights about how best to maintain health.

Recognize How Minority Health Disparities Intersect with Gay Men's Health Disparities

The study of health disparities among MSM owes a great deal to the pioneering work that has already been undertaken to resolve health disparities within racial/ethnic minority populations in the United States. It is likely that this cross-fertilization will continue for the foreseeable future, as many challenges are faced by researchers in both fields. Many issues cross-cut both fields: many MSM are, of course, members of racial/ethnic minority populations, and so deal with challenges to health as members of both groups. It is now self-evident that any attempts to resolve health disparities among MSM communities must address the health needs of racial/ethnic minority MSM as a central part of that endeavor. And racial/ethnic minority populations are, of course, affected by the health issues faced by MSM members of their communities. Challenges in sampling design confront both research agendas, as does the challenge of translating theory and prevention practice so that it is culturally relevant to these often "hidden populations." But the issue for which both groups have the greatest commonality is that of explaining the specific mechanisms by which the many specific dimensions of cultural marginalization affect the health of specific individuals. This is perhaps the core question that underlies endeavors to address health disparities among racial/ethnic minority and MSM populations, and those who seek to answer this question in both fields might well learn a great deal by cross-pollination of insights across these two fields. This sharing and collegiality will best occur if the efforts to study health disparities among sexual minority populations maintain strong connections with efforts to resolve health disparities with other populations.

Learn from Health Programs that Are Already Serving MSM

It is clear that health disparities among MSM are so substantial and varied that we cannot wait until such time that each is carefully characterized in the scientific literature before we attempt a response. This general understanding has existed among practitioners for at least the past 30 years in the case of some responses to specific health problems among MSM. Currently, a network of community-based organizations provide services to MSM and other LGBT populations across a wide variety of health problems. This network of organizations—and long working experience in providing public health services to these populations—provides the opportunity to gain important insights regarding how best to resolve health disparities among MSM.

Not all advances come from the application of abstract theory to programs in the field; advances to resolve health disparities can also come from hands-on work with populations in greatest need. The network of existing programs serving the health needs of MSM offers us the opportunity to create an inductively driven laboratory for the development of effective responses to gay men's health needs. Some of these insights can be gained through operational evaluation research to identify programs that seem to have the greatest effectiveness in the field, as well as the correlates of greatest reduction in risk behaviors or poor health in client populations. The findings and experience that we gain from ongoing program development may well help refine theory to explain the distribution of health among gay men as well.

Chart How Historical Changes in Societal Structures Affect the Health of MSM

We are living in a time when more than research on MSM is changing: significant cultural change is occurring in the societal understandings of MSM communities and in the place of MSM in American society. These changes are likely to continue over time and will provide a rich opportunity for natural experiments to shed light on how societal change affects the health of MSM.

One important societal change that is occurring in regard to LGBT communities concerns domestic partnerships and same-gender marriages. In the United States there is now wide variation in how same-gender partnerships are recognized by law, supported by private employer recognition and benefits, and/or recognized to exist in different social settings. The emergence of a legal and cultural discussion regarding MSM partnerships is very likely to change understandings of the meaning of same-gender relationships within the larger culture and LGBT communities alike. To the extent that same-gender marriage is widely recognized, we can hypothesize that changes will occur in terms of social isolation, sexual partner turnover, depression, substance abuse, and STI/HIV infection rates among MSM.

Some societal or technological changes may have both positive and negative effects. One example of this possibility is the use of the Internet to serve as a means for sexual minority communities to communicate, organize, and find sexual partnerships. Although increased communication and community involvement may well serve to combat social isolation among MSM, STD outbreaks have also been linked to the use of the Internet to find new sex partners (see Chapter 6 by Ronald Valdiserri, in this volume). Ongoing surveillance and use of quasi-experimental designs to describe differences in health profiles associated with different structural arrangements in the societal treatment of MSM (e.g., comparison of the health profile of MSM in legal jurisdictions in which same-gender relationships are recognized by law, compared to jurisdictions in which these relationships are not) may well provide important guidance in how best to support health among MSM and other LGBT communities.

Consider Translation of Proven Interventions to MSM Communities

The health disparities that challenge MSM communities are faced by other communities as well. In some cases, effective treatments and/or behavioral interventions exist to address these health problems. The question of whether these interventions can be translated for use among MSM should be considered. Put another way, even though we have strong evidence to show that a disproportionate number of MSM are addicted to tobacco, do we really need to develop and test from, the ground up, tobacco cessation interventions that have already been shown to work for other populations?

A good deal of the data to answer this question could be drawn from careful evaluations of programs with evidence of efficacy in other populations after they have been translated or adapted so that they are appropriate for MSM. Such work should be designed to determine not only whether translated programs yield similar effect sizes to those found among other populations, but also whether these translated programs would likely yield even stronger effects with further adaptations. Translated programs that fail to achieve similar effect sizes to those found in other populations should be considered as candidates for more basic, "ground up" development so that they can work among MSM populations.

Extend Findings and Expertise to Other LGBT Populations

At one level, the scope of this volume is artificial: a discussion of health disparities among MSM should also include findings that pertain to lesbian, bisexual, and transgender populations. Although this volume has focused on describing health disparities among MSM, it is clear that careful epidemiological research to better characterize the health profiles of other sexual minority populations is long overdue and needed.

Perhaps this volume should best be regarded as a promissory note for the day when we will know enough to produce analogous reviews for the other sexual minority populations. That work can start by creating collaborations with those who are interested in exploring and addressing health disparities in sexual minority populations beyond MSM. Efforts at such collaborations should work to share research methods, research tools, program practice insights, and other resources for critical review to gauge their value in these populations. As these tools are considered for use in these related populations, further insights as to their best use will be gained—insights that will doubtless add to the level of scientific rigor of research on MSM.

Provide Training Structures for New Generations of Scholars Interested in Health Disparities among MSM

The agenda to resolve health disparities among MSM will take many years, and probably generations, of research as well as program and policy advances. This agenda will include, as well, structural interventions to address the root causes of health disparities among MSM populations. However daunting that prospect may be, we should remember that our very ability to study health issues among MSM is in turn supported by generations of struggle for the civil rights and human dignity of LGBT people. The agenda to study gay men's health thus draws strength and historical continuity from this larger, generations-long struggle and provides an important context in which efforts to resolve health disparities among MSM can continue over time.

Because efforts to resolve health disparities among MSM are likely to take many years to realize, we must be able to transfer skills and scientific interest in health disparities research across generations of scholars. At present, very few organized training programs exist to facilitate training in the study of health issues among sexual minorities such as MSM. The lack of this organized structure risks losing the working experience and scientific focus that older scholars should bequeath to succeeding generations. Such training centers would also be an important force in sustaining an organized scientific focus on crucially important aspects of gay men's health issues. Creating sustainable settings where young scholars can move forward the study of health issues important to MSM and can collaborate with community-based practitioners to design, evaluate, and test new approaches to resolving health disparities is vital to resolving health disparities among MSM.

Conclusion: An Unexplored Continent

We are at an exciting time in the chronology of research into health disparities among MSM, as well as other LGBT populations. We have strong evidence showing that substantial health disparities affect these populations and recognize that additional research and improved public health practice will be necessary to resolve these disparities. We will chart out new areas of research, refine and develop theory to explain the distribution of health and illness in sexual minority populations, and create new interventions to prevent disease and sustain health in these populations. And in the process, we will help answer a question that has challenged scientists for the past two centuries: What are the specific mechanisms by which social and cultural marginalization result in poorer individual and community health? Answers to this fundamental question will be of value not only to LGBT populations, but to all those who suffer poor health as a result of marginalization and unequal access to care.

Thus, we are presented with an exceedingly rare and exciting opportunity in science: we have before us an "unexplored continent" to describe. Although the outlines of this unexplored continent are reasonably well known, we have good reason to believe that further exploration of the topic area of health disparities among MSM and other LGBT populations will yield numerous surprises and important findings. We also have good reason to believe that continued work in LGBT health will yield important insights toward improving the health of LGBT populations as well as other marginalized populations. We hope that the schema and suggested strategies outlined in this chapter will accelerate this work, and we look forward to participating with our colleagues in the further development of this critical field of endeavor.

Authors' Note

The findings and conclusions in this chapter are those of the authors and do not necessarily represent the views of the US Centers for Disease Control and Prevention or the US Department of Veterans Affairs.

References

1. Kilbourne A, Switzer G, Hyman K, Crowley-Matoka M, Fine J. Advancing health disparities research within the health care system: a conceptual framework. *Am J Public Health*. 2006;96:2113–2121.
2. Cochran S, Ackerman D, Mays V, Ross M. Prevalence of non-medical drug use and dependence among homosexually active men and women in the US population. *Addiction*. 2004;99:989–998.
3. Binson D, Michaels S, Stall R, Coates T, Gagnon J, Catania J. Prevalence and social distribution of men who have sex with men: United States and its urban centers. *J Sex Res*. 1995;32:245–254.

Index